PARKINSON'S DISEASE
The way forward!

An Integrated Approach
including Drugs, Surgery, Nutrition,
Bowel & Muscle Function,
Self-Esteem, Sexuality,
Stress Control & Carers

DR GEOFFREY LEADER
& LUCILLE LEADER

with contributions by
Professor Aroldo Rossi
& Professor Lia Rossi-Prosperi et al
Foreword by Professor Leslie Findley

DENOR
PRESS

ISBN: 0 9526056 8 6

British Library Cataloguing in Publication Data.
A catalogue record of this publication is available from the British Library.

American Library of Congress Register of Copyrights.

Published by Denor Press
PO Box 12913, London, N12 8ZR, United Kingdom.
Telephone: +44 (020) 8343 7368
Fax: +44 (020) 8446 4504
Email: denor@dial.pipex.com

Book cover, design and layout
Jonathan Phillips, Farnham, Surrey, United Kingdom.
Email: jon@toccatadesign.com
www.toccatadesign.com

Printed by Lightning Source UK Ltd
www.lightningsource.co.uk

Dr Geoffrey Leader and Lucille Leader

Dedication

To all People with Parkinson's Disease and their supporters,
Esther and Rachel with their indomitable spirits,
Patricia and Morris, Stella and Ernest.

Acknowledgements

Grateful thanks to the esteemed colleagues whom we invited
to join us in our vision of this book.
Their graciousness, generosity of time and expertise is very much appreciated.

♦

Much appreciation to Dr Serena Leader for her editorial skills and advice.

♦

Thanks to Wendy Susan Hart for her help with translation from Italian,
Tony Leather and Dorothy Churchman for contributing so personally to this book,
Marianne Rist-Ravenscroft for proof reading and help with biochemical analysis,
Researchers Muriel Hallatt and the team at the British Medical Association Library,
Barnet Carers Centre and Bridget McCall of the London PD Society, for information,
Dr Neil Ward for assistance with his research on minerals,
Professor Leslie Findley for his support,
Patrick Holford for biochemical information,
Paul Stanbridge for IT, Jo Clarkson for secretarial co-ordination,
Felicia Beder, Agnieszka Korolczuk and Bozena Dubiaga for technical help,
Tatiana Schenk of Midpoint Trade Books and Beverly Friedgood for publishing advice,
Professor John Hunt and Ian Panton for "sound-boarding,"
David and Eline Carman for invaluable assistance with indexing
and unstinting moral support,
Dr Herman Hagens, Dr Erich Segal and Karen Segal, for inspiration.

♦

Very special thanks to Alison Kiersz-Brownstone at Denor Press.
Her skills and dedication were invaluable in bringing this book to fruition.

♦

Thanks to our book designer, Jonathan Phillips,
for his creativity and excellent co-operation.

♦

Our appreciation to Joe Leader for his drawing skills and patience,
Felicia Beder and Brendan Beder for their faith in this book.

♦

Special Appreciation to Mary Baker MBE and Lizzie Graham of the European
Parkinson's Disease Association (EPDA) for their support and encouragement
of our team approach.

Contents

Why This Title?

By Dr Geoffrey Leader MB ChB FRCA **and Lucille Leader** Dip ION

People with Parkinson's disease have presented at our clinic with a variety of health-related problems. These problems have been associated with the disease itself or its specific medication. However, many symptoms have also been noted arising from an imbalance or dysfunction of non-neurological systems.

It has therefore been our aim to optimise the entire functional health of individuals so that they may function as best as they can. In so doing, they are able to enhance their mental and physical potential and derive a sense of wellbeing not often experienced by sufferers of Parkinson's disease.

We have always worked within a multidisciplinary framework, believing and experiencing that the integrated approach is the only WAY FORWARD! for the total support of people with Parkinson's disease and those associated with them.

With our ideal of the "'team approach" to health management, we have called upon a broad spectrum of specialists to contribute to this book, each with a special interest and expertise in the management of different aspects of Parkinson's disease. They share our vision.

Note

There are other recent therapeutic modalities such as the injection of stem cells. These should be discussed with the patient's own neurologist. There is also ongoing research and interest in the field of genetic manipulation. This subject has not formed part of the first edition of **Parkinson's Disease - The Way Forward!** as its design is to present only those strategies which have been in use for some time and found to be helpful. We do hope that future editions will be able to reflect the success of this highly exciting development.

About the Editors

Dr Geoffrey Leader MB ChB FRCA

Dr Geoffrey Leader has always believed in a multi-disciplinary approach to the assessment and treatment of patients with chronic illness. He is a consultant anaesthetist and Medical Director of The London Pain Relief and Nutritional Support Clinic, in London, UK, which functions in this way. His academic career has included anaesthesia, leadership of intensive care units and specialised pain clinics, lecturing, publishing in peer journals and writing. He has always been interested in the optimisation of movement related problems as they presented in the Pain Clinic as well as the biochemical effects of drugs. He has collaborated with Lucille Leader, clinical nutritionist, in planning this multi-faceted book and helped bring it to fruition. He co-edited it and contributed chapters to it, including those pertaining to general anaesthesia and intravenous nutritional protocols. He invited colleagues, who are leaders in their field, to contribute their specialised expertise to this project. Email: **denor@dial.pipex.com**   Telephone: **+44 (0)20 8445 4550**

Lucille Leader Dip ION

Lucille Leader is the Nutrition Director of The London Pain Relief and Nutritional Support Clinic, in London, UK. She has always promoted the idea of multi-disciplinary management of chronic illness. She is vitally interested in the biochemical aspects of disease and the specialised nutritional support of chronically ill patients. She is an experienced nutritionst, lecturer and author. Through her vision, together with the collaboration of Dr Geoffrey Leader and the input of esteemed colleagues, she is able to present multiple strategies in this book in order to optimise function and well-being in patients with Parkinson's disease. She and Dr Geoffrey Leader hope that this project will enable patients and their supporters to make informed choices and that the therapeutic spectrum will be enhanced. She has co-edited, contributed chapters and brought the book to fruition. Email: **denor@dial.pipex.com**   Telephone: **+44 (0)20 8445 4550**

Assistant Editor
Dr Serena Leader BSc MB BCh MRCP MRCGP

Dr Serena Leader has an appreciation of the pivotal role of the General Practitioner in coordinating team management of patients with chronic illness. Her medical background has been in hospital medicine in London, including posts at The Royal Free Hospital, The Brompton Hospital and The Hammersmith Hospital. Having obtained her membership of the Royal College of Physicians, she has now taken her medical skills into General Practice. Email: **drserene@hotmail.com**

About the Authors

Dr Geoffrey Leader MB ChB FRCA

Dr Geoffrey Leader is a consultant anaesthetist and the Medical Director of The London Pain Relief and Nutritional Support Clinic in London. He is a pioneer in the idea of a multi-disciplinary approach to the management of chronic illness. He has held senior academic posts in South Africa, the Netherlands (University of Erasmus, Rotterdam), and in the UK where his last academic appointment was Chairman of the Anaesthetic Department, Head of Intensive Care and Pain Clinic at Newham General Hospital, London and Senior Lecturer and Honorary Senior Consultant at The Royal London Hospital Medical College. He has published in anaesthetic peer journals and is the co-author with Lucille Leader of the book *Parkinson's Disease - The New Nutritional Handbook* (Denor Press, UK) as well as the Italian book **Morbo Di Parkinson** - Suggerimenti Nutrizionali (Pythagora Press, Milan, Italy) in collaboration with Professor Aroldo Rossi and Professor Lia Rossi Prosperi. He is particularly interested in the intravenous nutritional support of patients with Parkinson's Disease as well as the specialised details of their management during anaesthesia and sedation, and the detoxification of drugs. He presented a paper on the intravenous aspects of nutritional support in Parkinson's disease at the Parkinson's Disease Congress for Nutrition and Sexuality in Vienna in 1999 and will co-chair a workshop in specialised nutritional management in Parkinson's Disease at the International Congress of the European Parkinson's Disease Association in Lisborn, 2004.
Email: **denor@dial.pipex.com**   Telephone: **+44 (0)20 8445 4550**

Lucille Leader Dip ION

Lucille Leader is the Nutrition Director of The London Pain Relief and Nutritional Support Clinic in London, which pioneered the idea of a multi-disciplinary approach to the management of chronic illness. She is particularly interested in the biochemical aspects of nutritional support of patients with chronic illness. She is the co-author with Dr Geoffrey Leader of the book *Parkinson's Disease - The New Nutritional Handbook* (Denor Press, UK) as well as the Italian book *Morbo Di Parkinson* - Suggerimenti Nutrizionali (Pythagora Press, Milan, Italy) in collaboration with Professor Aroldo Rossi and Professor Lia Rossi Prosperi. She has delivered many lectures on nutritional aspects in Parkinson's Disease to Parkinson's Disease support groups, health professionals and nutrition students including Westminster and Middlesex Universities, London. She presented a paper on Nutritional Management in Parkinson's Disease at the Parkinson's Disease Congress for Nutrition and Sexuality in Vienna in 1999, has written articles for nutrition journals and has been interviewed by the media in South Africa and the UK. She is an Associate Member of The British Society of Allergy, Environmental and Nutritional Medicine, The Royal Society of Medicine and is a Member of the British Society for Nutritional Therapy (BANT). She will co-chair a workshop in specialised nutritional management in Parkinson's Disease at the International Congress of the European Parkinson's Disease Association in Lisborn, 2004.

Email: **denor@dial.pipex.com**   Telephone: **+44 (0)20 8445 4550**

PROFESSOR AROLDO ROSSI

Professor Aroldo Rossi is Associate Professor of Neurology in the Department of Neuroscience, University of Perugia, Italy. He is the author of 150 publications and has been Chairman at many national and international medical congresses. He is a contributory author in collaboration with Dr Geoffrey Leader, Lucille Leader and Professor Lia Rossi Prosperi of the Italian book Morbo Di Parkinson - Suggerimenti Nutrizionali (Pythagora Press, Milan, Italy) and provides information on neurological aspects and aging to the media. He is particularly interested in movement disorders, especially Parkinsonism, Parkinson's disease and tremor. He is associated with Dr Lia Rossi Prosperi in the Neurological -Nutritional Studio, Arezzo, Italy. He is a Member of the Movement Disorder Society.

Email: **aroldorossi@virgilio.it**

PROFESSOR LIA ROSSI PROSPERI

Professor Lia Rossi Prosperi graduated in Biological Sciences at the University of Florence and specialised in Alimentary Sciences on at the University of Perugia. She is Advisor to the Office of Health for Tuscany, to the province and commune of Arezzo and Sienna and is associated with the National Order of Biologists and European Communities Biologists Associations. She is President of the Italian Association of Restoration, Science Person Responsible for National Conferences and is a Member of the Scientific Committee of the centre "Francesco Redi" (social-health, environmental information and research centre). Dr Rossi Prosperi lectures on the nutritional aspects of neurological diseases at the University of Perugia, in Perugia, Italy. She is a contributory author in collaboration with Dr Geoffrey Leader, Lucille Leader and Professor Aroldo Rossi of the Italian book Morbo Di Parkinson - Suggerimenti Nutrizionali (Pythagora Press, Milan, Italy). Often a TV guest on nutrition and health programmes, she also writes for magazines which deal with health issues, has published several brochures of nutritional information and is author of the Italian book "Mangiare bene per crescere bene" ("Eat Well to Grow Well") for children, parents and teachers.

E-mail: **liarp@plugit.net**

PROFESSOR LESLIE J FINDLEY OLJ TD MD FRCP FACP MRCS DCH

Professor Leslie J Findley is a consultant neurologist and clinical lead at the Essex Neurosciences Unit, Oldchurch Hospital, Essex and Professor of Health Sciences (Neurology) at South Bank University, London. He is honorary consultant to the MRC Human Movement and Balance Unit at the Institute of Neurology, London and the West London Neurosciences Unit, Charing Cross Hospital. His major clinical and research interests are movement disorders, including tremor and Parkinson's disease, and fatigue syndrome. He is past Chairman of the Parkinson's Disease Society of the United Kingdom, UK Medical Adviser to the European Parkinson's Disease Association, UK Adviser to the International Tremor Foundation (USA), Chairman of the Committee of Trustees and Scientific Adviser of the National Tremor Foundation (UK). He is currently a member of the WHO Working Party on Parkinson's disease and Chairman of the Steering Group of the Global Parkinson's Disease Survey.
Email: ljfindley@uk-consultants.co.uk

DR MICHAEL PERRING MA MB BCHIR FCP(SA) DPM

Dr Michael Perring trained in general medicine at St Bartholemews, London, later specialising in psychiatry. He is a registered qualified psychotherapist and sex therapist. He has lectured in sexual medicine at Southamptom University, and Charing Cross Hospital, where he also taught communication and counselling skills. He is a founder member of the British Association of Sexual and Marital Therapists. Particular areas of interest include maintaining vitality and optimal sexual function in the 50+ age group, hormone replacement therapy for the older man and woman, and problems where medical and psychological concerns overlap. He finds much benefit through bringing a broad approach to the wide spectrum of conditions with which he works. He has practised psychotherapy both in the UK and overseas. His activities include teaching, writing and broadcasting. He is now in full-time private practice in London.
Email: mike@ophealth.demon.co.uk

DR DONALD GROSSET BSC (HONOURS) MB CHB MD FRCP

Dr Donald Grosset is Consultant Neurologist at the Institute of Neurological Sciences, Southern General Hospital, Glasgow, and Honorary Senior Lecturer in Neurology at the University of Glasgow. He is Director of the Movement Disorder Clinic, which is run as a joint venture with Dr Graeme Macphee, Consultant Physician in Medicine for the Elderly, thereby providing the joint skills of both Neurology and Medicine to patients with Parkinson's Disease and other movement disorders. Dr Grosset has dual training in Neurology and Clinical Pharmacology, hence his active research interests are in the application of new drug treatments, especially in Parkinson's disease patients. He passionately believes that more patients should be offered early opportunity of newer treatments that are being introduced in clinical research programs. His additional focus in clinical care of Parkinson's disease patients - ensuring maximum diagnostic accuracy - is reflected in recently completed research on brain scan imaging, referred to in his chapter of this book, and for which he held the position of Principal Investigator. He is on the Medical Advisory Panel of the UK Parkinson's Disease Society, holds the positions of Secretary and Treasurer of the Scottish Association of Neurological Sciences, and has published widely including the Lancet, British Medical Journal, Quarterly Journal of Medicine, British Journal of Clinical Pharmacology, Stroke, and Movement Disorders.

Email: gcl137@clinmed.gla.ac.uk   Telephone: +44 (0)141 201 2486

DR DOUGLAS MACMAHON MB MS LRCP MRCS MRCP FRCP

Dr Douglas MacMahon is a Consultant Physician with Special Responsibility for the Elderly with The Cornwall Healthcare Trust and Honorary Senior Lecturer in the University of Plymouth, UK. He has a particular interest in Parkinson's Disease and movement disorders as well as in community care and rehabilitation. Dr MacMahon has been chairman of the British Geriatrics Society (BGS) Policy Committee and the Parkinson's Disease special interest group. He has worked closely with the Parkinson's Disease Society to develop the role of the specialist nurse, chaired the Nurse Steering Group and has been an adviser on Parkinson's Disease to the World Health Organisation. He has lectured widely, published many articles on the above subjects and is a member of several advisory and editorial boards. His most recent publication is entitled 'Services for Older People – The 4 H Approach' and is the result of a Winston Churchill Fellowship that he was awarded.

Email: dgm@doctor.com

TIPU AZIZ MD FRCS

Mr Tipu Aziz is presently consultant neurosurgeon at the Radcliffe Infirmary, Oxford, UK, and Charing Cross Hospital, London, with an interest in surgery for movement disorders. He is also a neuro-physiologist at Oxford University, studying brain stem mechanisms in movement control. Mr Tipu Aziz entered medicine after studying neuro-physiology at University College, London. He was interested in pursuing a career in neuro-surgery and became interested in surgery for movement disorders. However, on completing his surgical training this was no longer in vogue so he studied parkinsonian mechanisms, in the laboratory, towards his doctorate. In 1990 he demonstrated that STN was a new surgical target for Parkinson's disease. This has been central to surgical resurgence in recent years. Tipu Aziz and his team publish extensively on all aspects of surgery for movement disorders.

Email: tipuaziz@btinternet.com

DR DAVID SHLUGMAN MB CHB FRCA

Dr David Shlugman is a Consultant Anaesthetist at the Radcliffe Infirmary, Oxford, UK, where he has been part of the Movement Disorders Team since its inception, publishing together with them on various aspects. Following medical qualification in

Cape Town, South Africa, he specialised in anaesthetics at Groote Schuur Hospital, Cape Town and Hammersmith Hospital, London.
Telephone: **+44 (0)1865 311188**

DR RALPH GREGORY FRCP

Dr Ralph Gregory is a Consultant Neurologist at the Radcliffe Infirmary in Oxford and Royal Berkshire and Battle Hospitals in Reading. He is an Honorary Clinical Senior Lecturer at Oxford University, UK. His particular interest is the management of advanced Parkinson's disease. He currently forms part of a multidisciplanary team with Consultant Neurosurgeon Tipu Aziz. He was formerly at Frenchay Hospital in Bristol with Consultant Neurosurgeon Steven Gill. Telephone: **+44 (0)1865 311188**

CAROLE JOINT RGN

Carole Joint is the Movement Disorder Nurse at the Radcliffe Infirmary, Oxford, UK, working as part of the multi-disciplinary Movement Disorder Group. She has worked as Infection Control Nurse and as an Operating Theatre Sister in Bristol and Oxford. Telephone: **+44 (0)1865 311188**

DR ANNA TURNER BA(HONS) DCLINPSY

Dr Anna Turner is a clinical psychologist who works with the neuro-psychology team in the Russell-Cairns Unit at the Radcliffe Infirmary, Oxford,UK. She qualified as a clinical psychologist at the University of East Anglia, Norwich. Prior to training she completed her undergraduate psychology degree at the University of Reading. In addition to the Movement Disorder work, her interests include oncology and dysexecutive functioning within the adult and paediatric populations. Telephone: **+44 (0)1865 311188**

DR DAVID PERLMUTTER MD

Dr David Perlmutter is a Board-Certified Neurologist who received his medical degree from the University of Miami School of Medicine where he was awarded the Leonard G. Rowntree Research Award. After completing residency training in Neurology at the University of Miami, Dr Perlmutter entered private practice in Naples, Florida where he is Medical Director of the Perlmutter Health Center, Naples MRI, and the Perlmutter Hyperbaric Center. Dr. Perlmutter also serves as Adjunct Instructor at the Institute for Functional Medicine in Gig Harbor, Washington, and has contributed extensively to international medical literature. Publications include papers in The Journal of Neurosurgery, The Southern Medical Journal, and Archives of Neurology. He is the author of the book BrainRecovery.com – Powerful Therapy for Challenging Brain Disorders, and is recognised internationally as a leader in the field of nutritional influences in neurological disorders. Dr Perlmutter has been interviewed on many United States nationally syndicated radio and television

programs including 20/20, The Faith Daniels Program, and Larry King Live.
Email: **perlhealth@aol.com**

Dr Dieter Volc MD

Dr Dieter Volc studied medicine at the University of Innsbruck/Austria. He specialised in Neurology & Psychiatry at the Hospital of Vienna-Lainz and the Psychiatric Hospital. He has established neuro-sonology laboratories and programs for treatment & prevention of stroke, assessment of risk factors of stroke and neurogeriatrics, especially Parkinson's disease, Alzheimer's disease and depressive disorders. In 1990-1994 he became associated with Prof Dr Walther Birkmayer, the founder of L-DOPA therapy in Parkinson's disease, and eventually took over his clinic for the treatment of Parkinson's disease and related disorders. He heads the Neurology Department of the CONFRATERNITÄT - Privatklinik Josefstadt, Vienna and is also the director of PROSENEX Ambulatoriumbetriebsges.m.b.H, a private outpatient facility for neurogeriatric disorders. He lectures and has published widely.
Email: **Prosenex@abacus.at**

Dr Rodney Adeniyi-Jones LRCP & SI MRCP (UK)

After winning the Silver prize for physiology and the Leonard Abramson prize for medicine as an undergraduate, Dr Rodney Adeniyi-Jones went on to specialise in diabetes and endocrinology at St Thomas Hospital in London where he did research on receptors and insulin function. Thereafter, he entered private practice, and since 1993 has been the medical director of the Regent Clinic in London, UK. In 1995, he underwent training in chelation therapy in the USA and is board certified. At his clinic, he focuses on functional and nutritional medicine with a special interest in integrative approaches to cardiovascular disease. He is a Member of The American College for the Advancement of Medicine.
Email: **info@regentclinic.co.uk**

Dr John McLaren-Howard DSc FACN

Dr John McLaren-Howard is internationally acknowledged as an authority on the use of nutrient-related laboratory investigations in medicine. He is the Laboratory Director of BioLab Medical Unit in London. In 1984 he established this state-of-the-art laboratory which specialises in all aspects of nutrition in medicine, together with its Medical Director, Dr Stephen Davies. Over the years, the laboratory facilities have continued to expand under Dr McLaren-Howard and many innovative test procedures have been developed. He is a fellow of the American College of Nutrition and has made many valuable contributions in the USA. Dr McLaren-Howard is author or co-author of numerous scientific papers, a number of which have introduced new medical tests including the Myothermogram.
Email: **info@biolab.demon.co.uk**

DR MONIKA BIRKMAYER

Dr Monika Birkmayer graduated in medicine from The Medical University of Vienna. She went on to specialise in Traditional Chinese Medicine (TCM) doing internships in Austria, Sri Lanka and China. She is the granddaughter of the late Professor Walter Birkmayer, international pioneer in the use of L-dopa therapy, who together with his son, Dr George Birkmayer, first used NADH in the management of Parkinson's disease. She practices as a General Medical Practitioner in Vienna.
Email: **denor@dial.pipex.com**

DR CHRISTIAN THUILE

Dr Christian Thuile graduated in medicine from The Medical University of Vienna. He is President of the International Medical Association for Energetic Medicine and is lector (Associate Professor) of Complimentary Medicine at The Medical University of Vienna. He practices medicine in Vienna as a General Practitioner specialising in Energy-based medicine. He is the author of various books: Practice of Magnetic Therapy (IGEM), Guide to MRS Therapy (IGEM), C.E.S. Cranial Electrotherapy Stimulation (IGEM), Leben mit Vergeßlichkeit (Neomedica Verlag, Wien), So hilft Ihnen das Magnetfeld (Haug-Thieme Verlag), Das Große Buch der Magnetfeldtherapie (Neomedica Verlag), Gefährliche Strahlungen (Molden Verlag), Heilsame Schwingungen (Molden Verlag).
Email: **denor@dial.pipex.com**

DAVID BELL FPODA DPM FAAAS DIPCHORTH DPODM

David Bell first graduated in the UK at The Manchester Foot Hospital and School of Chiropody in Chiropodial Orthopaedics and Chiropody. Postgraduate studies followed at The College of Chiropodial Orthopaedics in Manchester. Postgraduate specialisation included Radiography and Diagnostic Radiology at the University Hospital of Wales, Cardiff, UK, Skin Surgery at Chase Farm Hospital, Enfield, UK, Post-graduate Internal Bone Fixation, Manchester University Anatomy Department, UK, as well as completing the Post Graduate Anatomy Dissection Course at Owens College, Manchester Medical School, UK. He holds a Fellowship of the Podiatry Association, UK, a Doctorate of Podiatric Medicine in the USA, as well as the Fellowship of the Academy of Ambulatory Foot Surgeons in the USA. He then completed Podiatric Education in the USA also doing courses in Endoscopic Surgery. Until its recent closure, he worked at The Devonshire Hospital in London.
Email: **denor@dial.pipex.com**

HELEN KIMBER BSc(HONS) PGCE ECNP

Helen Kimber graduated with Honours from Huddersfield University in the UK in Catering and Applied Nutrition. She has since gained a Post-Graduate Certificate in Education (PGCS) specialising in Nutrition and Anatomy and is currently studying for a Masters Degree in Nutritional Medicine at the University of Surrey. Helen Kimber now leads a dedicated team who specialise in the development of nutritional supplements and the involvement and application of numerous diagnostic tests. She lectures frequently to health professionals and students on the subject of nutrition and is particularly interested in the nutritional aspects of detoxification.
Email: **denor@dial.pipex.com**

JOHN BIRD DO

John Bird is a Registered Osteopath and member of the General Osteopathic Council. He has lectured at The London School of Osteopathy (LSO), and has worked as part of an integrated neurological team. He also works in association with Dr Geoffrey Leader of The London Pain Relief and Nutritional Support Clinic. John Bird has his own osteopathic clinic in London.
Facsimile: **+44 (0)20 8909 2861**

PAM STANBRIDGE MCSP GRAD DIPPHYS SRP

Pam Stanbridge is Senior Physiotherapist in the Elderly Rehabilitation Team and Intermediate Care, as part of the Bedfordshire and Luton Community NHS Trust, UK. She is particularly interested in Parkinson's disease and the physical challenges posed in the home and general environment.
Email: **pamstanbridge@easicom.com**

ADRIENNE GOLEMBO DIP MASS DWR GICFFI DIP AROMIPTI

Adrienne Golembo has designed the "Building Better Backs and Bodies" system of exercises, which is used in various institutes in the UK. Her remedial exercises have been endorsed by Hilda Walsh, Lead Physiotherapist and Back Pain Specialist (City and Hackney Back Pain Programme), as well as by other health professionals. She is particularly interested in optimising musculoskeletal function in people with neurological illness. She works with patients on a one-to-one basis and in this respect, she is part of a multi-disciplinary team. Adrienne Golembo also runs the remedial programme for The Association for Spinal Injury (ASPIRE).
Email: **bbbacks@hotmail.com**   Telephone: **+44 (0)20 895 82626**

CATHERINE BURLEY MSc PGCE BSc AFBPS

Catherine Burley is a consultant clinical psychologist who works for Northwest Anglia Healthcare (NHS Trust) where she has the responsibility of managing the development of psychological services for the elderly in Peterborough and Fenland, UK. She supervises trainees for the PhD Clinical Psychology Training course at University of East Anglia. Her clinical interests are loss and bereavement, working with carers of people with dementia, developing multi-sensory environments and links between stress and cardiac rehabilitation. She is particularly interested in Parkinson's Disease and spoke at the PDNSA conference at Droitwich in 1999. A graduate of Bristol and Leicester Universities, she has her Masters degree in Psychopathology
Email: **theburleys@burley5.freeserve.co.uk**

CAROLYN NOBLE RGN

Carolyn Noble is a Parkinson's Disease Nurse Specialist and Neurological Rehabilitation Co-ordinator. After working for several years as a community nurse she set up the Parkinson's Disease Nursing Service in the Peterborough area. She has published on the role of the Parkinson's Disease Nurse Specialist (PDNS), has presented papers at many national and international conferences and has visited nurses in Stockholm to discuss the development of the role in Sweden. Carolyn Noble is a founder member of the Parkinson's Disease Nurse Specialist Association and is currently involved in research investigating the role of "nurse prescribing" within the PDNS practice framework. She is a member both of the Parkinson's Disease Society Primary Care Task Force and The Parkinson's Disease Society Nurse Development Committee.
Facsimile: **+44 (0)1733 874227**

S. CHRISTINE GLOVER MCSLT

Christine Glover is a member of the Adult Team of Speech and Language Therapists working in hospitals and the surrounding community in Peterborough, UK. She specialises in acquired degenerative and progressive neurological disorders. Christine Glover trained at the Central School of Speech Training and Dramatic Art in London, UK, has worked with children with cerebral palsey and also at the West Middlesex Hospital and Stoke Mandeville.
Email: **denor@dial.pipex.com**

RUTH ROBBINS

Ruth Robbins was a bereavement counsellor in Cape Town, South Africa. She was particularly interested in working with chronically ill people, their families as well as those who are bereaved.

Vera Diamond Dip AT MBAS MISSD

Vera Diamond is a psychotherapist and founder member of the British Autogenic Society. She has pioneered the use of autogenic training together with Dr Wolfgang Luthe's Creativity Mobilisation Technique. Vera Diamond has also worked with child abuse issues in conjunction with the obscene publications branch of New Scotland Yard, London UK. She is now particularly interested in training Parkinson's disease patients to use autogenic training techniques and works in association with the London Pain Relief and Nutritional Support Clinic.

Email: **vera.diamond@lineone.net**   Telephone: **+44 (0)20 7723 2184**

Esther Roos-Lohner DipPhys

Esther Roos-Lohner was the Senior Physiotherapist at The Heilbad, an integrated rehabilitation clinic in St Moritz, Switzerland. She is particularly interested in remedial exercise and has contributed to the book "Total Physical Preparation for Piano Playing" (Denor Press, London, UK) which concentrates on toning, stretching and mobilising of hands, as well as body posture.

Email: **denor@dial.pipex.com**

Dr Jack Levenson LDS RCS(Edin)

Dr Jack Levenson is President of the British Society for Mercury Free Dentistry. He is also Dental Advisor and Executive Committee Member of the Environmental Medicine Foundation and a member of the British Dental Editors Forum. He has been in dental practice and been responsible for the dental sections of the Allergy and Environmental Medicine Departments of The Wellington and Lister Hospitals in London. Jack lectures extensively on the subjects of mercury and safe amalgam removal, allergies and other environmental factors which affect the health of the teeth and supporting structures. Currently, he runs a practice at The Brompton Dental and Health Clinic in London, confined to testing patients for mercury toxicity, and advising both patients and dentists on protective procedures.

Telephone: **+44 (0)20 7370 0055**

Foreword

by Professor Leslie Findley OLJ TD MD FRCP FACP MRCS DCH

It is now one hundred and eighty three years since the first clinical description, of what we now know as Parkinson's disease, entered the medical literature. The last two centuries have seen clinicians and basic scientists define the condition and describe much of the structural pathology. In the middle of the last century, the importance of degeneration of the nigro striatal dopamine system, with resultant loss of the neurotransmitter dopamine, was recognised as a core change in the brain underlying the development of Parkinson's disease.

Central dopamine replacement then became, and remains, the mainstay of medical management. However, it soon became recognised that dopamine replacement, whilst improving the motor symptoms of Parkinson's disease, did not influence the continued progression of the disease, and in addition, resulted in the now well recognised motor and neuro-psychiatric complications of long term treatment. The response to this, in the last two decades, has been an increasing availability of dopaminergic and other drugs in attempts to improve pharmacological management. Likewise, there has been a renaissance of surgical techniques, ranging from lesioning and deep brain stimulation to brain implants of various types.

These last decades have been associated with a growing appreciation, by those responsible for care of people with Parkinson's disease, that control of motor symptoms is just one facet of any management programme. Those with Parkinson's disease may now expect to live their full term and the long term side-effects of dopaminergic medications, associated with complex effects of disease progression, including neuro-psychiatric and cognitive problems, continue to provide a challenge to all.

The practising clinician, who has responsibilities for diagnosing and managing Parkinson's disease, now recognises the need for access to multi-disciplinary teams to deal with the complexities of problems arising as a result of the disease and its treatment. In brief, the clinician has had to recognise that any programme of management must endeavour to improve the quality of life of the individual with Parkinson's disease, rather than simply suppress individual symptoms.

With these ideas in mind the editors of this volume have boldly drawn together health professionals of diverse skills and backgrounds to present an integrated picture of the management of Parkinson's disease. In addition to chapters on the diagnosis, medical and surgical management, which remain the core of many volumes published on the subject of Parkinson's disease, the editors have gone on to cover such diverse areas as nutrition, the role of various specialist therapists, psychology and behavioural programmes, sexual function, bowel function and most importantly, the needs and health of carers.

The format of this volume has been constructed to be of value and accessible, not only to physicians and other healthcare professionals, but to those with Parkinson's disease and their carers.

The individual chapters naturally represent the views of the individual authors and some may not be accepted by all. However, this volume contains a wealth of theoretical and practical knowledge which will be of benefit to all those in the world of Parkinson's disease.

Until we are able to prevent Parkinson's disease, and reverse the pathology in those who already have it, a regularly updated text covering the holistic management of this complex disorder will continue to be needed.

Leslie J Findley

Diagnosis of Parkinson's Disease

by Professor Aroldo Rossi

The diagnosis of Parkinson's disease is essentially clinical and is based on the natural history of the disease and the patient's clinical symptoms[1, 2, 3, 4, 5, 6].

Diagnosis during a person's lifetime is, however, always presumptive, with a variable degree of precision. A definite diagnosis is only possible through post mortem analysis of pathological findings[7].

A diagnosis, however, should be made as early as possible in order to assess symptoms that can be improved and initiate appropriate treatment.

Natural History of the Disease

1. Age of disease onset

About 80% of cases present between the ages of 40 and 70 years with a peak incidence occurring at about 60 years of age. Disease onset before the age of 35 or after 75 years is uncommon[8, 9].

Parkinson's disease at a young age is generally associated with a familial prevalence. These patients progress more slowly with excellent response to L-dopa but have a greater incidence of motor fluctuations.

2. Mode of onset

Parkinson's disease is usually of insidious and gradual onset, primarily affecting the upper extremities in an asymmetric fashion. Symptoms are initially unilateral for the first one to two years and bilateral over three to four years from the onset of symptoms[10].

Often the characteristic motor symptoms are preceded by non-specific disorders such as fatigue, myalgia, loss of smell, depression, constipation and sweating abnormalities[11].

3. Progression of the disease

The disease progresses slowly and continually without any sharp variations. Progression may be more rapid in the first years of the disease[12, 13].

4. Initial features

Resting tremor is the most common initial feature, even if the patient cannot always pinpoint the first symptom. The tremor increases in periods of anxiety and disappears during sleep and motor actions and it occurs more commonly in younger patients. Another first sign may be the loss of finger dexterity, which causes difficulty in handwriting. Relatively early signs may be: decreased associated movements and slowness of gait, reduced volume and monotonous speech. Sialorrhea, dysphagia, impotence, urinary disturbances, postural instability and cognitive impairment occur late in Parkinson's disease[14, 15].

Clinical Manifestations

In order to diagnose Parkinson's disease, the following should be taken into consideration: 1) cardinal signs, 2) secondary signs and 3) exclusion criteria[16, 17, 18].

1) **The cardinal signs are** (Table 1 page 4):

a) tremor at rest[19.]

b) bradykinesia (slowness of initiation of voluntary movement with progressive reduction of speed and amplitude of repetitive movement)[20, 21].

c) rigidity (muscular stiffness with some intensity in both extensor and flexor muscle; the degree of rigidity is an important determinant of patient's level of functional disability.

d) postural instability (loss of balance associated with propulsion and retropulsion not caused by vestibular, cerebellar, or propioceptive dysfunctions). Bradykinesia and rigidity occur in almost all patients and tremor in about 75%.

Although not included among the cardinal signs, a good or excellent response to levodopa given in suitable doses for an adequate period of time is present in all Parkinson's disease patients. It is important to evaluate not only the effect of a single dose (short-term effects) but also the effects of a single drug administered over a period of several days (long term effects)[22, 23].

2) **Secondary signs** (Table 1 page 4).

These are not generally present in the initial stages of the disease. Some, such as orthostatic hypotension or delay in gastric emptying may be caused by anti-parkinsonian drugs. The most frequent symptoms are depression, bradyphrenia, sexual and urinary disturbances, and seborrhoea[24].

3) **Exclusion criteria** (Table 2 page 5) .

These are clinical, which, when present, exclude the diagnosis of Parkinson's disease[25].

Degree of Certainty of Diagnosis[26]
Clinically possible if the patient shows one of the following features: tremor, rigidity or bradykinesia.

Clinically probable if the patient shows two of the cardinal signs (tremor, rigidity, bradykinesia and postural instability) or if these are asymmetrical.

Clinically definite if the patient shows three of the cardinal signs and if two of these are asymmetrical.

Differential Diagnosis
Before diagnosing Parkinson's disease it is necessary to exclude other causes of Parkinsonism (Table 3 page 5).

The most frequent causes are drug-induced and atypical neuro-degenerative disorders.

The latter form a group of degenerative diseases, which in adults are characterised by bradykinesia and rigidity. These include progressive supranuclear palsy (PSP), the multi system atrophies (MSA) and corticobasal ganglionic degeneration (CBGD)[27].

As opposed to Parkinson's disease resting tremor is uncommon, onset is symmetrical and response to the dopaminergic therapy is minimal or absent (see Table 2). Some signs are very typical and help us make a differential diagnosis. In PSP the most characteristic sign, although not a very early one, is a supranuclear gaze palsy (limited voluntary or pursuit vertical or horizontal eye movements with preservation of oculocephalic reflexes); early postural instability with frequent falls as well as difficulty in swallowing and speech are often present. In MSA the main characteristics are severe early autonomic dysfunction and early cerebellar symptoms (ataxia of stance and gait, dysmetria and dysartria)[28, 29, 30, 31].

In CBGD the most characteristic clinical signs are an initial asymmetric akinetic-rigidity syndrome with contra-lateral involvement of 1 to 2 years and cortical features such as alien-limb (patients do not consider the affected limb), apraxia and dysphasia[32].

Drug-induced Parkinsonism (DIP) is also very common: in fact a variety of drugs have the potential to produce Parkinsonism (see Table 5). DIP may be clinically indistinguishable from Parkinson's disease, so patients' therapeutic history should be carefully reviewed and a history should be taken to check ataxia, unsteadiness and inco-ordination of movement. Several clinical clues can help distinguish between the two disease entities.

In DIP the following are more common: asymmetrical presentation, a lower incidence of resting tremor and the presence of low frequency perioral tremor known as the "rabbit syndrome"[33, 34, 35].

Obviously these drugs should not be used to treat Parkinson's disease.

Table 1.
Clinical Manifestations of Parkinson's disease

1) **Cardinal signs**	- resting tremor - bradykinesia/akinesia - cogwheel rigidity - postural instability
2) **Secondary signs**	- cognitive - (bradyphrenia (slow thinking), dementia) - psychiatric (depression, agitation, sleep disturbances) - cranial nerve (decreased eye blinking, blurred vision, dysarthria, dysphagia) - autonomic (siallorhea, orthostatic hypotension, impotence, delayed emptying time, constipation, urinary bladder dysfunction) - sensory (cramps, paresthesias, pain, olfactory dysfunction) - skin (seborrhoea)

Table 2.
Exclusion Criteria for Parkinson's Disease (UK Parkinson's Disease Society Brain Bank, 1998)

	- History of repeated strokes, repeated head injury, and definite encephalopathies, and neuroleptic treatment
	- Oculomotor deficits
	- Pyramidal signs
	- Cerebellar signs
	- Early severe autonomic involvement
	- Early severe dementia
	- More than one affected relative
	- Strictly unilateral features after 3 years
	- Presence of cerebral tremor or communicating hydrocephalus on CT scan
	- Negative response to large dose of levodopa

Table 3.
Classification of Parkinsonism

Atypical neurodegenerative syndrome		
(Parkinson-plus Syndrome)	-	Progressive Supranuclear Palsy (PSP)
	-	Multiple System Atrophy (MSA)
	-	Corticobasal Ganglionic Degeneration (CBGD)
Secondary	-	Drug induced (DIP)
	-	Postencephalitic
	-	Atherosclerotic
	-	Repeated head injury
	-	Toxic

Table 4.
Features Suggestive of an Atypical Neurodegenerative Parkinsonism

Motor	-	Early instability and falls
	-	Rapid disease progression
	-	Absent or poor response to levodopa
	-	Pyramidal and/or cerebellar signs
	-	Early dysphagia and/or dysarthria
Oculomotor	-	Supranuclear gaze palsy
	-	Slowing and difficulty initiating saccades
Cognitive	-	Early dementia
	-	Cortical signs
Autonomic	-	Early autonomic failure unrelated to
	-	treatment

Table 5.
Drugs that may Induce Parkinsonism

	-	Typical neuroleptics
	-	Anti-emetic dopamine blocking agent including (metoclopramide, sulpiride)
	-	Dopamine depleting drugs (reserpine, tetrabenazine)
	-	Anticonvulsants (valproic acid, phenytoin)
	-	Calcium-channel blockers (cinnarizine, flunarizine)
	-	Other drugs (lithium, alpha-methyl-dopa)

References

1. Calne DB, Snow BJ, Lee C. *Criteria For Diagnosing Parkinson's Disease.* Ann Neurol 32 (Suppl): 125-127, 1992

2. Gelb DJ, Oliver E, Gilman S. *Diagnostic Criteria For Parkinson's Disease.* Arch Neurol 56: 33-39, 1999

3. Huges AJ, Ben-Schlomo Y, Daniel SE, Lees AJ. *What Features Improve The Accuracy Of Clinical Diagnosis In Parkinsons' Disease.* Neurology 42: 1142-1146, 1992

4. Huges AJ,Daniel SE, Kilford L, Lees AJ. *The Accuracy Of The Clinical Diagnosis Of Parkinsonis Disease: A Clinico-Pathological Study Of 100 Cases.* J Neurol Neurosurg Psychiatry 55: 181-184, 1992

5. Lalli F, Rossi A. *Semeiotica Del Morbo Di Parkinson.* Gallai V, Rossi A, Parnetti L (Eds): Update Sulle Malattie Extrapiramidali. ESI Napoli 93-107, 2000

6. Paulson HL, Stern MB. *Clinical Manifestation Of Parkinson's Disease.* Watts RL And Koller WC (Eds): *Movement Disorders: Neurologic Principles And Practice.* Mcgraw-Hill New York 183-199, 1997

7. Stern M. *The Clinical Characteristics Of Parkinson's Disease And Parkinsonian Syndrome: Diagnosis And Assessment.* In Stern MB, Hurtig HI (Eds): *The Comprehensive Management Of Parkinson's Disease.* New York: PMA Publishing Corporation 1988

8. Rajput AH, Offord KP, Beard CM, Kurland LT. *Epidemiology Of Parkinsonism: Incidence, Classification And Mortality.* Ann Neurol 16: 278-282, 1984

9. Tunner CM, Hubble CJ, Chan P. *Epidemiology And Genetics Of Parkinson's Disease.* : Watts RL And Koller WC (Eds): *Movement Disorders: Neurologic Principles And Practice.* Mcgraw-Hill New York 297-306, 1997

10. Hoehn MM, Yahr MD. *Parkinsonism: Onset, Progression And Mortality. Neurology* 17: 427-442, 1967

11. Op. Cit. N. 6

12 Op. Cit. N. 2

13. Op. Cit. N. 6

14. Op. Cit. N. 6

15. Quinn NP. *Parkinson's Disease: Clinical Features.* Bailliers, Clin Neurol 6: 1-13, 1997

16. Op. Cit. N. 1

17. Sely G. *Clinical Features.* Sterne G (Ed). *Parkinson's Disease.* London: Chapman And Hall Medical: 33-388, 1990

18. Gershanik OS. *Parkinson's Disease. Differential Diagnosis And Treatment Of Movement Disorders* Tolosa E, Koller WC, Gershanik OS (Eds): Butterworth-Heinemann, Boston 7-25,1998

19. Mancini ML, Rossi A. I Tremori. Gallai V, Rossi A, Parnetti L (Eds): *Update* Sulle Malattie Extrapiramidali. ESI Napoli 185-197, 2000

20. Bloxam CA, Mindall TA, Frith CD. *Initiation And Execution Of Predictable And Unpredictable Movements In Parkinson's Disease.* Brain 107: 371-384, 1984

21. Marsden CD. *Defects Of Movement In Parkinson's Disease.* Delwaide PJ, Agnoli A (Eds): *Clinical Neurophysiology In Parkinson's Disease.* Amsterdam: Elsevier Science Publisher, 1985

22. Costa DF, Sheehan LJ, Philips PA, Moore-Smith B. *The Levodopa Test In Parkinson's Disease.* Age Ageing 24: 210-212, 1995

23. Zappia M, Montesanti R, Colao R, Branca D, Nicoletti G, Aguglia U, Quattrone A. *Short Term Levodopa Test Assessed By Movement Time Accurately Predicts Dopaminergic Responsiveness In Parkinson's Disease.* Mov Disord 12: 103-106, 1997

24. Op. Cit. N. 18

25. Op. Cit. N. 18

26. Op. Cit. N. 1

27. *Movement Disorders: Neurologic Principles And Practice.* Watts RL, Koller CW (Eds): Mcgraw-Hill (Health Professional Division) New York 1997.

28. Op. Cit. N. 27

29. Golbe LI. *Progressive Supranuclear Palsy.* Watts RL And Koller WC (Eds): *Movment Disorders: Neurologic Principles And Practice.* Mcgraw-Hill New York 279- 295, 1997

30. Koller WC And Hbble JP. *Classification Of Parkinsonism.* Koller WC (Ed): *Handbook Of Parkinson's Disease.* Marcel Dekker, Inc. 59-103, 1992

31. Oertel WH, Quinn NP. *Multiple System Atrophy And Corticobasal Degeneration.* In: Differential In: Tolosa E, Koller WC, Gershanik OS (Eds): *Differential Diagnosis And Treatment Of Movement Disorders* Butterworth-Heinemann, Boston 39-51,1998

32. Op. Cit. N. 31

33. Hubble JP. *Drug Induced Parkinsonism.* Watts RL And Koller WC (Eds): *Movement Disorders: Neurologic Principles And Practice.* Mcgraw-Hill New York 325-330, 1997

34. Klawans HL, Bergen D, Bruyn GW. *Prolonged Drug-Induced Parkinsonism.* Cont Neurol 35: 368-377, 1973

35. Rossi A: Terapia Dei Parkinsonismi. Gallai V, Rossi A, Parnetti L (Eds): *Update* Sulle Malattie Extrapiramidali. ESI Napoli 289-301, 2000

Pharmacological Treatment in Parkinson's Disease

by Professor Aroldo Rossi

The primary aim of pharmacological treatment of Parkinson's disease is that of improving symptoms and quality of life.

It is, therefore, an exclusively symptomatic treatment that is unable to modify the natural history of the disease and is directed primarily at compensating the dopaminergic deficit found in the Parkinsonian brain.

There are still many unresolved questions. The principle debate centres around the optimum time at which to start pharmacological treatment. In fact, there are two contrasting opinions:

a) according to some people treatment should be started in the early stages, in order to ensure an immediate clinical improvement[1, 2, 3, 4, 5, 6].

b) others prefer to wait for the onset of motor complications. Before pharmacological treatment is instituted, in the pharmacological pre-treatment stage, the patient and his family can be given psychological, occupational, financial, physiotherapeutic and nutritional support[7, 8, 9, 10, 11, 12, 13].

If the second, preferable option is chosen, symptomatic therapy should be started only when symptoms are severe enough to cause functional disability. The level of disability will naturally be evaluated in each individual patient, taking into account various factors such as age, any working activity, the type of symptoms and their localisation. Rating scales exist, such as the ADL (Figure 1) (Activities of Daily Living) which is a submultiple of the Parkinson's disease (Figure 2) (Unified Parkinson's disease Rating Scale). It can help quantify this disability[14].

Generally speaking, administration of a single drug is preferable in the initial stages of the disease. Any increase in the dose and any addition of other drugs should be carried out only when there is an increase in functional disability with a worsening quality of life.

The criteria on which pharmacological treatment must be based are as follows: -
1. The symptoms can be attenuated but not abolished.

2. A patient should be made aware that the ideal pharmacological therapy does not exist at present and should be given realistic expectations of any treatment plan.

3. Pharmacological treatment should be started only when functional disability requires it.

4. Monotherapy should be used where possible.

5. The smallest number of drugs possible should be used at the minimum possible dose.

6. The therapy should be structured according to the patient's age. Treatment considerations are very different for a 50-year old patient, whose treatment horizon may span over 25-35 years, from those of a 70-year old patient.

7. The use of levodopa should be delayed as long as possible, especially in younger patients (< 50). In older patients (> 70), who have a shorter time horizon, levodopa is more clearly indicated. The risk of motor fluctuations and dyskinesias appear to be related to the duration and dose of the levodopa therapy.

8. Before starting treatment, patients should be evaluated for signs of cognitive impairment or depression. Cognitive disturbances of memory may, in fact, be worsened by anti-parkinsonian drugs, particularly by anticholinergics, selegiline and dopamine agonists.

9. Dopamine agonists may more easily produce hallucinations or delirium in those patients with underlying or pre-existing psychiatric disorders.

10. The presence of other diseases such as cardiac, renal or hepatic disorders should be carefully taken into account.

Drugs to be used are levodopa, dopamine agonists, anticholinergics, amantadine, MAO-B inhibitors and catechol-O-methyltransferase inhibitors.

Levodopa (L-Dopa)

This is the most effective drug in the symptomatic treatment of Parkinson's disease. Levodopa is, in fact, the precursor of dopamine, a substance that is lacking in the brain of Parkinson's disease patients[15, 16].

As dopamine is unable to pass through the blood-brain barrier, its precursor, levodopa, is able to reach the brain and has been used as a dopaminergic substitute treatment.

When using levodopa there are three critical points, which may limit therapeutic effectiveness:

1. Its absorption and transport to the brain

2. Its peripheral metabolism

3. Its short half-life.

1. Orally administered levodopa first passes through the stomach and is then absorbed by the small intestine. As a result, all factors that alter gastric motility reduce or delay the levodopa plasma peak, causing delay in or failure of the clinical response. Among the factors that reduce gastric motility are the disease itself as well as the drugs that are used such as anticholinergics and levodopa in particular, which relaxes the lower esophageal sphincter. An increase in pH in the stomach slows down emptying, in the same way as a decrease in the pH may prevent the tablet from dissolving completely so that it is only partially absorbed. Once the small intestine has been reached, levodopa has to pass through the gut wall into the circulation and the blood-brain barrier (BBB) in order to reach the brain[17, 18, 19.]

   The transport of levodopa across the gut wall and the blood-brain barrier is an active saturable transport system that, "if occupied by other substances" is unable to transport a sufficient quantity of levodopa to the brain. Substances that easily occupy these transport systems are the neutral amino acids, derived from the breakdown of dietary protein[20].

2. Once absorbed, levodopa undergoes peripheral transformation that diminish its therapeutic properties. There are two main ways of transformation.

a) The first predominant way takes place at an intestinal and hepatic level and is a process of decarboxylation, which leads to the formation of dopamine. We know that this substance is unable to pass through the blood-brain barrier and therefore, as it is unable to reach the brain, it is destined to remain outside this organ. Not only is this useless from a therapeutic point of view, it can cause serious peripheral side affects[21, 22]. The combination of levodopa with substances able to inhibit peripheral decarboxylation and which do not pass the blood-brain barrier, have resolved the majority of these problems. Levodopa is, in fact, found on the market in combination with peripheral inhibitors of decarboxylation, such as CARBIDOPA, administered in a dose of 25 mg to 250 mg of levodopa (ratio 1:10), and BENZERAZIDE, administered in a dose of 25 mg to 100 mg of levodopa (ratio 1:4).

b) Much of an oral dose of levodopa is metabolised by the enzyme catechol - o - methyl transferase (COMT) before it can cross the blood brain barrier and leads to the formation of 3-0-methyl dopa. This has a half-life of over twelve hours and is able to compete with levodopa across the blood brain barrier. In order to limit this transformation, COMT inhibitors can be used as an adjunct to levodopa, thereby increasing the amount of dopamine available in the brain[23, 24, 25].

3. In addition to problems of absorption and distribution, a further complication in the treatment with levodopa is due to its short half-life, which is approximately 60-90 minutes. This causes fluctuations in its plasma levels with peaks followed by fairly sharp drops. Similar fluctuations in dopamine levels occur in the brain leading to alternating hyper and hypo stimulation of the dopaminergic pathway. This is thought to be responsible for the decompensation stage when in the long run treatment with levodopa is no longer able to guarantee an adequate functional response[26, 27, 2,8 29].

For some time now, there has been a trend to delay the use of levodopa as long as possible and to introduce it only when other drugs are no longer able to guarantee sufficient personal autonomy. This is particularly important in younger patients with a far greater number of years on treatment.

In fact, after it has been used for a few years, it causes the onset of important, serious side effects in the majority of cases.

Two stages can be identified in Parkinson's disease. In the first, initial stage, also known as the "honeymoon stage", levodopa is able to effectively control symptoms. In the second stage or "L-dopa long term syndrome" which occurs within 5-10 years, levodopa is no longer able to guarantee adequate functional autonomy and well-being and serious motor complications begin to occur ("wearing-off" and "on-off" states) as well as dyskinesia). "Wearing-off" is a predictable variation in motor function related to levodopa ingestion. "On" refers to the condition of patients with good clinical motor status and "off" refers to patients who have lost that good motor status. "On-off" is an unpredictable functional status not related to levodopa intake.   Once treatment has begun with levodopa, it is essential to administer the least possible number of doses and maintain the total daily dose below 500 mg. It is easier to maintain doses at a low level if levodopa is used in conjunction with other anti-parkinsonian drugs, such as amantadine or dopamine agonists[30, 31, 32, 33].

It is always advisable to start with low doses: 50-60 mg/day during the first week and escalate very slowly until symptomatic relief is achieved. The final dose must be tailored to the individual patient.

Levodopa is more effective in controlling bradykinesia and rigidity whereas its effects on tremor are variable and unpredictable. It has no positive effect on postural instability.

Two drugs, Madopar and Sinemet, can be found on the market which differ in their peripheral decarboxylation inhibitor, benserazide and carbidopa, respectively.

There are no significant differences between the two products and the choice between one or the other depends on the physician's personal experience.

There are various types of formulations:

- Standard formulations which are the most commonly used.

- Controlled-release preparation (Madopar HBS and Sinemet CR): these have been developed to try to obtain longer lasting plasma levels. However, it should be underlined that absorption of these formulations is even more unpredictable than for standard formulations and it is doubtful whether their use gives significant advantages.

- Rapid absorption formulations (Madopar dispersible): these formulations are soluble in water and pass more rapidly into the circulatory stream, as they reach the absorption site in the small intestine more rapidly.

The most frequent side effects are nausea and orthostatic hypotension, which can be seen particularly at the beginning of the treatment. Less commonly and, especially in the advanced stages of the disease, hallucinations and psychosis may appear. Treatment of these problems will be discussed in a separate chapter.

Suggestions to Optimise Response to the Use of Levodopa

1. Introduce levodopa at a low dosage and then escalate very slowly.

2. Try to keep the dose of levodopa below 500 mg per day.
   Do not exceed a total daily dose of 1000mg.

3. L-dopa should be taken on an empty stomach. Patients should wait until the drug has properly "kicked in" before eating. If the ensuing meal has contained protein-rich food, they should wait two hours before further taking L-dopa. If the meal has only contained carbohydrates/fats, L-dopa may be administered earlier. (Details of drug-nutrient interactions and recommendations are to be found in the chapter "Nutritional management" in the section titled "Optimising Function by Nutritional Manipulation.)

4. Try to encourage gastric emptying with the diet and, if necessary, with prokinetic drugs.

5. Use the controlled release formulations preferably at night.

Dopamine Agonists(DA-agonists)

These compounds simulate the action of dopamine and are able to directly stimulate dopamine receptors.

The term agonist derives from the fact that these molecules have an affinity equal to or greater than that of dopamine for its receptor. Various classes of dopamine receptors have been identified: those, which are important for motor functions, are called D1, D2 and D3. Compared with levodopa, dopamine agonists offer several advantages.

Firstly, they act independently of the dopamine-producing neurones in the subtantia nigra, which have been shown to degenerate in Parkinson's disease.

Secondly, they do not use saturable carriers for their absorption and transportation in the brain, and therefore there is no interference with meals. They can be taken with or without food. Patients with nausea should take dopaminergic agents after a meal[34, 35, 36, 37].

Thirdly, they are characterised by a greater duration of action compared with levodopa and therefore each single dose of the drug ensures a longer period of L-dopa receptor stimulation.

This is very important as many of the motor complications of long-term treatment are caused by intermittent stimulation of the receptors. In fact, several studies[38, 39, 40, 41, 42] have demonstrated that dopamine agonists are associated with a lower incidence of motor fluctuations and dyskinesia than levodopa.

Dopamine Agonists appear to have a neuroprotective effect, as they are capable of both reducing the production and enhancing the elimination of free radicals[43, 44, 45, 46, 47, 48, 49]. They are, at least in part, able to slow down the progression of the disease[50, 51, 52, 53]. Neuroprotective treatment uses drugs that protect neurones of the substantia nigra by slowing down the degenerative process. Up until now Selegiline has been used but there are other promising compounds such as anti-apoptotics and trophic factors[54, 55, 56, 57].

For these reasons dopamine agonists are used ever increasingly today in the treatment of both the initial stage and the advanced stage of Parkinson's disease.

The general opinion is that in the initial stages of the disease and in patients under 65, first line therapy should be with a dopamine agonist alone. As monotherapy they are, in fact, able to offer a good therapeutic response which is maintained for 3-5 years in more than one third of the patients. To optimise this effect and maintain it as long as possible the doses have to be increased very slowly. This enables us to delay the use of levodopa for as long as possible and therefore delay the onset of the "long term L-dopa syndrome"[58, 59, 60].

Those available on the market are: bromocriptine, pramipexole, pergolide, ropinirole, apomorphine and cabergoline.

Although they differ in their pharmacological profile, clinical experience has shown they have similar therapeutic effects.

1. Bromocriptine: this is an ergot alkaloid dopamine receptor agonist with a high affinity for the D2 receptor. It was one of the first available dopamine agonists. Its half-life is 3 hours with a peak plasma level after about 1 hour. The clinical effect lasts for 3-4 hours and with larger doses can last up to 6 hours. It can be initiated at a dose of one half of a 2.5 mg tablet per day and increased slowly to a daily dose in the range of 20-50 mg per day. Potential side effects, that in 20% of the patients can be very serious, are nausea, vomiting, orthostatic hypotension, confusion, hallucinations and erythromelalgia: a painful reddish discoloration of the skin.

2. Pergolide: this is a semisynthetic ergot derivative that acts on both D1 and D2 receptors peak plasma levels are reached within 1-2 hours and its half-life is about 20-27 hours. The starting dose is half of a 0.05 mg tablet, with an initial target dose of 0.25 mg, three times daily (TID) achieved over 15-20 days. The mean recommended total dose is 3 mg divided throughout

the day. Its long half-life has the advantage of continually stimulating the dopaminergic receptors. Potential side effects such as nausea, vomiting, orthostatic hypotension, cognitive dysfunction, increased liver enzymes and peripheral edema are usually less intense than those caused by bromocriptine.

3. Ropinirole: this is a non-ergoline agonist with a high affinity for D2 receptors. It has a half-life of about 6 hours and the plasma peak is reached after about 1.5 hours in fasted patients and after about 4 hours when taken with a meal.

   The starting dose is 0.25 mg TID, with an initial target dose of 1 mg TID achieved over 1-2 months. The mean dose in the initial stages of the disease is about 6-8 mg per day and the maximum dose is 24 mg. Its original chemical formula is very similar to that of dopamine. It can be used in all stages of the disease, both as monotherapy and as an adjunct to levodopa, as shown by numerous clinical studies[61, 62, 63]. In the initial stages it has shown itself to be as effective as levodopa in controlling the symptoms of the disease. In the more advanced stages, in conjunction with levodopa, it reduces fluctuations in motor function and improves quality of life. Although side effects are similar to those of dopamine agonists, they appear less serious.

4. Pramipexole: this is a non-ergoline dopamine agonist with a high affinity for D2 and D3 receptors. Peak plasma level is reached in 2-3 hours and its half-life is 8-12 hours. It is introduced at a dose of 0.25 mg/day and escalated to an initial target of 1.5 mg/day over 1-2 months. The usual maximum dose is 3 to 4.5 mg/day. Although side effects are similar to those of other dopamine agonists, orthostatic hypotension is less frequent, whereas somnolence may be more common and may necessitate dose reduction or discontinuation. It is effective both as monotherapy in the initial stages and as an adjunct to levadopa in the more advanced stages[64, 65, 66, 67].

5. Cabergoline: this is an ergot derivative with a high affinity for D2 receptors. It has a long half-lifeof about 65 hours and can be administered once a day. The initial dose is 0.05 mg with a maximum of 5 mg/day. Side effects are the same as those of other DA-agonists. The interest shown in this drug is due to its long half-life, which guarantees stable stimulation of dopaminergic receptors. It is particularly effective in the advanced stages of the disease and when used as an adjunct to levodopa, it is able to significantly decrease motor fluctuations[68, 69].

6. Apomorphine: this is a synthetic derivative of morphine that effectively relieves all Parkinsonian symptoms; it is a non-selective D1 and D2 dopamine receptor agonist. It cannot be administered orally and is given subcutaneously. This onset of action is within 5 to 15 minutes and its effect lasts 30 to 120 minutes. It is used as a diagnostic test to assess dopaminergic responsiveness in patients with Parkinson's disease and also as a rescue agent for refractory off periods. It can be given by continuous subcutaneous infusion by a programmable pump. Its most serious side effect is that it induces vomiting and is therefore used together with an anti-emetic such as domperidone (50 mg/day)[70, 71, 72].

Suggestions for Optimising Response to Dopamine Agonists

■ Use as monotherapy in the initial stages of the disease and in patients under 65 years of age.

■ Give preference to non-ergoline derivatives such as ropinirole and pramipexole.

■ Give preference to those with the longest half-life: cabergoline (65 hours), pergolide (15-27 hours), pramipexole (8-12 hours), ropinirole (3-10 hours).

■ Associate with anti-emetics such as domperidone to reduce nausea and vomiting.

■ Administer after a meal in order to reduce their side effects.

■ Escalate the dose very slowly.

■ Administer the minimum effective dose.

■ Use them in conjunction with levodopa in the advanced stages to diminish motor fluctuations, especially dyskinesia.

■ Administer with great care in patients over 65 years of age.

Amantadine

This is an antiviral drug, which was found to improve parkinsonian symptoms when it was used to treated Asian influenza in 1960.

This drug has recently been reintroduced because it alleviates early parkinsonian symptoms. It also has a neuroprotective action[74, 75] and is also useful in controlling dyskinesias in the advanced stages of the disease.

Orally administered amantadine is rapidly absorbed with a plasma peak after about 3 hours and a half-life of about 24 hours. The dose ranges from 200 to 400 mg per day and must be used with great care in patients with renal disease.

As adjunctive therapy to dopamine agonists, it is effective in controlling dyskinesia in the advanced stages of the disease.

Anticholinergics

In the striatum the dopaminergic and cholinergic neurotransmission are in balance. In PD patients the striatum dopamine deficiency causes a relative cholinergic overactivity. The anticholinergic agents balance this cholinergic overactivity.

Currently, the use of these agents is generally limited to younger patients whose main symptom is tremor. They should not be used for elderly patients because they may worsen any cognitive deficit and cause mental confusion, hallucinations and memory impairment.

The most commonly used are Trihexyphenildyl-HCL-Benztropine Mesylate, Biperiden-HCL and Procyclidine-HCL.

Selegiline

This is a relatively selective, irreversible inhibitor of the enzyme monoamine oxidase type B (MAO-B). Monoamine oxidase inhibitors (MAO) are enzymes that play an important role in the catabolism of neuro-transmitters. MAO-B is important in the breakdown of dopamine, a biochemical process in which potentially harmful products such as free-radicals are formed.

By inhibiting the oxidative metabolism of dopamine, Selegiline improves the symptoms of Parkinson's disease and may have a neuro-protective effect[76]. Selegiline also has the capacity to clear free radicals[77, 78, 79, 80].

Selegiline is well absorbed when ingested orally and easily crosses the blood-brain barrier. Its plasma half-life time is 40 hours and its effect can persist for 3-4 months after it has been discontinued. The dose is 10 mg per day and is well tolerated. Sporadic side effects include raised liver enzymes and, when administered with levodopa, can exacerbate dyskinesias and hallucinations. A serotonin syndrome may occur if selegiline is used with some antidepressants such as serotonin re-uptake inhibitors and tryptophane. It is usually used at the onset of the disease either as monotherapy or as an adjunct to levodopa or dopamine agonists and can benefit patients with motor fluctuations in the advanced stages of Parkinson's disease.

Catechol-o-methyltransferease (COMT) Inhibitors

Levodopa is mainly metabolised by the enzyme dopa decarboxylase and catechol-O-methyltransferase (COMT). When levodopa is administered with a peripheral dopa decarboxylase inhibitor, such as benserazide or carbidopa, levodopa metabolism with COMT increases resulting in increased production of 3-O-methyldopa. This metabolite competes with levodopa for transport across the gut and blood-brain barrier and may decrease the absorption and efficacy of levodopa in the brain[81, 82].

The addition of a peripheral COMT inhibitor has several advantages with prolongation of the half life of levodopa by 30-50%, and thus more levodopa becomes available for transport across the blood-brain barrier.

Two COMT inhibitors are available: Tolcapone and Entacapone. Currently Entacapone is the only one available as the European Union, Canada and Australia have suspended the marketing of Tolcapone.

Entacapone is rapidly absorbed after oral administration and its half-life is approximately 2 to 3 hours. The dose is 200 mg with each dose of levodopa. Entacapone is metabolised by the liver and is contraindicated in patients with clinically significant liver impairment.

It facilitates higher and more uniform levels of levodopa in the brain. This in turn reduces the extent of motor fluctuations in both the early and late stages of the disease[83, 84].

Frequent Side Effects of Anti-Parkinsonian Drugs

1) Orthostatic Hypotension

A fall in blood pressure on standing is frequently found in patients with Parkinson's disease. It may be caused by the disease itself or, more often, by the drugs used, particularly dopamine agonists, commonly during the first week of treatment. If severe, it can cause syncope by reducing cerebral perfusion. For this reason it is advisable to measure the blood pressure both lying and standing.

There are generally two approaches to managing orthostatic hypotension[85, 86].

a) Non-pharmacological measures:

■ Change posture frequently

■ Get up slowly

- Sit with the feet over the bed ten minutes before getting up in the morning

- Avoid large meals and alcohol

- Avoid extreme heat

- Ensure adequate fluid intake

- Sleep with the bed raised at the foot end

- Wear compressive garments if appropriate

b) If these measures are not sufficient, it is necessary to employ one or more pharmacological agents:

- Fludrocortisone, a salt-retaining steroid, can be started at 0.1 mg per day and increased to 0.3 mg TID. The patients should be monitored for supine hypertension and symptoms of congestive heart failure[87].

- Midodrine, a new - adrenoreceptor agonist, at a dose of 5 to 10 mgs, three times daily (TID), is particularly effective in some patients. Potential side effects are pilo-erection, urinary retention and supine hypertension[88, 89].

2) Nausea and Vomiting

Although nausea and vomiting are not symptoms of Parkinson's disease per se, they are a frequent side effect of all dopaminergic agents and constitute the major limitations to their use.

In order to avoid these side effects, treatment with levodopa and dopamine agonists must be introduced gradually.

If this precaution is ineffective, a peripheral dopamine receptor blocker, which does not cross the blood-brain barrier, such as domperidone, may help symptoms without worsening Parkinson's disease. Dopamine blocking agents with central effects, such as chlorpromazine and metoclopramide, should be avoided, as these drugs worsen Parkinson's disease and reduce the efficacy of dopaminergic agents.

3) Neuropsychiatric Problems

The major neuropsychiatric problems include: cognitive impairment, agitation, depression, delirium, hallucination psychosis and sleep disorders.

Cognitive Impairment

Cognitive impairment in patients with Parkinson's disease, especially memory loss or confusion, can be the result of anti-parkinsonian drugs such as anticholinergic agents and amantadine. This effect appears to be more evident in the elderly.

The treatment consists of reducing and eliminating the offending drugs.

Agitation

Agitation can occur as a reaction to Parkinson's disease or can be induced by any anti-parkinsonian drugs, in particular by selegiline, anticholinergic agents and amantadine.

If reducing the dosage of these drugs is ineffective, it may be necessary to use anxiolytics. Preference should be given to the short-acting benzodiazepines, such as alprazolam (0.5 to 1 mg TID) and lorazepam (1 to 2 mg TID). Reduced doses are indicated for patients with cognitive impairment.

Depression

Depression is extremely frequent in Parkinson's disease and occurs in upto 40% of patients. The selective serotonin re-uptake inhibitors (SSRIs), paroxetine (20 mg/day), fluoxetine (20 to 40 mg/day) and sertraline (50 to 100 mg/day) are the mainstay of treatment for patients who are apathetic, anergic and passive[90, 91].

Worsening of parkinsonian symptoms during SSRI therapy is unusual. Since there is a potential adverse interaction between SSRIs and selegiline, concurrent use is discouraged. Tricyclic antidepressants are indicated for their sedative properties and are useful for patients with sleep disorders, but their use may be limited by anticholinergic and orthostatic side effects[92, 93, 94, 95].

It is best to use those with a short half-life and little anticholinergic activity, such as desipramine (initial night-time dose 10 to 25 mg) or nortriptyline (initial night-time dose 20 to 40 mg)[96, 97].

Hallucinations and Psychosis

Psychiatric adverse effects may occur when a patient with predisposing factors such as cognitive impairment, advanced age and pre-morbid psychiatric illness, is treated with anti-parkinsonian drugs[98].

Anticholinergic agents, amantadine, selegiline, dopaminergic agents and levodopa may induce hallucinations and psychosis in the order listed. In the event of an acute confusional state, an organic cause should be sought such as electrolyte imbalance or a septic focus[99].

The first step in the management of the patient receiving several anti-parkinsonian drugs is to decrease or discontinue the drug with the least anti-parkinsonian activity and with the most psychosis-inducing potential. In order of importance these drugs are anticholinergics, amantadine, selegiline, dopamine agonists and levodopa[100].

When psychosis persists despite the maximally tolerated reduction of anti-parkinsonian drugs, this can be treated with neuroleptics, such as clozapine (6.25 mg as the starting dose at bedtime and final dose of 75 mg/day) and olanzapine (2 to 5 mg/day). These drugs do not worsen Parkinsonian symptoms[101].

Agranulocytosis, the most serious adverse effect of clozapine, occurs in approximately 2% of the patients. For this reason weekly white cell monitoring is required for all patients whilst on treatment[102].

Sleep Disturbances

The most common sleep abnormalities are insomnia and excessive daytime somnolence. Insomnia may be idiopathic or drug induced.

Pharmacological treatment options for idiopathic induced insomnia are tricyclic antidepressants and benzodiazepines. The latter are not recommended for long term use because physical dependence and frequent cognitive side effects.

Selegiline and amantadine may produce insomnia. Dose reduction and discontinuation should be considered.

Excessive daytime somnolence is defined as a tendency to fall asleep during the day. In patients with Parkinson's disease, this is most commonly drug induced by sedating drugs and agents such as pramipexole as the dopamine agonist.

Editors' Notes
for Patients and Carers

Dr Serena Leader BSc MB BCh MRCP DRCOG MRCGP
Lucille Leader Dip ION

As you no doubt know, people with Parkinson's disease often present primarily with the symptoms of tremor, rigidity, unsteadiness and slow movement. The reason for impaired control of movement has been attributed to a deficiency of the neuro-transmitter (brain chemical messenger), dopamine. Dopamine is "manufactured" from L-dopa by neurones (brain cells) in the substantia nigra area of the brain. The body synthesises L-dopa from dietary protein.

There may be many different reasons for the insufficient production of dopamine - genetic, drugs, environmental toxicity including organophosphates and organochlorines, free radical damage, cell death (apoptosis), disease, mitochondrial inadequacy (lack of cell energy), precursor problems (steps in body metabolism which lead up to the production of dopamine), or for no particular reason.

Professor Aroldo Ross presents the two approaches to pharmaceutical treatment of Parkinson's disease:
a) postponing drug therapy until patients are unable to function adequately for their daily needs
b) commencing drug treatment immediately after diagnosis in order to relieve symptoms in the early stages

These two different approaches are being debated as treatment with levodopa (L-dopa including "Sinemet" and "Madopar") can lead to problems after several years. These include a reduced response to L-dopa therapy and increased fluctuations in motor function.

Professor Rossi writes that it may be preferable to delay starting L-dopa therapy in younger patients and rather to commence treatment with dopamine agonists. He also recommends non-pharmacological measures including nutritional management. Cellular energy production as well as the body's own metabolism of dopamine and adrenaline use nutrients as co-factors and co-enzymes. The integrity of cell membranes depend on dietary essential fatty acids.

He recommends psychological support as well as remedial exercises, from the early stages of Parkinson's disease. Stretching, toning and exercising the body as well as doing voice exercises will help to maintain function.

There are various means (rating scales) of monitoring the progress of the illness by neurologists. These are presented by Professor Rossi in the next chapter. There are also nutritional biochemical tests available to monitor the nutritional status of cells so that an appropriate nutritional support programme can be prescribed for the individual.

There are diverse drugs on offer for the pharmaceutical support of people with Parkinson's disease. These include anticholinergics, dopamine agonists, receptor stimulators, COMT inhibitors and L-dopa with decarboxylase inhibitors ("Sinemet" and "Madopar"). In this chapter you will find indications for their use, their benefits and their side effects. Professor Rossi gives recommendations for the optimum administration of L-dopa in relation to food and dosage, and suggests that agonists be taken after a meal if nausea is a problem. He also presents strategies for sufferers of orthostatic hypotension.

Brief Glossary

agonist	- *a drug which binds to a receptor and produces a response similar to that caused by the neurotransmitter.*
apoptosis	- *cell death*
apraxia	- *inability to carry out coordinated, skilled, purposive motor activity*
ataxia	- *unsteadiness, incoordination, disorganisation of movements*
blood brain barrier	- *a barrier of special capillaries which controls the passage of substances from the blood into the brain and cerebrospinal fluid*
dysarthria	- *a speech disorder*
dyskinesia	- *movement disturbance characterised by involuntary, irregular, incoodinated movements*
dysphagia	- *difficulty in swallowing*
organophosphates	- *toxic chemicals in pesticides and herbicides amongst other products*
serotonin syndrome	- *includes symptoms of facial flushing and diarrhoea*

References

1. Agid Y, Chase TN, Marsden CD. *Adverse Reaction To Levodopa: Drug Toxicity Or Progression Disease?* Lancet 351: 851-852, 1998

2. Fahn S. *Parkinson's Disease, The Effects Of Levodopa And The ELLDOPA Trial.* Arch Neurol 56: 529-535, 1999

3. Koller WC, Tolosa E (Eds). *Current And Emerging Therapies In The Management Of Parkinson's Disease.* Neurology 50(Suppl 3) 1-57, 1998

4. Markham CH, Diamond SG. *Evidence To Support Early Levodopa Therapy In Parkinson's Disease.* Neurology 31: 125-131, 1981

5. Mizuno Y (Ed). *Second International Symposium On The Treatment Of Parkinson's Disease.* Neurology 51(Suppl 2): 1-40, 1998

6. Stern MB (Ed). Th*e Changing Standard Of Care In Parkinson's Disease: Current Cocepts And Controversies.* Neurology 49(Suppl 1): 1-62, 1997

7. Poewe W. *Should Treatment Of Parkinson's Disease Be Started With A Dopamine Agonist.* Neurology 51 (Suppl 2) S 21-24, 1998

8. Fahn S, Bressman SB. *Should Levodopa Therapy For Parkinson's Disease Be Started Early Or Late? Evidence Against Early Treatment.* Can J Neurol Sci 11: 200-205, 1984

9. Fahn S. *Controversies In The Therapy Of Parkinson's Disease.* Adv Neurol 69: 477- 486, 1996

10. Pilemer K, Suitor JJ. *"It Takes One To Help One": Effects Of Similar Others On The Well-Being Of Caregivers.* J Gerentol Soc Sci 51 B:S250-257, 1996

11. Conella CL, Stebbins GT, Brown-Toms N, Goetz CG. *Physical Therapy And Parkinson's Disease: A Controlled Clinical Study.* Neurology 44:376-378, 1994

12. Kempster PA, Wahlquist ML. *Dietary Factors In The Management Of Parkinson's Disease.* Nutr Rev 52: 51-58, 1994

13. Kurodat T, Tatara K, Takatorigne T, Shimsho F. *Effect Of Physical Exercise On Motility In Patients With Parkinson's Disease.* Acta Neurol Scand 86: 55-59, 1992

14. Fahn S, Elton R, *Members Of UPDRS Development Committee.* In Fahn S, Marsden CD Calne DB, Goldstein M (Eds). *Recent Developments In Parkinson'S Disease.* Vol 2. Florham Park, NJ. *Mcmillan Health Care Information* Pp 153-163, 293-304, 1987

15. Hoehn MMM. *The Natural History Of Parkinson's Disease In The Pre-Levodopa And Postlevodopa Eras.* Neurol Clin 10: 331-339, 1992

16. Op. Cit. N. 5

17. Wade DN, Mearrik PT, Morris JL. *Active Transport Of L-Dopa In The Intestine.* Nature 242:463-465, 1973

18. Nutt JG, Fellman JH. *Pharmacokinetics Ol Levodopa.* Clin Neuropharmacol 7: 35-49, 1984

19. Rossi A., Lalli F., Tambasco N., Mancini M.L., Gallai V. Studio Degli Effetti Di Un Farmaco Procinetico Sui Livelli Plasmatici Di L-Dopa E Sulle Fluttuazioni Motorie Nel Morbo Di Parkinson. Atti XXIV Riunione L.I.M.P.E. *"Indicatori Storia Naturale Terapie Delle Malattie Extrapiramidali"*, Perugia, 9-11, 243-51, 1997.

20. Gancher ST, Nutt JG, Woodwart WR. *Peripheral Pharmacokinetics Of Levodopa In Untreated, Stable And Fluctuating Parkinsonian Patients.* Neurology 37: 940-944, 1987

21. Op. Cit. N. 18

22. Op. Cit. N. 20

23. Nutt JG, Woodward WR, Gancher ST, Merrick D. *3-O-Methyldopa And The Response To Levodopa In Parkinson's Disease.* Ann Neurol 21: 584-588, 1987

24. Nutt JG, Holford NH. *The Response To Levodopa In Parkinson's Disease: Imposing Pharmacological Law And Order.* Ann Neurol 39: 561-573, 1996

25. Zappia M, Olivieri RL, Montesanti R, Rizzo M, Bosco D, Plastino M, Crescibene L, Bastone L, Aguglia U, Gambardella A, Quattrone A. *Loss Of Long-Duration Response To Levodopa Over Time In PD: Implications For Wearing-Off.* Neurology 52: 763-767, 1999

26. Op. Cit. N. 24

27. Op. Cit. N. 25

28. Caraceni T, Scigliano G, Musicco M. *The Occurence Of Motor Fluctuations In Parkinsonian Patients Treated Long Term With Levodopa: Role Of Early Treatment And Disease Progression.* Neurology 41: 380-384, 1991

29. Agid Y. Levodopa: *Is Toxicity A Myth?* Neurology 50: 858-863, 1998

30. Op. Cit. N. 29

31. Myawaki E, Lyons K, Pahwa R, Troster AI, Hubble J, Smith D, Busenbark K, Mcguire D, Michalek D, Koller WC. *Motor Complications Of Chronic Levodopa Therapy In Parkinson's Disease.* Clin Neuropharmacol 20: 523-530, 1997

32. Fahn S. Adverse Effects Of Levodopa. In: Olanow CW, Lieberman AN (Eds). *The Scientific Basis For The Treatment Of Parkinson's Disease.* Lanes, UK: Parthenon Publishing Group 89-112, 1992

33. Koller WC, Hubble JP. *Levodopa Therapy In Parkinson's Disease.* 40 (Suppl 3): S184- 195, 1990

34. Op. Cit. N. 3

35. Op. Cit. N. 5

36. Op. Cit. N. 6

37. Olanow CW 8ed). *Cell Death And Neuroprotection In Parkinson's Disease.* Ann. Neurol 44 (Suppl 1): S1-S196, 1998

38. Jenner P. Teh *Rationale For The Use Of Dopamine Agonist In Parkinson's Disease.* Neurology 45 (Suppl 3): S 6-12, 1995.

39. Watts RL. *The Role Of Dopamine Agonist In Early Parkinson's Disease.* Neurology 49 (Suppl 1): S 34-48, 1997.

40. Ogawa N, Tanaka K, Asanuma M. *Bromocriptine Protects Mice Against &-Hydroxyl Free Radical In Vitro.* Brain Res 657: 207-213, 1994

41. Przuntrk H, Welzel D, Gerlach M. *Early Institution Of Bromocriptine In Parkinson's Disease Inhibits The Emergence Of Levodopa Associated Motor Side Effects. Long Term Results Of PRADO Study.* J Neural Transm 103: 699-715, 1996.

42. Piccoli F, Ruggeri RM. *Dopaminergic Agonist In The Treatment Of Parkinson's Disease: A Review.* J Neural Transm 45(Suppl): 187-195, 1995

43. Op. Cit. N. 5

44. Op. Cit. N. 40

45. Op. Cit. N. 42

46. Kondo T, Ito T, Sugita Y. *Bromocriptine Scavenges Methamphetamine- Induced Hydroxyl Radicals And Attenuates Dopamine Depletion In mouse Striatum.* Neurobiology 738: 22-229, 1994

47. Yoshikawa T, Minamiyama Y, Naito Y. *Antioxidant Properties Of Bromocriptine, A Dopamine Agonist.* J Neurochem 62: 1034-1038, 1994

48. Nishibayashi S, Asanuma M, Koho M. *Scavenging Effects Of Dopamine Agonist On Nitric Oxide Radicals.* J Neurochem 67: 2208-2211. 1996

49. Felten DL, Feltens SY, Fuller RW. *Chronic Dietary Pergolide Preserves Nigrostriatal Neuronal Integrity In Aged.* Neurobiol Aging 13. 339-351, 1992

50. Op. Cit. N. 5

51. Op. Cit. N. 41

52. Op. Cit. N. 47

53. Op. Cit. N. 49

54. Tatton WG, Ju WY, Holland DP, Tai C, Kwan M. *Deprenyl Reduces PC12 Cell Apoptosis By Inducing New Protein Synthesis.* J Neurochem 63: 1572, 1994

55. The Parkinson Study Group. *Impact Of Deprenyl On The Progression Of Disability In Early Parkinson's Disease.* N Engl J Med 321: 1364-1371, 1989

56. Offen D, Ziv I, Gordin S, Panet H, Melamed E. *Dopamine Melanin Induces Apoptosis PC 12 In Neuronal Cells: Possible Implications For Therapeutic Approaches In Parkinson's Disease.* Mov Disord 11: 45, 1996

57. Przedborski S, Jackson-Lewis V, Fahn S. *Antiparkinsonian Therapies And Brain Mitochondrial Complex I Activity.* Mov Disord 10: 312-317, 1995

58. Op. Cit. N. 3

59. Op. Cit. N. 5

60. Op. Cit. N. 6

61. Liberman A, Olanow CW, Sethi K, Swanson P, Waters CH, Fahn S, Hurtig H, Yahr M And The Ropinirole Study Group. *A Multicenter Trial Of Ropinirole As Adjunct Treatment Foe Parkinson's Disease.* Neurology 51: 1057-1062, 1998

62. Rascol O On Behalf Of The Study Group. *A Double-Blind L-Dopa Controlled Study Of Ropinirole In De Novo Patients With Parkinson's Disease.* Mov Disord 11(Suppl 1): 130, 1996

63. Wheadon DE, Wilson-Lynch K, Gardiner D, Kreider MS. Ropinirole, *A Non Ergolinic D2 Agonist, Is Effective In Early Parkinsonian Patients Not Treated With L-Dopa.* Mov Disord 11(Suppl 1): 162, 1996

64. Op. Cit. N. 3

65. Op. Cit. N. 5

66. Op. Cit. N. 6

67. Guttman M And The Pramipexole-Bromocriptine Study Group. *Double Blind Comparison Of Pramipexole And Bromocriptine Treatment With Placebo In Advanced Parkinson's Disease*.Neurology 49:1060-1065, 1997

68. Inzelbrg R, Nisipeanu P, Rabey JM, Orlov E, Catz T, Kippervasser S, Schechtman E, Korczyn AD. *Double-Blind Comparison Of Cabergoline And Bromocriptine In Parkinson's Disease Patients With Motor Fluctuations*. Neurology 47:785-788, 1996

69. Hutton JT, Morris JL, Brewer MA. *Controlled Study Of The Antiparkinsonian Activity And Tolerability Of Cabergoline*. Neurology 43:613-616, 1993

70. Bonuccelli U, Piccini P, Del Dotto P, D'Antonio P, Muratorio P. Apomorphine *Test In De Novo Parkinson's Disease*. Funct Neurol 7: 295-298, 1992

71. Bonuccelli U, Piccini P, Del Dotto P, Rossi G, Corsini GU, Muratorio P. *Apomorphine Test For Dopaminergic Responsiveness: A Dose Assessment Study*. Mov Disord 8: 15-164, 1993

72. Schelosky L, Hierholzer J, Wissel J, Cordes M, Poewe W. *Correlation Of Clinical Response In Apomorphine Test With D2- Receptor Status As Demonstrated By 123I-IBMZ-SPECT*. Mov Disord 8:453-458, 1993

73. Hauser R, Zesiewicz T. *Parkinson's Disease. Questions And Answers*. Merit Publishing International, Hampshire, England (Second Edition): 55-77, 1997.

74. Danysz W, Parsons CG, Kornhuber J, Schidt WJ, Quack G. Aminoadamatanesasnmda *Receptors Antagonists And Antiparkinsonian Agentes – Preclinical Studies*. Neurosci Biobehav Rev 21: 455-468, 1997.

75. Kornhubej, Weller M, Shoppmeyer K, Riederer P. Amantadine And Nemantine *Are NMDA Receptor Antagonist With Neuroprotective Properties*. J Neurol Transm 43(Suppl): 91-104, 1994.

76. Tatton WG, Chalmers-Redmond RME. *Modulation Of Gene Expression Rather Than Monoamine Oxidase Inhibition: Deprenyl-Related Compounds In Controlling Neurodegeneration*. Neurology 47 (Suppl 3): S171-183, 1996

77. Op. Cit. N. 3

78. Op. Cit. N. 5

79. Op. Cit. N. 6

80. Op. Cit. N. 76

81. Bonifati V, Meco G. *New, Selective Catechol-O-Methyltransferase Inhibitors As Therapeutic Agents In Parkinson's Disease*. Pharmacol Ther 81 (1): 1-36, 1999

82. Rabasseda X. *Prospectives In The Treatment Of Parkinson's Disease: COMT Inhibitor Open Up New Treatment Strategies*. Drugs Today 35 (9): 701-717, 1999

83. Op. Cit. N. 81

84. Op. Cit. N. 82

85. Rossi A: Terapia Dei Parkinsonismi. In: Gallai V, Rossi A, Parnetti L (Eds): *Update Sulle Malattie Extrapiramidali*. ESI Napoli 289-301, 2000

86. Bannister R, Ardill L, Fentem PA. *An Assessment Of Various Methods Of Treatment Of Idiophatic Orthostatic Hypotension.* Q J Med 38: 377-395, 1969

87. Hickler RB, Thompson GR, Fox LM, Hamlin JT. *Successful Treatment Of Orthostatic Hypotension With 9-Alpha-Fluorohydrocortisone.* N Engl J Med 261: 788-791, 1959

88. Mctavisc D, Goa KL. *Midodrine. A Review Of Its Pharmacological Properties And Therapeutic Use In Orthostatic Hypotension And Secondary Hypotensive Disorders.* Drugs 38: 757-777, 1989

89. Freeman R, Young J, Landsberg L, Lipsitz L. *The Treatment Of Postprandial Hypotension In Autonomic Failure With 3,4-DL-Threo-Dihydroxyphenylserine.* Neurology 47: 1414-1420, 1996.

90. Cummings JL. *Depression And Parkinson's Disease: A Review.* Am J Psychiatry 149: 443-454, 1992

91. Jansen Steur ENH. *Increase Of Parkinson's Disability After Fluoxetine Medications* Neurology 43: 211-213, 1993

92. Liebermann A. *Managing The Neuropsychiatric Symptoms Of Parkinson's Disease.* Neurology 50 (Suppl 6): S33-38, 1998

93. Corkeron MA. *Serotonin Syndrome: A Potential Fatal Complication Of Antidepressant Syndrome.* Med J Austral 163: 481-482, 1995

94. Palhagen S, Heindmen EH, Hägglund J And The Swedish Parkinson's Study Group. *Selegiline Delays The Onset Of Disability In De Novo Parkinsonian Patients.* Neurology 51: 520-525, 1998

95. Sternbach H. *The Serotonin Syndrome.* Am J Psichiatr 148: 705-713, 1991

96. Niremberg DW, Semprebon M. *The Central Nervous System Serotonin Syndrome.* Clin Pharmacol Ther 84-88, 1993

97. Laitenen L. *Desipramine In The Treatment Of Parkinson's Disease.* Acta Neurol Scand 45: 109-113, 1969.

98. Andersen J, Abro E, Gulman N, Hjelmested A, Pedersen HE. *Anti-Depresive Treatment In Parkinson's Disease: A Controlled Trial Of The Effect Of Nortriptyline In Patients With Parkinson's Disease Treated With L-Dopa*: Acta Neurol Scan 52: 210-219, 1980

99. Sanchez-Ramos JR, Ortoll R, Paulson GW, *Visual Hallucination Associated With Parkinson's Disease.* Arc Neurol 53: 1256-1268, 1996

100. Moskovitz C, Moses H, Klavans HL. *Levodopa Induced Psychosis: A Kindling Phenomenon.* Am J Psychiatry 135: 669-675, 1978

101. Greene P, Cote L, Fahn S. *Treatment Of Drug-Induced Psychosis In Parkinson's Disease With Clozapine.* Adv Neurol 60: 703-706, 1993

102. Ruggeri S, Depandis MF, Bonamartini A, Vacca L, Stocchi F. *Low Dose Of Clozapine In The Treatment Of Dopaminergic Psychosis In Parkinson's Disease.* Clin Neurpharmacol 20: 204-209, 1997

CHAPTER 1.3

Monitoring in Parkinson's Disease

by Professor Aroldo Rossi

Standardised methods are available to quantify disease severity, monitor response to treatment and assess quality of life.

There are three commonly used rating scales.

Hohen and Yahr Staging Scale[1,2,3].

This scale is used widely and is useful to monitor the progression of Parkinson's disease. The scale divides patients into five different stages of severity:

1. unilateral disease only;

2. bilateral disease, with or without axial involvement;

3. mild to moderate bilateral disease, with first signs of deteriorating balance;

4. severe disease requiring considerable assistance;

5. confinement to wheelchair or bed unless aided.

The advantage of this scale is that it is simple and easy to use; its disadvantage is its lack of sensitivity because it is able to evaluate only major changes of severity.

Unified Parkinson's Disease Rating Scale (UPDRS)[4,5]

This scale assesses the severity of the disease and contains six sections.
The first section is a limited evaluation of mental state in patients with depression or cognitive disorders and will often be subjected to other specific tests.

The second section assesses the activities of daily living in both the "on" and "off" state, and the third is a detailed examination of motor performance.

The fourth contains the assessment of levodopa-related complications, focusing principally on fluctuation and dyskinesias.

The fifth and sixth sections contain a modified Hohen and Yahr Scale on the Schwab and England Scale.

Schwab and England Scale[6,7]

This provides an accurate assessment of patients' ability to perform routine activities of daily living considering their speed and independence.

It contains an 11 level recording system, ranging from a 100% completely independent patient to a 0% completely helpless patient.

When evaluating the Parkinson's disease patient in the advanced stage of the illness, it is useful to keep a daily journal where the patients themselves report on their own motor situation alongside a record of their current therapy (see the chapter on "Assessment Diary Chart").

References

1. Hoehn MM, Yahr MD. *Parkinsonism: Onset, Progression and Mortality.* Neurology 17: 427-442, 1967
2. Hoehn MM. *The Natural History of Parkinson's disease in the pre-levodopa and post-levodopa eras.* Neurol Clin 17: 331-339, 1992
3. Lang AE. *Clinical Rating Scales and videotape analysis.* In Paulson GW, Koller WC (eds): Therapy of Parkinson's disease. New York, Marcel Decker, 1995
4. op.cit.n.3
5. Fahn S, Elton RL and Members of UPDRS Development Committee. *Unified Parkinson's Disease Rating Scale.*
6. op.cit.n.3
7. op.cit.n.4

Bibliography

Fahn S, Marsden CD, Goldestein M, Calne DB (eds): *Recent developments in Parkinson's Disease.* New York, McMillan, 1987

CHAPTER 2

Cerebral Imaging as a Diagnostic Aid

*By **Dr Donald Grosset** BSc (Hons) MB ChB MD FRCP*

The original description of what we now refer to as Parkinson's disease was made by James Parkinson on the basis of a group of patients having similar signs to each other, raising the possibility of a localised nervous system disorder. It remains true to this day that the primary method of diagnosing Parkinson's disease is based around the same set of clinical observations.

The use of cerebral imaging tests and other diagnostic techniques (such as challenge tests with dopaminergic medication) is considered when the clinical diagnosis is uncertain because of the presence of clinical features which do not match clearly to the clinical diagnostic categories. Cerebral imaging should be considered in two major separate categories namely structural imaging, such as with computed tomography (CT) and magnetic resonance imaging (MRI) and the alternative type of cerebral imaging, namely functional imaging. The latter is a technique of examining brain chemical function and in Parkinson's disease and other parkinsonian syndromes this is primarily based around the measurement of dopaminergic activity. Accordingly only some patients undergo some of these tests.

Many patients with a clinically clear-cut diagnosis and treatment response do not undergo such tests, some patients with co-existent disease in the brain or elsewhere may require structural or functional imaging to improve diagnostic accuracy, and a few patients with a complicated clinical course may undergo a combination of structural and functional imaging of different types. The decision to proceed with structural and or functional imaging is made during continued clinical observation of the patient. In other words, the tests may be undertaken, in some cases, at initial presentation but in many cases, later on, during the course of the illness. These would then take place if additional features or complications develop which need further enquiry to guide the next step in treatment or to give information about the expected prognosis.

It has been known for some decades that diagnostic accuracy in Parkinson's disease falls short at times. In the Brain Bank study, which involved a study of 100 patients considered throughout life to have Parkinson's disease, three quarters of patients had the diagnosis confirmed at post-mortem examination[1].

Of the remaining quarter, about half had a parkinsonian disorder either Multiple System Atrophy (MSA) or Progressive Supranuclear Palsy (PSP). Subsequent to this work (which was shown to be very similar in North American study[2]), clinical diagnostic criteria were established which have certainly improved the diagnostic accuracy in patients presenting with Parkinson's disease or similar disorders. It should also be recognised that the treatment approach for patients with Parkinson's disease or MSA or PSP is often the same at initial presentation, as the primary issue is to determine whether the patient is responsive to dopaminergic medication. Later on, maintaining or increasing treatment is appropriate if there is a continued therapy response but treatment should be discontinued if there is no response and only the production of side-effects. It is with this background that the use of structural and functional imaging should be considered.

Structural Imaging in Parkinsonism and Related Disorders

Cerebral Computerised Tomography (CT) and a Magnetic Resonance Imaging (MRI) show cerebral atrophy in patients with Parkinson's disease which is considered to be more prominent, even when corrected for age, than in patients without Parkinson's disease or similar brain disorders. The Parkinson's Plus disorders, namely PSP and MSA also show atrophy on structural imaging and this is often more prominent in the brain stem and cerebellum than elsewhere.

However, structural imaging with CT scanning is usually not a useful diagnostic test, as atrophy is variable with age and with other conditions. Also, structural imaging does not usually distinguish between Parkinson's disease, MSA and PSP, as there is an overlap in the observations made and the degree of atrophy seen. MRI scanning is more sensitive to the atrophic change particularly in the posterior fossa. In multiple system atrophy basal ganglia changes have also been reported with atrophy in the putamen and a hyper-intense rim adjacent to the putamen. One distinct problem in attempting to use structural imaging to separate Parkinson's disease from the Parkinson's Plus disorders is that the structural changes are much less prominent in the early stages of the disease. In a practical sense, this means that conducting structural imaging at initial diagnosis has no benefit in guiding the future development of the condition. In other words, it does not tell whether the patient with mild, early parkinsonian symptoms is going to remain a case of idiopathic Parkinson's disease or develop later into a case of Parkinson's Plus such as MSA or PSP.

There are times when structural imaging will identify an alternative diagnosis to Parkinson's disease or the Parkinson's Plus disorders referred to above. These findings are grouped together loosely under the term structural parkinsonism. The presence of parkinsonism with principally walking difficulties in association with early mental impairment and bladder dysfunction may raise the possibility of hydrocephalus (an increase in size of the fluid-filled spaces in the brain), which is readily identified on structural imaging. Hydrocephalus, however, would not be considered in a patient with a typical Parkinson's onset in one arm with tremor and a degree of stiffness over a number of months, progressing to the leg on the same side of the body and subsequently progressing to the other side of the body.

Another important alternative diagnosis to consider is one of cerebral vascular disease. Like Parkinson's disease, cerebral vascular disease increases in the older population and a certain form of cerebral vascular disease may present as a form of parkinsonism. This is rather distinct from stroke events or transient ischaemic attacks, which result in focal recovering neurological deficit. It results from small vessel changes in the deep sub-cortical brain areas and this is more common in patients with hypertension and additional risk factors, which are diabetes, high cholesterol and cigarette smoking. The clinical picture of parkinsonism in patients with cerebral vascular disease is often quite different from that in patients with Parkinson's disease itself. The predominant problem in cerebrovascular parkinsonism is in the legs, which show rigidity and stiffness resulting in a short steppage gait. By contrast the arms may be unaffected or barely affected. This differs considerably from idiopathic Parkinson's disease where the onset is in the arms initially and where the arm symptoms tend to remain more prominent than leg symptoms throughout the course of the illness. In describing these variations, it should again be recognised that there are patients with less clear-cut separations in their clinical features and it is in this group that structural and or functional imaging should be considered. Structural imaging will show evidence of small vessel damage, usually a fairly symmetrical pattern in the deep brain areas, at times small areas of lacunar infarction, sometimes referred to as periventricular low attenuation. It should be recognised that in an older population that Parkinson's disease itself and cerebral vascular disease may co-exist. Indeed, the Brain Bank study conducted in the 1980's in London showed that cerebral vascular disease and Parkinson's disease often co-existed in the same patient, but it also showed that cerebral vascular disease alone had been responsible for a clinical syndrome of parkinsonism in a separate group of patients[3].

Alternative diagnosis to parkinsonism sometimes has to be considered for patients with a more tremulous disorder. Essential tremor in its clear cut form, this is easy to distinguish clinically from Parkinson's disease and parkinsonism, but at times it has a rather asymmetric onset and sometimes the exclusion of other clinical features is difficult. Particularly in the older patient there may be a loss of arm swing or a degree of general slowing raising the possibility of bradykinesia in association with the tremor and hence raising the possibility of Parkinson's disease or atypical parkinsonism. Accordingly, this is a further group of patients in whom structural and functional imaging can be considered - structural imaging will be normal in cases of essential tremor and the functional imaging of the basal ganglia will also be normal, as discussed below.

Functional Imaging Studies

Positron emission tomography (PET) and Single Photon Emission Computed Tomography (SPECT) are the two main types of functional neuro-imaging to be considered in Parkinson's disease diagnosis. Both techniques use tracer material to highlight the activity of brain areas. PET is primarily a research tool and has contributed to significant advances in our understanding of Parkinson's disease and related disorders. SPECT scanning on the other hand has recently become a more available technique generally, which can assist in routine clinical practice.

PET Studies with Fluoro-Deoxy-Glucose

FDG PET is a technique used to measure glucose metabolism in regional brain areas. This test shows reduced metabolism in the basal ganglia areas and frontal cortex in patients with MSA but not in Parkinson's disease or control subjects.

18F-DOPA PET

Dopa decarboxylase activity is a marker of dopaminergic activity and therefore the uptake of 18F-DOPA matches the turnover of endogenous dopamine. Reduced uptake of 18F-DOPA occurs in patients with hemi-parkinsonism in the contralateral putamen initially. More prominent changes have been observed in patients with PSP, and intermediate changes in patients with MSA.

11C-Raclopride PET

This PET technique is designed to measure dopamine receptor density. In the initial untreated stages of Parkinson's disease 11C-Raclopride binding is normal or slightly raised. In patients with MSA, PSP and later treated Parkinson's disease when there is a fluctuating responsiveness, binding is reduced. There is some indication that the changes are more prominent in the putamen area of the brain in patients with Parkinson's disease, while in multiple system atrophy there is reduced binding in both the caudate and putamen areas.

11C-Nomifenisine PET

11C-Nomifenisine PET is a technique to image dopamine transporters. Uptake is reduced in the striatum particularly in the putamen in Parkinson's disease. Changes are noted more prominently in the more clinically affected cerebral hemisphere.

SPECT STUDIES

IBZM-SPECT

This SPECT technique highlights the post-synaptic dopamine area, which is the area responsible for receiving the signal from dopamine released from the pre-synaptic nerve terminal. In Parkinson's disease the pre-synaptic area is abnormal due to gradual loss of these nerves, while the post-synaptic area remains normal throughout the course of the illness. By contrast, in PSP and MSA, both the pre and post-synaptic areas degenerate. Accordingly IBZM-SPECT which highlights the post-synaptic area is normal in patients with Parkinson's disease and abnormal in patients with PSP or MSA. The results from a series of patients with parkinsonism have been compared for IBZM-SPECT to the results of single high dose challenge tests with Apomorphine and to the response in the patient to long term oral dopaminergic therapy[4]. The results generally show good correlation. A comparative study of IBZM-SPECT and 11C-Racropride PET suggested that the techniques were broadly comparable[5]. However it should be recognised that the PET study is more detailed and provides absolute values while the SPECT technique always provides relative indication of brain function in certain areas compared to brain function elsewhere.

The correlation of IBZM-SPECT readings to therapy response is very good but not perfect, and a few patients may have a normal IBZM uptake but a poor response to treatment.

123I-FP-CIT and 123I-CIT

These SPECT techniques measure dopamine transporter activity. Initial changes in Parkinson's disease occur in the putamen, on the more clinically affected side and progressive loss of dopamine transporter activity is noted as the disease progresses. These progressive changes are illustrated in the figure which shows a normal uptake in the putamen and caudate at A, a reduced uptake in the putamen and to a lesser extent caudate on one side, and a more marked impairment of uptake on the other side at B. At C, there is bilateral loss of putamen uptake and reduced intensity of uptake in the caudate. At D, there is significant impairment of uptake bilaterally with no putamen uptake and minimal caudate uptake. It will be seen that the changes are symmetrically abnormal at C and D but are asymmetric between right and left brain at B. This tends to match the clinical progression of Parkinson's disease, although often there will remain a difference in severity with the initial onset in Parkinson's disease showing more prominent symptoms throughout the lifetime of the illness. Therefore a correlation between tracer uptake and clinical severity measured by motor and performance scores has been shown for both the ß -CIT[6] and FP-CIT[7]. Interestingly the severity of tremor has not shown such a clear cut correlation[8], and this along with other evidence about therapy response to anti-parkinson's drugs for the tremor raises the possibility of the tremor control mechanisms being partly outside the dopaminergic system (see Fig. 1 left).

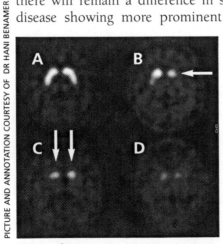

PICTURE AND ANNOTATION COURTESY OF DR HANI BENAMER

Figure 1

Because changes occur in the pre-synaptic area in PSP and MSA, pre-synaptic imaging does not usefully differentiate these disorders. Patients with PSP and MSA tend to have more symmetrical changes in the basal ganglia and in the clinical features than patients with Parkinson's disease who usually have a unilateral onset of the disease progressing within a period of one to three years to the other side[9]. Accordingly some clue as to the presence of Parkinson's disease compared to Parkinson's Plus disorders may come from pre-synaptic SPECT imaging and the calculation performed in the asymmetry index. Patients with a high degree of asymmetry between right and left brain on SPECT imaging are therefore more likely to have Parkinson's disease than a Parkinson's Plus disorder but this is only an inference rather than a definite diagnostic statement.

There is a practical difference in the use of ß-CIT compared to FP-CIT. Because ß-CIT is taken up slowly in the brain after it is injected (usually by intravenous injection into the arm), the patient needs to attend hospital on one day for the injection and to re-attend to the hospital on the next day for their imaging test. By contrast the FP-CIT study is undertaken on the same day as it is taken up in the brain areas much faster than ß-CIT. There are additional tracers under development, which have similar characteristics to ß-CIT and FP-CIT. However FP-CIT is the only licensed investigative tracer (European License for using this test was obtained in 2000).

Diagnosis of Essential Tremor

This condition is often misdiagnosed as Parkinson's disease or parkinsonism. This has been a long standing observation in the medical literature (recently confirmed by a study from North Wales[9]) in which essential tremor was one of the two commonest conditions leading to diagnostic confusion and the inappropriate diagnostic label of Parkinson's disease was applied in these cases. Pre-synaptic dopamine imaging is expected to be normal in patients with essential tremor. This has been studied in patients with clinically definite essential tremor and the results show a very clear match between the cases defined as clinically definite (who have normal FP-CIT imaging) and patients with clinically definite Parkinson's disease (who have abnormal FP-CIT imaging)[10]. However, two issues must be recognised. Firstly that the clinical diagnosis even once symptoms are well established is not 100% accurate. Secondly, that the clinical usefulness of the test is clearly far greater in the earlier stages of the disease process when symptoms are mild or limited rather than at the advanced stage. Accordingly, there is ongoing research into patients at the earlier stages of presentation, either with very mild and rather non-specific symptoms and signs, or with rather atypical or mixed clinical features which raise significant diagnostic doubt in the doctor's mind.

Projecting to the Future

There is, at present, intense interest in the exploration of treatments, which may modify the progression of Parkinson's disease. This is in contrast to the present treatments which are effective in treating the symptoms but do not alter the underlying course of the disease. The treatments which may help to slow the progression of the disease are often grouped together under the label of "possible neuro-protective" drugs, or alternatively as "disease modifying" drugs. At the time of writing there are no proven neuro-protective or disease modifying drugs, and it is clear that the next turning point in the management of Parkinson's disease will be the development of such an agent. Functional imaging has a potential role in monitoring the effects of such treatments by measuring residual dopamine activity in the brain at specific time points. Repeated cerebral imaging over a period of some years may therefore give additional information to clinical observations about progression while patients are on treatments which may delay disease progression.

References

1. Hughes AJ, Daniel SE, Kilford L, Lees AJ (1992). *Accuracy of clinical diagnosis of idiopathic Parkinson's disease*: a clinico-pathological study of 100 cases. J Neurol Neurosurg Psychiatry, 55:181-184.

2. Rajput AH, Rozdilsky B, Rajput A (1991). *Accuracy of clinical diagnosis in parkinsonism - A prospective study*. Can J Neurol Sci, 18:275-278.

3. Hughes AJ, Daniel SE, Kilford L, Lees AJ (1992). *Accuracy of clinical diagnosis of idiopathic Parkinson's disease: a clinico-pathological study of 100 cases*. J Neurol Neurosurg Psychiatry, 55:181-184.

4. Schwarz J, Tatsch K, Gasser T, Arnold G, Oertel WH (1997). [123]*IBZM binding predicts dopaminergic responsiveness in patients with parkinsonism and previous dopaminomimetic therapy*. Mov Disord, 12:898-902.

5. Schwarz J, Antonini A, Tatsch K, Kirsch CM, Oertel WH, Leenders KL (1994). *Comparison of ^{123}I-Iodobenzamide-SPECT and 11C-raclopride PET finding in patients with parkinsonism*. Nucl Med Commun, 15:806-813.

6. Seibyl JP, Marek KL, Quinlan D, Sheff K, Zoghbi S, Zea-Ponce Y, Baldwin RM, Fussell B, Smith EO, Charney DS, Hoffer PB, Innis RB (1995). *Decreased single-photon emission computed tomographic [123I] ß-CIT striatal uptake correlates with symptom severity in Parkinson's disease*. Ann Neurol, 38:589-598.

7. Benamer HTS, Patterson J, Wyper DJ, Hadley DM, Macphee GJ, Grosset DG. (2000) *Correlation of Parkinson's disease severity and duration with ^{123}I-FP-CIT SPECT striatal uptake*. Mov Disord, 15:692-698.

8. Benamer HTS, Patterson J, Grosset DG (2000), and the ^{123}I-FP-CIT Study Group. *Acccurate differentiation of parkinsonism and essential tremor using visual assessment of ^{123}I-FP-CIT SPECT imaging*. Mov Disord 15: 503-510.

9. Meara J, Bhowmick BK, Hobson P (1999). *Accuracy of diagnosis in patients with presumed Parkinson's disease*. Age and Ageing 28:99-102.

10. Benamer HTS, Patterson J, Grosset DG (2000), and the ^{123}I-FP-CIT Study Group. *Acccurate differentiation of parkinsonism and essential tremor using visual assessment of ^{123}I-FP-CIT SPECT imaging*. Mov Disord 15: 503-510.

CHAPTER 3

Older People
Special Features of Parkinsonism

by Dr. Douglas MacMahon (Lond) LRCP MRCS (Eng) MRCP (UK) FRCP (L)

Introduction

Idiopathic Parkinson's disease is a relatively common, age-related, disabling neuro-degenerative disorder. There is often much media attention on younger patients with the disease, and whilst it can occur at any age, it becomes very much more common in older age groups, with peak incidence in the seventh decade, and a prevalence of at least 2% in the ninth decade[1]. Many epidemiological studies have confirmed that Parkinson's disease is found throughout the world and confirm that its prevalence increases exponentially with age[2, 3]. There has been continued controversy around whether the disease in older people differs from that in younger ones, indeed, whether there are two diseases or just one with different expression at extremes of age. This chapter examines these issues and uses the four-stage structure of the 'Pathways' Paradigm to highlight them[4].

Diagnosis

The diagnosis of Parkinson's disease can often be difficult - it is often difficult to distinguish the features from normal ageing, or a number of other causes of Parkinsonism, most of which have different, often worse prognoses.

Parkinsonism

Parkinsonism is a term used to describe the clinical features of Parkinson's disease – bradykinesia, rigidity, and tremor. It may be surprising how frequently these features are found among people over the age of 65. In one American study, the overall prevalence of Parkinsonism rose from 14.9 percent for people 65 to 74 years of age, to 29.5 percent for those 75 to 84, and up to 52.4 percent for the oldest group aged 85 and older. It is not an innocent finding - the mortality for those with Parkinsonism was 78%, and was 49% for those without in the mean follow-up period of 9.2 years. When adjusted for age and sex, the overall risk of death among people with Parkinsonism was double that of those without (95% confidence interval, 1.6 to 2.6). The clinical implications are that the presence of gait disturbance is strongly associated with an increased risk of death[5].

Misdiagnosis is also common. In a community-based study in Wales, designed to review the diagnostic accuracy of Parkinson's disease, people on anti-parkinsonian medication were examined using clinical diagnostic criteria to establish the likely diagnosis. Parkinsonism was confirmed in 74% and clinically probable Parkinson's disease in 53%. The commonest causes of misdiagnosis were essential tremor, Alzheimer's disease and vascular pseudo-parkinsonism. Over one-quarter of subjects did not benefit from anti-parkinsonian medication[6]. Several other papers and audits confirm that idiopathic disease represents the cause of approximately three quarters of cases of parkinsonism – the others being either Parkinson's-plus syndromes such as multi-system atrophy and progressive supranuclear palsy, cerebrovascular disease, or drug-induced. The commonest drugs include the vestibular sedatives used to counteract dizziness or vertigo-prochlorperazine (Stemetil), cinnarizine (Stugeron), and anti-emetics such as metoclopramide (Maxalon). These should be avoided in older patients if at all possible, and discontinued in the event of Parkinsonism developing. Domperidone is a safe anti-emetic that does not cross the blood-brain barrier, and can be used in Parkinsonism.

Do younger and older patients present differently?

A controversy still exists around the distinction between younger and older onset cases. One of the few trials that have compared old-onset patients with young-onset disease showed many similarities and also several clinical differences. Those with a mean age at onset of below 47 were compared with those with age at onset above 70 (the mean for the whole group +/- one standard deviation). The most important distinctions were that the old-onset Parkinson's disease patients were found to have greater tendency to develop psychotic complications. They more often had tremor both as presenting and dominant symptoms of their disease. In contrast, the young-onset Parkinson's disease more often displayed bradykinesia as the dominant clinical feature, and their susceptibility to dyskinesia induced by levodopa was considerably higher. In addition, paraesthesia was more commonly a presenting feature in the younger onset cases whereas this was rare in the old onset group[7].

A longitudinal study in Australia showed that older patients presented earlier after the onset of symptoms, deteriorated more rapidly, and were significantly more likely to develop dementia and impairment of balance than younger ones. They also found that increasing age and symmetrical disease predicted the new appearance of imbalance, but in contrast to Friedman, age of onset did not predict dyskinesia or end of dose failure[8]. An American longitudinal disability study showed that patients with younger onset of Parkinson's disease (under 50 years of age) appeared to have a more favorable prognosis than those whose symptoms appear in later years[9].

Although most cases can be diagnosed sufficiently well on clinical grounds, CT or MRI scans are useful in atypical cases to exclude vascular lesions or normal pressure hydrocephalus, and the definitive test is imaging from PET scans or SPET scans. Similarly, most cases will not require many haematological or biochemical tests, but occasionally there is a need to examine serological tests for syphylis and other routine assays.

The time of diagnosis can be quite traumatic for patients of any age. This distress needs careful handling by an experienced multidisciplinary team[10]. In addition, depression frequently co-exists with anxiety at this time, and has a major impact on quality of life. Many older patients will be as upset as younger ones on being told the diagnosis, and may well have experiences of earlier generations when less effective treatment was available. It is therefore important to ascertain prior experiences, and this is best achieved by a joint medical and nursing assessment and follow up[11, 12].

Arteriopathic Pseudoparkinsonism
Cerebrovascular disease can mimic many other neurological disorders, and parkinsonism is no exception. This has several similarities to Parkinson's disease but is usually distinguishable from idiopathic disease by the absence of tremor and the predominance of signs in the legs - so called 'Lower Body Parkinsonism'. Consequently, the greatest functional effect is on gait, and facial expression, and manual dexterity is usually preserved.

Progressive Supranuclear Palsy
(Steele-Richardson-Olszewski Syndrome)
When the presenting feature is falling, one needs to consider this diagnosis. The most frequent clinical features are of early postural instability and falls (often causing fractures), optical supranuclear palsy (initially upward, but later also downward and laterally), a symmetric akinetic-rigid predominant parkinsonian disorder unrelieved by levodopa, and ultimately pseudobulbar palsy, and primitive frontal reflexes. Prognosis is much worse, typical survival time being 5 years. Onset of falls during the first year, early dysphagia, and incontinence predict a shorter survival time[13].

Recognition and Referral - Medical Care
In the British Health Service, the General Practitioner is usually the first person to be consulted and starts the process of diagnosis. In view of the diagnostic difficulties most authors recommend early referral of those suspected of having Parkinsonism for specialist assessment and for the establishment of a plan for future treatment and care[14, 15]. Referral patterns vary, with the younger patients almost universally being referred to a neurologist and many older ones and those

with complex needs, to geriatricians, although this varies with local policies, priorities, practices, and resources.

Early Treatment – Does Age Make a Difference?

The treatment of Parkinson's disease has advanced considerably in recent years. Treatment Strategies now include the following components: -

- Information and Education
- Health Maintenance / Promotion
- Nutrition
- Exercise
- Activity
- Neuro-rehabilitative Education and Training Strategies (OT and PT)
- Drugs
- Surgery (for advanced cases)

Drug Management

The only general agreement about the treatment of Parkinson's disease is that there is no single way to treat and manage Parkinson's disease. There are controversies both around initial treatment and supplementary regimens required when the initial treatment needs augmentation. To some extent guidelines and treatment algorithms can provide aids to assist decision making and suggest options. However, ultimately, decisions are individual, pragmatic, and require negotiation between patients and their doctor, often assisted and informed by carers and other health professionals such as specialist nurses[16].

The disabling effects of the disease can be limited with modern drug therapy. The choice of drug and the timing of its initiation remain individual decisions. Most specialists advocate that drug treatment be reserved until symptoms cause significant problems, or if there is difficulty in maintaining independence, employment or social activities. Pragmatically, this may be at presentation for older patients in whom a shorter life expectancy may be anticipated.

The UK guidelines on the management of Parkinson's disease that were produced make no specific distinction based solely on age[17]. Most practitioners would consider biological age rather than chronological age, taking into account cognitive state, co-morbidities -which are age-associated, and concurrent medication before discussing with both patient, and where relevant, the partner or carer.

Essentially, the choice of initial treatment lies between levodopa preparations, or other drugs such as direct agonists. Whilst in younger patients anticholinergics may provide an option, older ones rarely tolerate the side effects of dry mouth, constipation, memory loss, and hallucinations.

If levodopa is chosen, most recent papers would advocate the use of as low a dose as can be commensurate with adequate clinical control. There are a range of pharmaceutical preparations of co-careldopa and co-beneldopa, but usually the conventional (immediate release) version is perfectly adequate.

The alternative strategy is the early use of a dopaminergic agonist. Typically, patients treated with agonists will not develop dyskinesia or troublesome end of dose failure until levodopa-carbidopa is added, and not only is the prevalence of dyskinesia less than patients given levodopa-carbidopa alone, they are often less severe. However until recently, efficacy has been limited, with few patients able to remain on monotherapy for even a year, although the same study suggested that lower dosages of levodopa-carbidopa adequately controlled symptoms and delayed the appearance of dyskinesia and end of dose failure for about two years longer than conventional doses[18]. Patients need to understand that the benefits of less dyskinesia may be attainable by using lower doses of levodopa, or by a levodopa avoidance strategy, primarily using a modern dopaminergic agonist

More recent studies with the newer agonists shows greater efficacy, for example early Parkinson's disease has recently been shown to be successfully managed for up to five years with a reduced risk of dyskinesia by initiating treatment with Ropinerole monotherapy supplemented with levodopa when it became necessary - which it did in the majority - 68%[19]. These results were little different between younger and older patients, although they were, of course, carefully screened clinical trial patients. Similar data is now accumulating for other agents, such as cabergoline, pramipexole, and pergolide. However, caution should be applied if there is any evidence of cognitive impairment and especially hallucinations, and care should be taken and patients warned of the risks of somnolence with all these drugs, especially if this should occur when driving.

Maintenance Therapy

The aims in this phase are for morbidity relief, prevention of complications, and the promotion and maintenance of good health. Many patients in this stage will access their hospital consultant occasionally (e.g. six- or twelve-monthly), but the availability of telephone contact has been shown to be highly beneficial in general terms, and specifically in Parkinson's disease. As far as possible patients should be encouraged to develop coping strategies that minimise the impact of the disease. Specialist nurses have valuable inputs at this stage often supporting the primary care team, and consulting the hospital specialist if suspicions of complications are raised, heralding the next, complex phase.

COMPLICATIONS OF PARKINSON'S DISEASE AND ITS TREATMENT

Treatment Effects

Fading Effect and Motor Fluctuations (end of dose; see-saw; on-off; freezing; dyskinesias; exacerbated tremor)

Dystonias

Neuropsychiatric

Depression, Anxiety, Panic attacks

Hallucinations, Psychosis

Dementia

General Effects

Constipation, Weight Loss, Incontinence, etc.

Complex Care

In this phase, increasingly complex arrays of potentially toxic drugs will be deployed to counteract the advancing effects not only of the disease, but also of its complications, many of which are at least in part, iatrogenic.

Drug options include the direct agonists and levodopa (if not already established), the mono-amine oxidase inhibitor selegiline, COMT ihnhibitor (entacapone), more rarely amantadine, apomorphine, and very rarely anticholinergics.

Ultimately, if the elderly patient is otherwise fit, and in the absence of cognitive changes, surgical options may be required from a specialist neurosurgical team. In addition, throughout, a range of ancillary therapies will be required, including physiotherapy, occupational therapy, speech and language therapy, nutrition, chiropody, social care, advocacy and advice.

Co-morbidities may well be a problem in the older patient. Compliance issues also need to be considered.

Palliative Care

The needs of patients in the final, palliative care stage are often very difficult and hence often underestimated. In older people, it is often not the Parkinson's disease but other co-existent diseases that herald the onset of the final stage. The main aims in this phase are to relieve symptoms and distress for both patient and carers whilst retaining dignity. At the time at which their needs are at a maximal level, a visit to a hospital specialist may be difficult because of immobility, and it may also be difficult to assess their needs in a typical out-patient environment.

For these reasons, Day Hospital attendance may be easier, or domiciliary based services, which have the additional advantage of not only facilitating a better assessment of the domestic circumstances and current problems, but also allowing the discussion of practical advice and guidance. This is especially true where the patient is in institutional care and as such the need for training staff in this sector cannot be underestimated.

To achieve these aims, there is often a need to progressively reduce, and eventually even to withdraw dopaminergic drugs. There may be needs for other palliative measures such as analgesia, sedation, and other therapies such as physiotherapy. The place of residence may need adaptation, and in some cases, often when social factors arise in addition to the medical ones, residential, or nursing home admission may be necessary.

Parkinson's Disease in Nursing Homes

Whilst the majority will be able to cope at home for many years with the illness, older patients are more likely to suffer cognitive problems and carry a higher risk of admission to residential or nursing home care. Usually this is as a result of both physical and mental decline and carries a high risk of mortality in such institutions – an American study showed that hallucinations were the strongest predictor of admission[20]. Those Parkinson's disease patients admitted to nursing homes showed a mean survival of less than one year, and all had died within two years[21].

Parkinson's disease is therefore a common cause of admission to institutional care, accounting for up to 10% of all nursing home-dwellers[22] and it should also be noted that it can also develop in residents, particularly if medication is not carefully vetted for drugs such as tranquilisers and vestibular sedatives that may cause drug induced parkinsonism. The prevalence of Parkinson's disease in Nursing Homes has been variously estimated as between 5-10% of residents. From diagnosis, one quarter of all patients in the Sydney study had been admitted to nursing homes by 10 years[23].

Dementia is the major concern in older ages, in one longitudinal series the cumulative proportion of patients with Parkinson's disease who developed dementia exceeded 50% at ten years[24]. An earlier paper published on this cohort (at 5 years) showed that age of onset, duration of Parkinson's disease, and disability all correlated with the development of dementia. In addition, those who demented had minor intellectual changes at inclusion, suggesting that even slight reduction in a generic mental test score (in this case a Folstein mini-mental test score of 25-29/30) may signify the likely later development of dementia.

Conclusion

There is mounting evidence that patients can help themselves by taking a positive, optimistic outlook right from the first diagnosis. Their prospective carers should do similarly, for themselves, and for their partners. Both patients and carers will need to develop their mutual relationship, aided and abetted by the caring professionals with whom a positive relationship should be encouraged. It is strongly suspected, even though not scientifically proven, that a sensible approach to nutrition, exercise, activity and psychological support will do much to alleviate the impact of the disease at any age. Well chosen drug treatments and accessibility of a range of therapies in a coordinated service for patients with Parkinson's disease will help minimise the physical and mental impact of this disease. This approach will improve not only the quality of life, but also the individual adaptation to one of the commoner insults primarily attack older people at the dawn of this new millenium.

References

1. Mutch WJ, Dingwall-Fordyce I, Downie AW, Paterson JG, Roy SK. *Parkinson's disease in a Scottish City*. Br Med J 1986;292:534-6
2. op. cit. n. 1
3. Ben-Shlomo Y *The epidemiology of Parkinson's disease*. Baillieres Clin Neurol 1997 Apr;6(1):55-68
4. MacMahon DG, Thomas S *Practical Approach to quality of life in Parkinson's disease*. J Neurol (1998) 245[suppl 1]: S19-22
5. Bennett DA; Beckett LA; Murray AM; Shannon KM; Goetz CG; Pilgrim DM; Evans DA. *Prevalence of parkinsonian signs and associated mortality in a community population of older people* N Engl J Med 1996 Jan 11;334(2):71-6
6. Meara J, Bhowmick BK and Hobson P. *Accuracy of diagnosis in patients with presumed Parkinson's disease Age & Ageing* 1999;28:99-102
7. Friedman A *Old-onset Parkinson's disease compared with young-onset disease: clinical differences and similarities*. Acta Neurol Scand 1994 Apr;89(4):258-61
8. Hely MA; Morris JG; Reid WG; O'Sullivan DJ; Williamson PM; Broe GA; Adena MA. *Age at onset: the major determinant of outcome in Parkinson's disease*. Acta Neurol Scand 1995 Dec;92(6):455-63
9. Diamond SG; Markham CH; Hoehn MM; McDowell FH; Muenter MD *Effect of age at onset on progression and mortality in Parkinson's disease*. Neurology 1989 Sep;39(9):1187-90
10. Findley L, Global Parkinson's Disease Steering Committee. *Investigating factors which may influence quality of life in Parkinson's disease. Parkinsonism and Related Disorders* 1999;5(suppl):146.
11. op. cit. n. 4
12. op. cit. n. 10

13. Litvan I; Mangone CA; McKee A; Verny M; Parsa A; Jellinger K; D'Olhaberriague L; Chaudhuri KR; Pearce RK *Natural history of progressive supranuclear palsy* (Steele-Richardson-Olszewski syndrome) *and clinical predictors of survival: a clinicopathological study.* J Neurol Neurosurg Psychiatry 1996 Jun;60(6):615-20

14. *The Parkinson's Disease Task Force. "Parkinson's Awareness in Primary Care"* Parkinson's Disease Society of the United Kingdom, London 1998 (revised 1999)

15. Bhatia K, Brooks DJ, Burn DJ, Clarke CE, Playfer J, Sawle GV, Schapira AHV, Stewart D and Williams AC. *1998 Guidelines for the management of Parkinson's disease.* Hospital Medicine 59(6): 469-480.

16. MacMahon D, Brooks D, Smith R. *Parkinson's Disease: integrating the primary and secondary care guidelines.* The Practitioner. 2000;244(1609):370-8

17. op. cit. n. 15

18. Hely MA; Morris JG; Reid WG; O'Sullivan DJ; Williamson PM; Rail D; Broe GA; Margrie S *The Sydney Multicentre Study of Parkinson's disease: a randomised, prospective five year study comparing low dose bromocriptine with low dose levodopa-carbidopa.* J Neurol Neurosurg Psychiatry 1994 Aug;57(8):903-10

19. Rascol O; Brooks DJ; Korczyn AD; De Deyn PP; Clarke CE; Lang AE *A five-year study of the incidence of dyskinesia in patients with early Parkinson's disease who were treated with ropinirole or levodopa.* 056 Study Group. N Engl J Med 2000 May 18;342(20):1484-91

20. Goetz CG, et al. *Risk factors for nursing home placement in advanced Parkinson's disease.* Neurology. 1993 Nov;43(11):2227

21. Goetz CG, et al. *Mortality and hallucinations in nursing home patients with advanced Parkinson's disease.* Neurology. 1995 Apr;45(4):669-71

22. Larsen JP. *Parkinson's disease as community health problem: study in Norwegian nursing homes. The Norwegian Study Group of Parkinson's Disease in the Elderly.* BMJ. 1991 Sep 28;303(6805):741-3.

23. Hely MA; Morris JG; Traficante R; Reid WG; O'Sullivan DJ; Williamson PM *The Sydney multicentre study of Parkinson's disease: progression and mortality at 10 years.* J Neurol Neurosurg Psychiatry 1999 Sep;67(3):300-7

24. Hughes TA, Ross HF, Musa S, Bhattacherjee S, Nathan RN, Mindham RH, Spokes EG: *A ten year study of the incidence of and factors predicting dementia in Parkinson's Disease:* Neurology 2000 April 25; 54 (8): pps. 1596-1602

CHAPTER 4

Assessing How Often to take L-Dopa

by Dr Geoffrey Leader MB ChB FRCA *and Lucille Leader* Dip ION

Many patients do not understand when they should ideally take their L-dopa medication. Doctors, patients and carers need to take several important factors into account:

a) Symptoms of dyskinesia and other exacerbated movement disturbance can sometimes be the result of too high a level of L-dopa in the blood due to the adjunctive use of supportive drugs for example Cabergoline[1], Ropinerole[2], Entacapone[3]. Drug companies recommend that with the addition of these drugs, the existing dosage of L-dopa should be reduced.

b) The neutral amino acids in protein can compete with L-dopa for absorption at intestinal receptor sites and at the blood brain barrier[4, 5]. This impedes absorption and it has been observed clinically that dyskinesia and tremor can be exacerbated with inappropriate diet in relation to L-dopa medication (see the section "L-dopa and Protein" in the chapter Nutritional Management).

c) Parkinson's disease is a fluctuating illness and there are many triggers which can exacerbate movement disturbance. Some of these include stress, medication, the "wearing off" and prior to "kick-in" of L-dopa, surgery, environmental pollution and drug-nutrient interactions. Taking an extra dose of L-dopa to counterbalance these extra disturbances, whilst the level of L-dopa in the blood is still high, does not solve the problem and can exacerbate symptoms.

We have devised a patient Assessment Diary to aid health professionals in assessing at what intervals L-dopa medication may best be prescribed. (see the Patient Assessment Diary overpage) The day on which assessment takes place should include a diet which is compatible with the absorption of L-dopa so that the physician will be able to more accurately assess the efficacy of the medication. (see the "Specialised Diet Day" on page 53). For practical purposes the assessment day should be based on the patient using standard L-dopa because the slow release formula is less predictable, lasting longer than the standard. It is, therefore, difficult to assess when patients are able to eat protein which contains the competitive neutral amino acids.

Taking into account the fluctuating nature of Parkinson's disease, it should be remembered that guidelines are helpful but there are no hard and fast rules that will always be successful. Regular intermittent assessment of patient performance, with the help of diary charts, can be useful in drug and dietary management. Symptom charts can be utilised in recommending the timing of subsequent doses of L-dopa in order to smooth out the on / off discomfort.

The diary chart can also be used to establish baselines for health care professionals.

See the following pages for the Assessment Diary and Diet.

DIARY SCHEME

© London Pain Relief and Nutritional Support Clinic, PO Box 12913, London, N12 8ZR

DATE: NAME: DOB: WEIGHT: TEL/FAX:

TIME 24-hour diary	MADOPAR (L-dopa) Dosage and Type	SINEMET (L-dopa) Dosage and Type	OTHER DRUGS, NUTRIENTS AND HERBS Dosage (Oral - IV - IM)	FOOD AND DRINK DETAIL	BOWEL / URINE	LIFESTYLE & EMOTIONAL REACTIONS	SYMPTOMS		
							Type	Time of Relief	Time of Recurrence
WAKE At									
TIME									
TIME									
TIME									
TIME									
Time continued									

OTHER NOTES:

50

How to fill in your diary

The following are examples of the detail required in each section, reading from left to right on the chart:

1. **TIME**
   Example: 7am

2. **MADOPAR**
   Example: Madopar Standard

3. **SINEMET**
   Example: Sinemet - Plus

4. **OTHER DRUGS, NUTRIENTS AND HERBS**
   (taken orally or administered intravenously (IV) or intramuscularly (IM))

   Example: Selegeline 5mgs, Astralagus (Solgar),
   Zinc citrate 15mgs elemental value
   Vitamin C (IV), Vitamin B complex (IM)

5. **FOOD AND DRINK**
   Example: Tea (caffeine), wholemeal toast, cod fish, wine,
   rice bread, chocolates

6. **BOWEL / URINE**
   Example: Bowel - straining, diarrhoea, pain, spasm, blood, mucus
   Urine - difficult starting, incontinence, pain, burning

7. **LIFESTYLE AND EMOTIONAL REACTIONS**
   Example: Swimming, Walking, Cinema - happy
   Work   - stress
   Movement difficulties   - stress
   Personal   - stress / happy

8. **SYMPTOMS**
   Example: Tremor, Stiffness, Dystonia,
   Feeling of unease, Dyskinesia commences/ends
   Flexible movement, Feeling cohesive, Coping well
   Hungry, Tired, Nervous, Agitated
   Speech difficulties, Uncontrolled movements

SPECIALISED DIET DAY COMBINED WITH DIARY CHART

Introduction

This "assessment day" uses standard preparations of L-dopa, not slow release. This is because the slow release formula is less predictable and dopamine levels last longer than with standard L-dopa. It is therefore difficult to know when to eat protein, which contains the competitive neutral amino acids that undermine absorption.

The accompanying diet should be used on the day that the Assessment Diary is filled in as the foods recommended are compatible with L-dopa absorption. Breakfast and lunch do not include protein-rich food. The evening meal does, however, contain protein-rich food and people should wait one hour after taking their L-dopa (Sinemet /Madopar) before eating dinner. Thereafter, ideally, there should be a two hour interval before taking L-dopa again if needed.

Note to Patients and Carers

Assessing the Diary Chart afterwards will show approximately how long the L-dopa (Sinemet/Madopar) works for the individual. The conclusion could well be that a person may be helped by taking L-dopa 45 minutes - 1 hour before anticipated symptoms set in. The attending neurologist/GP will advise you after studying the diary chart together with you. However, the optimum dosage pattern depends on the choice of foods, which are compatible with L-dopa absorption. This is because competitive amino acids found in dietary protein, if taken at an inappropriate time in relation to L-dopa, can often exacerbate dyskinesia and tremor (see the section "Optimising Function by Nutritional Manipulation" in the chapter Nutritional Management).

Taking into account the fluctuating nature of Parkinson's disease, it should be remembered that guidelines are helpful but there are no hard and fast rules that will always be successful. Regular intermittent assessment, with the help of diary charts, can be useful in drug and dietary management. Symptom charts can be utilised in recommending the timing of subsequent doses of L-dopa in order to smooth out the "on / off" discomfort.

THE ONE DAY DIET

About the drugs

1. If on *Sinemet*, you must wait 45 minutes - 1 hour before eating breakfast. Take a glass of water with your medication.

2. If on *Madopar*, you must wait 45 minutes - 1 hour before eating breakfast. Take a glass of water with your medication.

3. If on *Madopar Dispersible*, you may eat after it has "kicked in".

Eat the diet prescribed below for the whole day and evening. Take your drugs as usual but replace any slow release L-dopa with standard L-dopa, just on this day. Fill in your diary most precisely.

Breakfast
Choice of:
EnerG Brown Rice or EnerG Tapioca bread, toasted / corn bread or other gluten free bread (toasted gluten free breads seem to taste best) or rice crackers.
Butter and St Dalfour Jam or other sugar free jam with no artificial sweetening
Camomile herb tea made with still mineral water / still mineral water
Fruit (not grapefruit)
Kallo or other Puffed Rice Cereal or Corn Flakes (without gluten grains added)
Rice Dream (vanilla or plain flavour) as a milk substitute. This is rice milk

Between Meals
Prunes (at least 6), if constipated, or rice cracker with salad
2 glasses of still mineral water
(for ease, sip them between meals) / or herb tea

Lunch
Fruit (not grapefruit)
Jacket potato with a little butter (if desired)
Salad or vegetables
Warm sauce made with cold pressed olive oil, onion, tomato, Heinz Tomato Sauce (if required for taste), courgette, garlic (if desired)
Herbal peppermint tea / glass of still mineral water

Between Meals
Prunes (at least 6), if constipated, or a rice cracker with salad or vegetable soup
Glasses of still mineral water (for ease, sip them between meals)

Dinner

Piece of fruit (no grapefruit) as a starter
Filet of cod or haddock (not smoked) cooked with cold pressed olive oil
and other herbs/tomato
Sweet potato steamed / ordinary potato
Broccoli, green beans or other green vegetable but not cooked spinach
A glass of still mineral water

Later in the evening, if hungry

A bowl of liquidised soup (made from sweet potato, courgette, leek), fruit
or fruit juice (no grapefruit), camomile tea, still mineral or purified water

Optional
Still mineral water or herb tea, at any time

References

1. ABPI Compendium of Data Sheets and Summaries of Product Characteristics: p.1169: 1999 - 2000: Datapharm Publications Limited, London, UK

2. ABPI Compendium of Data Sheets and Summaries of Product Characteristics: p.1610: 1999 - 2000: Datapharm Publications Limited, London, UK

3. ABPI Compendium of Data Sheets and Summaries of Product Characteristics: p.1104: 1999 - 2000: Datapharm Publications Limited, London, UK

4. Dietary Factors in the Management of Parkinson's Disease: PA Kempster MD MRCP FRACP, MC Wahlqvist MD FRACP, Nutrition Reviews Vol 52, No. 2, 1994.

5. Parkinson's Disease - The New Nutritional Handbook: pps. 2 & 20: Dr Geoffrey Leader MBChB FRCA and Lucille Leader Dip ION: 1996: Denor Press, London, UK

Notes

CHAPTER 5

Surgical Neurology
A Multi-disciplinary Approach

by *Mr Tipu Aziz* MD FRCS, *Dr David Shlugman* MB CHB FRCA,
Dr Ralph Gregory FRCP, *Dr Anna Turner* BA(HONS) DCLINPSY, *Carole Joint* RGN
(The Oxford Movement Disorder Group)

Introduction

In recent years there has been a large increase in stereotactic functional surgery for Parkinson's disease (PD). This reflects the realisation by the medical community that the drug therapy, which was so promising in the late 1960's and 1970's, was not the panacea that it was originally thought to be. Prior to the introduction of L-Dopa therapy for Parkinson's disease by Cotzias in 1969, surgery was the mainstay of the management of the condition. Charcot had introduced anti-cholinergic therapy for parkinsonism in the late 1890's when he observed that dancers of the Moulin Rouge developed dry mouths when they took belladona to increase their appeal by inducing pupillary dilatation. Since many patients with Parkinson's disease suffer from drooling, he tried it in them but also noted that tremor was somewhat improved. Apart from this, there were no other effective therapies.

Surgery for the condition had its origins in the observation by James Parkinson in 1817 that a stroke abolished contralateral tremor. Given this, in 1908, Sir Victor Horsley excised the motor cortex in a boy with dystonia, alleviating the dystonia but causing epilepsy. After that, many open brain and spinal cord operations were devised to alleviate this crippling disease by either excising or sectioning nervous tissue. The theory behind this effort was that creating a hemi-paresis was essential to alleviate a movement disorder.

The major change came about with the findings of Meyer in 1938 that excision of deep brain gray matter could alleviate parkinsonism without causing a paralysis, but death from such major surgery was of the order of 15%. Nevertheless it did establish that the basal ganglia structures were involved in the disease. Cooper and Speigel in the USA, Mundinger in Europe, and Narabayashi in Japan virtually concurrently began to target the pallidum for lesioning to alleviate the symptoms of Parkinson's disease. The methodology to do this was pioneered by Speigel and Wycis in 1947 when they described the use of a stereotactic frame to guide needles deep into the human brain. This technique was pioneered by Horsley and Clarke in studying the cerebellar nuclei in monkeys in the late 1890s.

There followed an explosion in the use of pallidotomy for parkinsonism but these lesions alleviated rigidity more than tremor, which was more visible. Given that the pallidum projects to the ventro-lateral thalamus, thalamic lesions were tried and found to be much better at alleviating both symptoms. Even so, although most patients could expect to lose tremor and rigidity after surgery, few could actually do more because of the most disabling feature of Parkinson's disease, slowness of movement or bradykinesia. However, in 1969, L-Dopa was found to alleviate all cardinal signs of the disease without surgery and it seemed that there could be no place for such procedures. Such was the wave of optimism that attended its success that patients with other tremulous disorders were no longer offered surgery in the hope that a new drug was around the corner.

With long term experience of L-Dopa therapy in the treatment of Parkinson's disease, it became apparent that side effects, such as unpredictable motor fluctuations and involuntary movements known as dyskinesias, would become a problem for many patients. Lack of understanding of the mechanisms within the brain, that underlay the symptoms, held back any hope of safe and effective surgical treatment.

However, in 1979, a drug addict developed parkinsonism after intravenous injection of a home made drug, and several other cases were to follow. The condition was clinically indistinguishable from the true disease and the drug was identified as MPTP. In 1983, when administered to monkeys, a parkinsonian state identical to that in man was induced. Using this invaluable model, critical studies clarified the neural mechanisms that caused the symptoms. Essentially, there is loss of dopamine producing cells in the substantia nigra. Lack of dopamine, which normally acts as a 'brake' within the basal ganglia circuit, leads to excessive activity of the subthalamic nucleus (STN) which in turn drives the medial pallidum to over inhibit the motor thalamus and upper brain stem and thus induce the symptoms of Parkinson's disease. Within this framework, destroying all or part of the STN should alleviate parkinsonism and this was found to be the case in monkeys. It followed that surgery should be re-explored for people with Parkinson's disease.

At this time the main target of surgical interest was not the STN but the medial pallidum. The reasons for this were varied. Senior surgeons who had experience of the pallidum as a target were comfortable in resurrecting the procedure. Also, re-evaluation of the procedure in the post L-dopa era showed it still to be profoundly beneficial and it was relatively safe since the development of new technologies that enable these small targets within the brain to be located very accurately. STN surgery had theoretical risks of inducing severe involuntary movements known as chorea and the monkey studies implied a high risk of haemorrhage. Numerous publications confirmed that pallidotomy done on one side offered considerable benefits with regard to improvements in rigidity, tremor, slowness of movements and dyskinesias but predominantly on the side opposite to the surgery. Doing both sides carried a greater risk of side effects, limiting the overall benefits, and never became widely practised.

Given the fact that lesional surgery had the potential to cause irreversible side effects, deep brain stimulation was extensively studied by Benabid's group in France, initially with thalamic stimulation for tremor, and in 1993, using stimulation of the STN. Their work has led to a strong case for arguing that STN stimulation is the treatment of choice for Parkinson's disease.

Management of parkinsonian patients in the context of surgery should ideally be within a multi-disciplinary framework. This chapter incorporates short pieces by members of such a team describing their roles within the Oxford Movement Disorders Group and the management of patients in surgical neurology.

The Neurologist

The majority of patients with idiopathic Parkinson's disease can have their symptoms adequately controlled by medication. Despite all the new drugs that have been licensed for the treatment of the condition in recent years, L-dopa remains the most effective therapy, and is the mainstay of treatment for practically all patients. In the short term this drug can largely abolish all Parkinson's disease symptoms, but after 5 to 10 years patients begin to develop unpredictable motor fluctuations and drug induced dyskinesias. The dyskinesias usually occur at peak doses of L-dopa, and the patient therefore has the choice of being slow, rigid and tremulous, or mobile but with wild thrashing movements, which in some cases can involve the whole body. Neurologists have therefore attempted to develop strategies to try and delay the onset of these "complications", such as using dopamine agonist drugs at the time of diagnosis, rather than starting with L-dopa. Fluctuations can sometimes respond to a continuous infusion of drug called apomorphine, but this is a cumbersome, uncomfortable, and expensive option. Even the most sceptical neurologists have become converted to the idea that surgery can have a role in selected cases, but many remain concerned about the logic of destructive brain lesions in patients with a progressive degenerative condition and therefore favour the use of deep brain stimulation.

The crucial key to success is patient selection. Younger patients who have retained an excellent, albeit short-lived, response to L-dopa, have the most to gain from these procedures, particularly involving the STN. Parkinson's disease is not a "surgical" disease, and it is therefore important that the neurologist is closely involved at all stages of the process. All forms of surgery have risks, even in the most experienced centres, and it is therefore preferable that all medical options have been tried first. If patients on referral are not under active neurological or Parkinson's disease specialist follow-up, then the neurologist on the surgical team should assess them to ensure that alternative therapeutic strategies are not possible. However, surgery should not be delayed until the very advanced stages of the disease. It can be tempting to offer surgery to any patient no matter how severe their disease, because "there is nothing to lose". The consequences of this practice are often disastrous, and the neurologist can help in the counselling of such patients. Intra-operatively, target confirmation depends on the control of the patient's symptoms, which are best assessed by the physician who has assessed the patient pre-operatively. Post-operatively, the patients still require medical management of their Parkinson's disease, and it is preferable that they are nursed on a neurological, rather than neurosurgical ward. Selecting the best stimulation parameters can be extremely difficult, and is often best done by the neurologist and specialist nurse. The neurologist must therefore be fully involved, and work closely with the surgeon to ensure an optimum outcome.

The Clinical Neuro-psychologist

The clinical neuropsychologist working within a multi-disciplinary Movement Disorder Team is uniquely placed to assess and evaluate the complex cognitive, functional, emotional and social issues associated with neurodegenerative disease. The clinical assessment, therefore, should assimilate a detailed background history and information regarding the functional/emotional impact of the patient's illness upon everyday life (from patient and carer perspectives), in addition to a comprehensive neuropsychological review.

The aims of psychological assessment are fourfold:

- To screen patients for diagnosis on Axis I of DSM IV for various anxiety disorders, depression and suicidal ideation.

- To complete a global assessment of neuropsychological functioning, enabling general cognitive decline (such as dementia), or specific impairments (such as those involving speech-motor apparatus) to be identified.

- The semi-structured interview, completed with the patient and carer, allows for greater understanding of psychosocial issues relevant to post-operative care and individual expectations of surgery. Where appropriate, follow-up support can be organised, such as on-going psychological support or respite care.

■ Pre-operative assessment serves as a baseline measure of social, emotional and neuropsychological functioning, against which to any post-operative change can be evaluated. Cognitive changes may occur (both deficits and improvements) that may or may not be related to the surgical procedure. Having access to a baseline enables clarification of these issues both for the Movement Disorder Group as a whole, and for the patient and their relatives.

Depending upon individual circumstances, any of the above mentioned factors might contraindicate surgery.

Pre and post-operative neuropsychological assessment usually takes place during the in-patient admission to hospital, and can take 3-4 hours. Post-operative review usually takes place at 6 months, with further review possibly at 18 months-2 years. The heterogeneity and severity of presenting symptomology require a flexible approach to assessment. Parkinson's disease patients often experience considerable physical discomfort, so they may struggle to sit and concentrate for any length of time. Speech-motor problems may make communication a challenge, and motor skills can be poor. Thus, sensitivity to the individual's needs is paramount in the selection and administration of the test battery. A number of methodological factors need to be considered when interpreting results, such as practice effects and disease related neurodegeneration. It is important to ensure that testing is carried out with patients on optimal medication and during the 'on' state.

Areas of neuropsychological functioning assessed might include: pre-morbid and current levels of general intellect, memory/new learning, speech and language (articulation, naming and fluency), visuo-spatial scanning, processing speed, attention and hand-eye co-ordination. For evaluative purposes, the neuropsychological battery usually remains unchanged across testing. The remainder of the protocol takes the form of a semi-structured interview with the patient and carer (where possible). A patient-rated questionnaire measures psychological symptomology and quality of life, in addition to patient and carer rated questionnaires of functional disability.

Pre and post-operative neuropsychological assessment therefore forms a routine component of the multi-disiciplinary Movement Disorder Group clinic. The primary reasons being the need to audit outcome closely in order to compare the efficacy of different surgical procedures in a rapidly evolving field.

The Movement Disorder Nurse

The development of the nurse specialist role has been driven, in part, by a requirement to co-ordinate the care of the patient within the multi-disciplinary team and to contribute towards the collection of data about the outcome for patients following functional surgery. However, a stronger influence on the role has been the recognition of the specific needs of these patients and their families. A key function of the Movement Disorder Nurse is to provide nursing care, support and information through the whole of patients' experience in surgical neurology, with regard to both the medical and surgical aspects of their care.

If the Movement Disorder Team, the patient and their family agree that surgery is a possible option for them, arrangements are made for admission to hospital for a two to three day assessment period. These assessments are performed during an in-patient stay since they require manipulation of anti-parkinson medication, and also because it is important that the patient is seen throughout the whole spectrum of their Parkinson's disease, bearing in mind the degree of fluctuations in symptoms experienced by most people during the day. All patients are cared for in specialist neurology wards where the multi-disciplinary team has expertise in the management of Parkinson's disease, and specifically, in meeting the complex needs of people who are undergoing the rigorous assessment programme required before surgery and also during the operative period itself. Since each person with Parkinson's disease will experience a different pattern of symptoms and response to their medication, care is planned with them not for them. One of the key issues is to establish their involvement in timing of medication, preferably by the use of a self- medication protocol. It is recognised that timing is crucial to the relief of symptoms and therefore to independence for the patient.

Assessments used at this stage include objective measures of signs and symptoms of Parkinson's disease experienced by the patient, a full neuropsychological assessment, and also the effects of Parkinson's disease on their quality of life. The requirement for some of the assessments and investigations to be performed in the 'off-medication' state causes considerable disruption to normal routine. This can be particularly distressing to someone whose independence depends on strict timing of medication. Despite the fact that most patients are very willing to put up with the disruption, the specialist nurse will endeavour to minimise the effects by careful planning of the assessment timetable.

During this admission period, the patient and their family can again discuss the surgical procedure itself. The operation is performed with the patient awake, so that their parkinsonian signs and symptoms are apparent and they are able to co-operate with the surgical team. Some people may feel that they couldn't cope with this, but most are highly motivated to co-operate if there is an opportunity to gain an improvement in quality of life, and will accept the situation if an explanation of the reason for this is given. The Movement Disorder Team ensures that the patient and their family clearly understand the risks and benefits of the proposed procedure, and are realistic about the possible desirable and undesirable outcomes. The decision about whether surgery is appropriate for a patient is based on the outcome of the assessments, and is made by the whole Movement Disorder Team in conjunction with the patient themselves and their family. The date for readmission to hospital for surgery will usually be confirmed prior to discharge home.

Care during the operation and post-operative period: The Movement Disorder Nurse accompanies the patient throughout the operation and immediate recovery period, to provide nursing care and assist with assessment of the patient during surgery. Post-operatively, early mobilisation is encouraged and the goal is for the patient to resume or improve on the level of pre-operative independence as soon as possible. However, the surgical procedure is very tiring and it is important that patients rest when they are tired, at least during the initial post-operative period. Those who have been severely disabled may benefit from physiotherapy and occupational therapy at this stage, so that their body can be re-educated to function within the reduced level of disability.

The Movement Disorder Nurse works closely with the nursing and medical team on the ward to plan care for the patient during the hospital stay, and also works towards discharge home. Information and advice about what to expect following their operation is given to the patient and their family both verbally and in writing before they leave hospital.

The Peri-operative Period:

Pre-operative investigations include laboratory testing of blood to screen for any abnormalities that might cause a problem during or after the procedure, for example anaemia or an abnormal clotting profile. An MRI brain scan is performed one or two days before the operation date, usually with patients having been given some intravenous sedation to enable them to lie completely still. A CT brain scan is also required, but this is carried out at the time of surgery with a stereotactic frame applied to the patient's head to allow the surgeon to calculate the target within the brain.

The Anaesthetist

Pre-operative assessment: An assessment by the anaesthetist, followed by discussion with the surgical team, dictates whether the procedure will be carried out entirely under local anaesthetic or with a general anaesthetic during application of the stereotactic frame and for the CT scan. Since it can be quite uncomfortable to have the frame applied, and the patient must lie completely still for the scan, local anaesthesia with sedation is rarely used for this first part of the procedure and is confined to those who are medically unfit.

At the pre-operative visit it is important to get an accurate drug history as many of the anti-parkinsonian drugs have anaesthetic implications. Most if not all the patients will be on some form of L-dopa. One of the effects of this drug is to reduce blood pressure and this may result in some patients having a low blood pressure. Because the drug is stopped the day before surgery, pre-operative blood pressures bear little resemblance to the blood pressure on the day of surgery, as the latter is always significantly raised. To counter this effect, an anti-hypertensive is prescribed with the premedication especially in the older patient. A drug to reduce gastric acid secretion is prescribed as a pre-medication (H2 receptor antagonist) but the patient is not given sedation so as to be able to co-operate fully during surgery, and also to ensure that parkinsonian signs are not suppressed. This may present a problem if they are anxious about the forthcoming events.

Anaesthesia: Since most people with Parkinson's disease find being in the 'off' state distressing, it is usual for their operation to be scheduled early on the operating list so that the amount of time that they have to wait is minimised.

The most suitable general anaesthetic drugs for this type of procedure are those that can be easily antagonised (midazolam, vecuronium, alfentanyl). Propofol is given by infusion using a target controlled infusion pump. A low target plasma concentration is chosen for maintenance of anaesthesia, relying on an adequate dose of midazolam and nitrous oxide for hypnosis. An arterial line is placed on the contra-lateral side to surgery to facilitate constant blood pressure monitoring. A flexible laryngeal mask airway is used in preference to an endotracheal tube, as it is less stimulating to the upper airway and less likely to result in coughing or straining on removal. Following the CT scan the patient is returned to the operating room. Whilst the surgical team calculates the target co-ordinates from the CT and MRI data, the patient is allowed to wake up gently from the anaesthetic. Supplementary oxygen is given via nasal cannula.

Once awake, the patient can have their false teeth inserted and sips of water are given to help them to feel comfortable and to talk freely. During the waking phase and once awake, there is a tendency for the blood pressure to rise steadily. It is important to counteract this trend, as the surgical procedure involves passing a wire deep into the brain. Should a blood vessel be damaged en route, any intracerebral bleeding will be aggravated in the presence of hypertension. Direct acting vasodilators such as sodium nitroprusside are avoided as they increase cerebral blood flow, as do most of the anti-hypertensive agents to a greater or lesser extent. Intra-nasal nifedipine 10-20mg, and intravenous labetolol have been found to the most suitable.

At the end of the procedure, the patient is transferred to the recovery room. The arterial line is left in situ, and arterial pressure monitored closely. This will be removed before the patient returns to the ward. A dose of L-dopa is given to alleviate Parkinson's disease symptoms and has the added effect of restoring the blood pressure to pre-operative levels. The patient is also carefully observed for any signs of intra-cerebral bleeding over the following few hours.

The Surgical Procedure

Once the target is calculated, a small hole is made in the skull and a wire is passed into the brain to the target site. Since the brain has no sensory nerve endings, this procedure is not painful for the patient. An electrical pulse transmitted down the wire allows the Neurologist and the Movement Disorder Nurse to assess the effect of interfering with this specific area of the brain whilst causing no permanent damage. The point is found at which the symptoms of Parkinson's Disease are alleviated without causing any unwanted effects, and then this tiny area is either destroyed by heating the tip of the wire, or the permanent stimulation wire is implanted and secured to the skull using a small metal plate. Patients who have had a lesion made will have the scalp wound closed and are taken to the recovery area for a short time before being returned to the ward. Those patients who are having a stimulator implanted will have a short general anaesthetic to allow implantation of the connecting wires and stimulator battery, since this part of the procedure would be uncomfortable under local anaesthesia. If the beneficial effects on parkinsonian symptoms are not clear during the surgical procedure for stimulator implant, the brain electrode may be brought out onto the skin to allow a trial of stimulation for a week before a final decision is made on whether to fully implant the system.

Post-Operative Care

Patients are usually re-established on their anti-Parkinson medication as soon as possible after surgery although, following some types of procedure, the dose may be reduced. It is usual for patients to be ready for discharge from hospital a few days after their operation. If Deep Brain Stimulators have been implanted, it is common for the signs and symptoms of Parkinson's disease to be reduced immediately following surgery even without the stimulator being switched on. This is due to a 'stun' effect of implanting the wires in the brain, and in this case the stimulator will be left switched off for a few weeks following surgery to allow any swelling around the wires to subside. The patient will be readmitted to hospital to have the stimulation parameters set once their symptoms have returned.

The Movement Disorder Team provides on-going support for patients and their families following functional surgery. General Practitioners can help to arrange services such as physiotherapy or speech therapy, in the community, if these are required. The patients and their carers are encouraged to contact the Movement Disorder Nurse or the ward if they are concerned by any untoward events that occur once they at home. This allows their progress to be monitored and any problems to be resolved before they become a major source of anxiety. Referrals to other professionals can be made if necessary. Liaison with the community Parkinson's Disease Nurse will often have been made before the patient has come into hospital, and can be continued post-operatively to ensure continuity of care and support. Contact with the Movement Disorder Team will be maintained subsequently, as often as is needed by the patient and their family.

Conclusions

There is still reason to debate whether there is truly one best target for alleviation of symptoms in Parkinson's disease. It would appear that if there were no budgetary restraints, in an ideal world, deep brain stimulation would offer the best surgical treatment for Parkinson's disease, the choice of target depending on the patient's predominant symptoms. It is considered preferable now to offer deep brain stimulation if bilateral procedures are required. Thalamotomy or thalamic stimulation can abolish contralateral tremor, pallidotomy or pallidal stimulation is extremely effective for dyskinesias, contralateral rigidity and sometimes tremor, but neither has a sustained impact on any of the other parkinsonian symptoms. Many clinicians are enthusiastic about the prospect of stimulation of the STN. This area of the brain is very small and the procedure is proving technically much more difficult to perform than thalamic or pallidal surgery. It remains to be seen whether this labour intensive and expensive option will become a widely available treatment option.

Regardless of which procedure is chosen, the care of the patients must be provided within a multi-disciplinary team. The neurologist ascertains that the patients referred have exhausted all possibilities of medical therapy prior to considering surgery, the neuropsychologist ensures that there are no mental contra-indications to surgery, ensures that the patient and carer understand what surgery can achieve, and clarifies what their expectations are. The neurophysiologist is central to studying the effects on motor function before, during and after surgery in order that we understand what is achieved and to indicate future possibilities. The anaesthetist ensures that patients go through surgery safely and comfortably, and since much of the surgery is done with the patient awake, that this is as pleasant as possible. To organise such a large group and to maintain patient contact, to make their voice and concerns always heard, the specialist nurse is critical. She provides educational information that is user friendly, is the port of call to the patient and care body, and educates colleagues and interested parties in the aims and achievements of the group.

The procedures discussed here do not offer a cure for Parkinson's disease, nor do they free the patient from taking medication, making regular hospital visits, and the knowledge that as the disease continues to advance, any benefits will wane. Neurologists, like their surgical colleagues, hope that alternative medical strategies or 'restorative' surgery will replace the need for this type of procedure in the future.

Bibliography

Movement Disorder Surgery. (2000) AM Lozano (Ed): In "Progress In Neurological Surgery". Editor: LD Lunsford. Vol 15. Karger

Electrical Stimulation Of The Subthalamic Nucleus In Advanced Parkinson's Disease. (1998) Limousin, P.; Krack, P.; Pollak, P.; Benazzouz, A.; Ardouin, C.; Hoffmann, D., And Benabid, A. L. N Engl J Med. Oct 15; 339(16):1105-11.

A Multi-Disciplinary Approach To Tremor. (1996) Aziz T.Z And Bain P.G.. British Journal Of Neurosurgery: 10(5):435-437

Is There A Single Best Surgical Procedure For The Alleviation Of PD. (2001) Tipu Aziz, Simon Parkin, Carole Joint, Ralph Gregory, Peter Bain, John F Stein, And Richard Scott: In

Basal Ganglia And Thalamus In Health And Movement Disorders, Kristy Kultas- Ilinsky And Igor A. Ilinsky, Eds., Kluwer/Academic/Plenum Press, NY.

Pros And Cons Of Various Stereotactic Procedures For Parkinson's Disease. (2000) MI Hariz. Pan Arab Journal Of Neurosurgery: Vol4. No2. October

CHAPTER 6

Anaesthesia
for
General Operative Procedures
in Parkinson's Disease Patients

by Dr Geoffrey Leader MB ChB FRCA

Planning is of particular importance, not only because Parkinson's disease patients react adversely to stress, but also because of the specific drug regime that most Parkinson's disease patients are on, together with any potential drug interactions that must be considered.

General Considerations

Unless Parkinson's disease patients are following a specific exercise regime of fitness, toning and stretching, they tend to be less mobile and their vital capacity may be reduced. They therefore need early mobilisation and breathing exercises post-operatively so as to minimise the chance of respiratory complications. Also, any technique chosen should be aimed at quick recovery.

Drug Considerations

- In order to maintain control of stiffness and tremor, it is important that the Parkinson's disease patient is well stabilised on a drug regime, and also that this regime is maintained until just before the scheduled operation time and continued immediately post-operatively, so as to maintain L-dopa and other drug levels.

- A protein meal should ideally have been consumed the evening *prior* to the day of operation in order to avoid any drug-protein interaction and maximise L-dopa absorption.

- Four hours pre-operatively, a high calorie drink should be taken, for example "Ultrafuel" (Twin Lab), which contains long chain glucose polymers.

- Central sedatives (for example diazepam) and neuroleptic agents are best avoided.

- If an anti-cholinergic agent is needed, then Atropine or Robinul may be used. Scopolamine may be too sedative.

- Metoclopramide, phenothiazines and butyrophenones are contra-indicated as they may aggravate symptoms.

Anaesthesia

1. Pre-medication should be as light as possible to facilitate early recovery - only atropine, where indicated, to reduce excess salivation, and also ondansetron as an anti-emetic when the Parkinson's disease patient is using a drug such as apomorphine, which has a significant side effect of nausea.

2. General anaesthesia is preferable in order to control tremor and rigidity, and also to minimise stress. (Stress can exacerbate tremor post-operatively because of raised adrenaline levels).

- Induction with a short-acting agent such as propofol, is desirable.

- Maintenance with N2O-O2 and sevoflurane/desflurane/propofol infusion, for example in order to facilitate quick recovery.

- Muscle relaxants used may be of intermediate duration eg atracurim, which has also been proven to be safe for the elderly too, and is broken down in the plasma independently of liver or renal function. As well as providing muscle relaxation for laparotomy, muscle relaxants will also help to reduce the dose of inhalation agent/propofol infusion used, together with a short acting opiate such as alfentanyl and a small dose of hypnotic agent such as midazolam. However, opioids should be used with care and in small doses as they may precipate rigidity[1]. Appropriate antagonists are given, when necessary.

3. If local anaesthesia is indicated, adrenaline is best omitted, and sedation with for example midazolam and a propofol infusion may be added, in order to reduce anxiety and tremor.

Notes

- Patients on L-dopa may have a lower or unstable blood pressure because of impaired autonomic responses or because of a dopaminergic effect on the peripheral vasculature[2]. Hypotension may occur especially with long term L-dopa usage due to replacement of nor-adrenaline by dopamine in peripheral sympathetic nerves[3]. If present, it may be best treated with a direct perhiperally acting vasopressor such as phenylephrine 100-500mcg IV.

- Cardiac irritability may occasionally lead to arrhythmias, so that avoidance of halothane, ketamine and local anaesthetics containing adrenaline is prudent.

- Muscle relaxants usually show a normal response.

- Ensure a good fluid balance peri-operatively to prevent dehydration. Maintain normal temperature with a warming mattress or hot air blanket so as to prevent cooling and help to promote elimination of anaesthetic drugs.

- Specific drugs used in the management of Parkinson's Disease:

  Most of these drugs tend to produce nausea. In the case of L-dopa, domperidone may be most useful as an anti-emetic, as it is a dopamine antagonist which does not cross the blood brain barrier and interfere with the central action of L-dopa. For other drugs used, a selective 5HT receptor-antagonist such as ondansetron may be indicated.

  Selegiline may interact with pethidine, causing hypertension[4]. A single dose of 10mgs Selegiline may last up to 24-hours.

  Amantidine may cause sinus tachycardia, cardiac arrhythmias or hypertension[5].

  Cabergoline may cause hypertension by stimulating dopamine receptors[6,] and also nausea.

  Pergolide may also produce hypertension[7] and also nausea.

  Apomorphine and Ropinerole often cause troublesome nausea.

  Antibiotics such as metronidazole may cause muscle inco-ordination[8].

Nutrients and Herbs - Cautionary Note

Patients should avoid taking vitamins C and E and Essential Fatty Acids for at least two weeks before surgery. This is to reduce the risk of bleeding as these nutrients reduce platelet aggregation and can predispose to excessive bleeding intraoperatively and postoperatively. The herb Bromelain can also have this effect and other herbs and nutrients should always be checked for similar effects.

Post-operatively

- Ensure early mobilisation and breathing exercises, especially where there is stiffness of the chest wall, so as to help to prevent deep vein thrombosis and atelectasis.

- Pain relief may be provided with eg a diclofenac suppository 100mgs or an opiate in small doses.

- Nausea may be treated with for example ondansetron.

- At the end of anaesthesia, an infusion of B vitamins and vitamin C may help to aid detoxification of anaesthetic drugs and speed up complete recovery from anaesthesia[9].

- It may also be prudent to add other anti-oxidant nutrients to the infusion. This concept of enhancing detoxification is an important one for general anaesthesia and particularly in Parkinson's disease patients. This is because of the possible compromised cytochrome P450 liver detoxification pathway[10, 11, 12]. (For details of liver detoxification processes, see the section "Optimal Liver Function - A Nutritional Approach" by Helen Kimber in the chapter "Nutritional Management" on page 144.)

References

1. *Parkinsonism and The Anaesthetist:* Br J Anaesth, vol 61: pps. 761-770: A M Severn: 1988

2. *Drug Interactions in Anaesthesia:* p. 235: N Ty Smith, R D Miller, A N Corbascio: 1981: Lea & Febiger, Philadelphia, USA

3. *Cardiovascular reactions to anaesthesia during treatment with levodopa* (vol. 28): Anaesthesia: pps. 29-31: D R Bevan, P S Monks, D B Calne: 1973

4. *ABPI Compendium of Data Sheets and Summaries of Product Characteristics:* p. 1105: 1999 - 2000: Datapharm Publications Limited, London, UK

5. *ABPI Compendium of Data Sheets and Summaries of Product Characteristics:* p. 79: 1999 - 2000: Datapharm Publications Limited, London, UK

6. *ABPI Compendium of Data Sheets and Summaries of Product Characteristics:* p. 1169: 1999 - 2000: Datapharm Publications Limited, London, UK

7. *ABPI Compendium of Data Sheets and Summaries of Product Characteristics:* p. 734: 1999 - 2000: Datapharm Publications Limited, London, UK

8. *ABPI Compendium of Data Sheets and Summaries of Product Characteristics:* p. 549: 1999 - 2000: Datapharm Publications Limited, London, UK

9. *Dietary Regulation of cytochrome P450: Annual review of nutrition vol 11:* Ke Anderson, A Kappas: pps. 141-67: 1991

10. *Abnormal Liver Enzyme-mediated Metabolism in Parkinson's Disease - A Second Look - Neurology* 41(5 suppl 2): pps. 89 - 91: Discussion p. 92: C M Tanner: May 1991

11. *Metabolic Biomarkers of Parkinson's Disease - Actor Neurologica Scandinavica - Supplementum* 136: pps. 19 - 23: A Williams, S Sturman, G Steventon, R Waring: 1991

12. *Liver Enzyme Abnormalities in Parkinson's Disease: Geriatrics* 46 Suppl 1: pps. 60 - 63: August 1991:

CHAPTER 7

The Podiatric Surgeon in Parkinson's Disease

*by **David Bell** FPodA DPM FAAAS DipChOrth DPodM*

The role of the podiatric surgeon in patients with Parkinson's disease includes assessment of the musculo-skeletal dynamics of the feet, together with any corrective measures which may be necessary. These are remedial exercises, orthotics and surgery.

We have conducted a small study of patients at The London Pain Relief and Nutritional Support Clinic and have worked on increasing the stretching of muscle bellies to avoid contraction. This is inevitable, particularly in the posterior group of muscles of the lower leg the triceps surae. These consist of the gastrocnemeus, soleus and plantaris muscles. In all ten patients assessed, shortening of the calf muscles was found.

Contraction in this group of muscles reduces the ability to dorsi-flex the ankle. This is an essential part of smoothly co-ordinated human gait after heel strike, as the lower leg needs to be able to bend forward 10 degrees to unlock the sub-talar joint and allow for pronation to absorb the shock of body weight and accommodate for uneven terrain. This is followed by external rotation of the lower limb to produce supination for a powerful push off.

In the absence of ankle dorsi-flexion, this action is obtained at the mid-tarsal joint causing osteoarthritic changes with the resulting flattened arch.

Deep in the calf complex is the flexor digitorum longus muscle and the flexor hallucis longus muscle group which is responsible for the plantar flexion of the toes distal to the metatarso phalangeal joint. The tightness of this group results in the accompanying clawing of all the toes including the hallux.

It is therefore vitally important to educate patients to use a stretching programme, (diagram opposite) to try and lengthen the triceps surae muscle belly group to limit the resulting damage within the foot. However, exercising is extremely boring for patients and in particular stretching, where there is no immediate obvious benefit to patients. One must encourage motivation, in order to optimise walking.

The clawing of the toes, which is secondary to the flattening of the arch and the contracture of the posterior group of muscles, can be attended to by initially providing splinting in the form of a removable silicone splint to prevent this clawing worsening and give the toes a "bolster" to grip. This enables patients to grip the floor with their toes to provide sufficient thrust forward and avoid any further problems in the toes.

When this process is too far advanced, surgery is the only option. Tendon surgery has a very poor long-term prognosis and the author finds that fusion of the inter-phalangeal joints is the solution, which gives the best relief. Arthroplasty of the inter-phalangeal joints is doomed to failure due to the continuing contraction of the flexor group of toe muscles.

Finally, the pronation which occurs at the mid-tarsal and subtalar joints can be corrected by orthoses which are semi-rigid. This will help to limit the damage to the foot caused by muscle contraction.

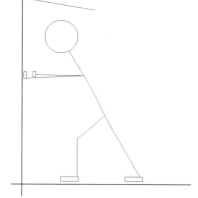

**Stretching Exercise
for Calf Muscle**

1. **Arms:**   Parallel to floor, shoulder height, palms of hands flat on the wall

2. **Front leg:** Foot pointing straight ahead and knee slightly bent

3. **Back Leg:** Foot pointing straight ahead and with locked knee

4. **Heels:**   Flat on the ground

5. Push forward and hold for a minimum of 20 seconds, without bouncing

6. Repeat 3 times with each leg and perform exercise twice daily

CHAPTER 8

The Patient's Diary

by Geoffrey Leader and Lucille Leader

Filling in this diary chart will provide a snapshot of patient performance over a 24 hour period. It provides helpful information for patients, carers and their healthcare professionals which may determine which aspects of daily activity and therapeutic management may need attention, in order to optimise function.

How to fill in your diary

The following are examples of the detail required in each section, reading from left to right on the chart:

1. **TIME**
    Example: 7am

2. **MADOPAR**
    Example: Madopar Standard

3. **SINEMET**
    Example: Sinemet - Plus

4. **OTHER DRUGS, NUTRIENTS AND HERBS**
    (taken orally or administered intravenously (IV) or intramuscularly (IM))

    Example: Selegeline 5mgs, Astralagus (Solgar),
                    Zinc citrate 15mgs elemental value
                    Vitamin C (IV), Vitamin B complex (IM)

5. **FOOD AND DRINK**
    Example: Tea (caffeine), wholemeal toast, cod fish, wine,
                    rice bread, chocolates

6. **BOWEL / URINE**
    Example: Bowel - straining, diarrhoea, pain, spasm, blood, mucus
                    Urine - difficult starting, incontinence, pain, burning

7. **LIFESTYLE AND EMOTIONAL REACTIONS**
    Example: Swimming, Walking, Cinema   - happy
                    Work   - stress
                    Movement difficulties   - stress
                    Personal   - stress / happy

8. **SYMPTOMS**
    Example: Tremor, Stiffness, Dystonia,
                    Feeling of unease, Dyskinesia commences/ends
                    Flexible movement, Feeling cohesive, Coping well
                    Hungry, Tired, Nervous, Agitated
                    Speech difficulties, Uncontrolled movements

DIARY SCHEME

© London Pain Relief and Nutritional Support Clinic, PO Box 12913, London, N12 8ZR

DATE: NAME: DOB: WEIGHT: TEL/FAX:

TIME 24-hour diary	MADOPAR (L-dopa) Dosage and Type	SINEMET (L-dopa) Dosage and Type	OTHER DRUGS, NUTRIENTS AND HERBS Dosage (Oral - IV - IM)	FOOD AND DRINK DETAIL	BOWEL / URINE	LIFESTYLE & EMOTIONAL REACTIONS	SYMPTOMS		
							Type	Time of Relief	Time of Recurrence
WAKE At									
TIME									
TIME									
TIME									
TIME									
Time continued									

OTHER NOTES:

Optimising Function
by Nutritional Manipulation

by Lucille Leader Dip ION

Why Nutritional Management?

Amino acids are derived from the breakdown of dietary protein. Dopamine (the neurotransmitter which is deficient in Parkinson's disease) is synthesised from one such amino acid, phenylalanine, which metabolises further to tyrosine, L-dopa and then dopamine (see figure 1 on page 78).

If a human being were to be "analysed" in a laboratory, it would be demonstrated that the body is composed of nutritional factors. These are protein, carbohydrates, fats, vitamins, minerals and water. Excesses or deficiencies of nutrients which may possibly be the cause of health problems, can be biochemically demonstrated on a cellular level.

Biochemical assessment[1] of people taking dopaminergic drugs, as well as those who do not, may demonstrate nutritional deficiencies, which if not addressed, compromise energy and other cellular functions. As such, it would seem totally logical to include nutritional assessment and management as part of health care. Besides addressing nutritional status, there are many other aspects in the management of Parkinson's disease which benefit from judicious and dynamic nutritional manipulation and can optimise function and wellbeing.

During the past decade, the field of biochemically based nutrition has entered the pharmacopoeia of medicine. Thanks to advances in molecular biology and the electron microscope, it has become possible to evaluate the significant roles of amino acids, carbohydrates, essential fatty acids, vitamins and minerals in cellular metabolism. All these elements influence brain biochemistry and metabolism. There is fascinating academic research published which demonstrates the significance of dietary factors as precursors of dopamine, the effects of alcohol and caffeine on dopamine transmission and turnover in the basal ganglia and other brain regions, and the consequences of diets, either rich or deficient in antioxidant nutrients, in relation to the development of Parkinson's disease. Joint studies undertaken by various university departments of Neurology, Human Nutrition, Epidemiology and Social Medicine, supported by the German Federal Ministry for Research and Technology have prompted the statement: "Ultimately insights into mechanisms that link nutrition with Parkinson's disease risk may give rise to new treatment approaches and preventative recommendations"[1a]. Nutritional therapy is now accepted as an effective and essential new player in the Parkinson's disease management team.

People with Parkinson's disease often present initially with symptoms of tremor, rigidity, unsteadiness and bradykinesia (slow movement). The reason for impaired muscular control and function has been attributed to a deficiency of the neurotransmitter dopamine. Dopamine is manufactured by neurones in the substantia nigra area of the brain. Parkinson's disease is not just a disease of the elderly. In the UK there are more than 120,000 sufferers ranging from teens through to old age. In the USA it is thought that there are more than 1million people with this illness.

There are possibly many contributory reasons for insufficient production of dopamine: degeneration of cells, cell death (apoptosis), mitochondrial and general metabolic inadequacy, dietary factors, enzyme malfunction, deficient cellular nutrition, disease, free-radical destruction, environmental toxicity, pesticides[2, 3, 4] and insecticides, genes, drugs, stress or idiopathic manifestation.

To date, treatment is mainly based on administration of the drug L-dopa (levodopa as in "Sinemet", "Madopar" or equivalent drug). L-dopa is the precursor of dopamine and therefore can replenish endogenous low levels of dopamine. Other drugs are available which potentiate the bioavailability of L-dopa. There are also surgical techniques, which can aid in the control of symptoms.

Specialised nutritional support includes dealing with the following aspects:

- intestinal problems including those of digestive enzymes, gut permeability, malabsorption and bowel function

- general dietary recommendations.

- specialised dietary recommendations:

    - defining the problems, with solutions, for the drug-nutrient interactions
      protein with L-dopa
      vitamin B6 with L-dopa
      tyramine rich foods with monoamine oxidase inhibitor drugs
    - specialised feeding for those with swallowing/chewing/malabsorption problems
    - identification of allergy and food intolerance

- support of detoxification pathways
- control of blood sugar levels
- optimisation of cellular energy
- antioxidant therapy (protection against excess free radicals)
- specialised cooking methods to reduce free radicals
- nutritional guidance for pregnancy

■ biochemical tests (nutritional and general)
■ oral nutritional supplementation when applicable
■ intravenous nutritional support where malabsorption is a problem
■ weight control
■ the possibility of environmental factors influencing genetic expression.

The nutritionist can direct awareness to identifiable hazards for example, the herbicide 1-methyl-4-phenyl-1,2.3.6-tetrahydropyrinine[5] (MPTP) is implicated in both stiffness and weakness in Parkinson's disease. Water contaminants (hexachlorobenzene) have been shown to have nervous system effects[6] and other herbicides have also had nervous system effects including tremor[7]. MPTP was responsible for the onset of symptoms of Parkinson's disease in young drug addicts in California USA who had taken synthetic heroin which contained MPTP. Dr Jeffrey Bland and Sarah Benum in their book Genetic Nutritioneering (Keats Publishing), have described how, although genetic inheritance does play a part in defining risks to most age related diseases, the way that people relate to their genes through diet and lifestyle may be vital to genetic expression.

How Dopamine is Metabolised from Dietary Protein

Figure 1

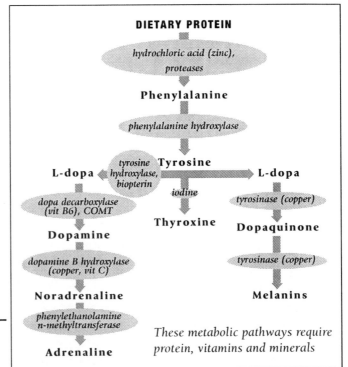

DIETARY PROTEIN

hydrochloric acid (zinc), proteases

Phenylalanine

phenylalanine hydroxylase

Tyrosine

L-dopa ← *tyrosine hydroxylase, biopterin* → **L-dopa**

iodine

dopa decarboxylase (vit B6), COMT   *tyrosinase (copper)*

Dopamine   **Thyroxine**   **Dopaquinone**

dopamine B hydroxylase (copper, vit C)   *tyrosinase (copper)*

Noradrenaline   **Melanins**

phenylethanolamine n-methyltransferase

Adrenaline

These metabolic pathways require protein, vitamins and minerals

ENERGY PRODUCTION

Energy is produced in the mitochondria (the "powerhouse") in body cells during a process called the Citric Acid Cycle[8, 9] or the Krebs Cycle. (See Figures 2 & 3) This energy is adenosine triphosphate (ATP). ATP is produced by cells' use of glucose, which can be metabolised from carbohydrates, proteins and fats together with specific nutrients including vitamins B2, B3, NADH, vitamin C, CoQ10, iron, copper, magnesium, manganese and biotin. The cycle requires oxygen. Mitochondrial energy is used for all physiological functions.

People with Parkinson's disease often have compromised energy. The process known as Complex I is impaired[10a,10b]. Some drugs also undermine certain processes of the Krebs Cycle[11, 12, 13].

Recommendations

Nutritional biochemical tests are useful in assessing whether mitochondrial support of energy production is necessary. Nutrients necessary in the manufacture of cellular energy (ATP) may be deficient and supplements needed to address specific deficiencies. If absorption is a problem, nutritional supplements are ideally taken as "sublinguals" These are vitamins and minerals which are manufactured in a specialised form and are held under the tongue where they are absorbed through the oral mucosa and bypass a compromised intestinal tract. Nutrients can also be given intravenously and the author's clinical observation is that people benefit most from this form of supplementation.

Figure 2. **Summary of ATP (Energy) Production**

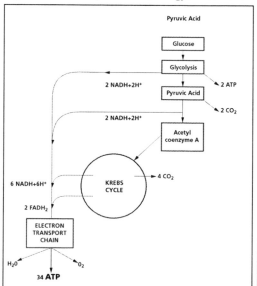

Figure 3. **Cell with Mitochondria**

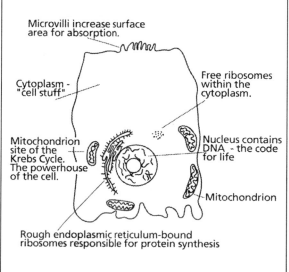

FREE RADICALS AND THEIR CONTROL

Free radicals are a reactive oxygen species necessary in normal metabolism. Over and above the natural formation of free radicals in the body for immune and physiological purposes, free radicals are generated by exposure to radiation both natural (for example the sun) and medical (for example x-rays). They are also generated by exposure to environmental pollution such as petrol and gas fumes, wood preservatives, fragrant sprays, organophosphates and organochlorine compounds found in pesticides. Drugs (medical and street) and surgery generate free radicals. They are also generated by trauma, both emotional and physical, as well as by heating polyunsaturated oil and margarine during cooking.

Antioxidants are specific vitamins and minerals. There are also antioxidant enzymes including superoxide dismutase (SOD) - two forms, of which one contains zinc and copper and the other manganese. Other anti-oxidant enzymes are glutathione peroxidase, which is dependent on selenium and catalase. During the normal course of events, when they have performed their physiological tasks, free radicals are quenched by antioxidants in the body. However, when an excess of free radicals is generated during oxidative stress including those instances mentioned above, antioxidants become depleted. This results in an ongoing cascade of free radicals which then causes damage to cells.

We now know that free radical damage plays a role in the development of degenerative diseases including Parkinson's disease[14] and cardiovascular disease.

On a scientific note, a free radical has become unstable by having an unpaired electron in its outer shell. It seeks stability by stealing an electron from elsewhere thus creating another free oxidising molecule. A chain of destruction ensues. DNA molecules and cell membranes, containing many double bonds, are targeted.

Recommendations

It is essential to ensure adequate antioxidant support which includes the nutrients alpha lipoic acid, vitamin A, the caroteens, vitamins C[15] and E, selenium, N-acetyl-cysteine and other specialised nutrients. Glutathione can also be administered intravenously (see the section "Intravenous Nutritional Support" in this chapter). As cell membranes are affected by oxidation, in order to enhance cell membrane stability, essential fatty acids (Omega 6 and Omega 3) should also be supplemented. Omega 6 is found in primrose and borage oils and Omega 3 in fish oil. Biochemical testing provides information about cellular nutritional status in order to prescribe supplementary antioxidant nutrients.

- It is important to reduce exposure to oxidative stress as much as possible.

- It is better to cook with a limited amount of cold pressed olive oil or a little butter (if cardiovascular health permits) or water. Food can be steamed, roasted or sautéed on a low heat.

- Organophosphates and organochlorines are sprayed on fruit and vegetables so that the choice of organic fresh foods is preferable. If these are not available, peeling fruit and vegetables is necessary.

- If patients are undergoing surgery and X-rays it may be prudent to have extra antioxidant support. Antioxidants may include vitamins A, C, E, lipoic acid and selenium. Around surgery, vitamins E and C should be limited as these may thin the blood too much.

- Medical drugs such as L-dopa[16] and "Viagra"[17] have been shown to generate free radicals. N-acetyl-cysteine, a powerful antioxidant, has been shown to reduce the formation of the free radical nitric oxide. Extra anti-oxidant protection might well be prudent when using these drugs.

REMOVAL OF DENTAL MERCURY FILLINGS AND CHELATION

Research shows that mercury exposure may play a role in Parkinson's disease[18, 19, 20, 21]. (For details, see the chapter "Mercury in Dentistry", by Dr Jack Levenson.)

Recommendations
- Patients with Parkinson's disease are advised to ask for mercury-free fillings.

- Only if it is medically necessary to consider removal of old mercury fillings, should Parkinson's disease patients do this. With their compromised ability to detoxify, they should not have all of them removed in one session.

- It is essential that removal of amalgam fillings should be accompanied by chelation therapy. The chelating agent binds the mercury and it is then able to be excreted. Nutrients used for chelation include vitamin C and selenium amongst others. Chelation therapy should always be supervised by a specialist healthcare professional.

Protocols for chelation are presented by Dr Jack Levenson in his book "Menace in the Mouth?" (Brompton Health, London, UK) and general advice about mercury free dentistry can be obtained British Society for Mercury Free Dentistry[22].

L-DOPA (LEVODOPA) - "SINEMET", "MADOPAR" OR EQUIVALENT WITH PROTEIN

In clinical practice we often find that patients on L-dopa medication have increased movement disturbance after eating. This is because they have unwittingly eaten concentrated proteins too close to the time of taking L-dopa, which compete with L-dopa medication for absorption. For this reason, the effect of the L-dopa medication ("Sinemet", "Madopar" or equivalent) is undermined.

These are Commonly Eaten Protein-rich Foods

- Meat, Poultry, Fish, Eggs (good sources of whole protein)
- All dairy products including Milk, Cheese, Yoghurt but not Butter
- Soy and Pulses (soy is a good source of whole protein)
- Wheat which includes Couscous and Bulgar
- Rye, Oats, Barley, Spelt, Sago
- Coconut
- Nuts, Seeds
- Avocado, Asparagus

There is competition for the absorption sites in the proximal small bowel, as well as competition for active transport across the blood brain barrier between most of the neutral amino acids and the drugs containing L-dopa[23]. The neutral amino acids (constituents of dietary protein) are tyrosine, phenylalanine, valine, leucine, isoleucine, tryptophane, methionine and histadine.

Recommendations

The timing of taking L-dopa medication in relation to eating protein-rich foods can be of help in controlling reactive symptoms. *However it is vital to eat good sources of protein at least once a day as protein is essential for anabolic function and provides "building blocks" for the body.*

Scheme

- Take L-dopa medication

- Then wait **ONE HOUR** before eating any of the above protein rich foods

- Thereafter wait **TWO HOURS**, if possible, before taking L-dopa medication again

---

IMORTANT NOTE: Some patients are unable to wait for 2 hours after eating protein before needing their L-dopa again and as a result are experiencing exacerbated movement disturbance. They can be helped by replacing protein-rich food with predigested amino-acid drinks or complete elemental feeds which are predigested, such as Peptamen (Nestlé Clinical Nutrition). Predigested amino acid and peptide based drinks and supplements are rapidly absorbed and are helpful when wishing to avoid competition with L-dopa medication within 2 hours of taking protein.

L-DOPA (LEVODOPA) "SINEMET", "MADOPAR" OR EQUIVALENT WITH CARBOHYDRATES AND FATS

If, after taking L-dopa ("Sinemet" or "Madopar"), people would like to eat food which is not protein-rich, this is the recommendation:

Scheme

- Take L-dopa

- Wait approximately 45 minutes (or until the drug has "kicked in"). Then eat food containing predominately carbohydrates and/or fats.

- Patients do not have to wait 2 hours as they might do after eating concentrated protein* before taking L-dopa again. This is because carbohydrates and fats will not compete with this medication. Experience will show how long it is necessary to wait, as each individual can differ in rate of digestion, gastric emptying and absoprtion.

*meat, poultry, fish, eggs, dairy, soy, wheat which includes couscous and bulgar, rye, oats, barley, spelt, sago, coconut, nuts, seeds, avocado, asparagus and pulses

---

Polyunsaturated oils such as flaxseed oil, pumpkin seed oil, unrefined sunflower seed and corn oils can be used cold as food dressings. All oils should be kept refrigerated. Polyunsaturated oils, margarine and hydrogenated fats should never be heated (unhealthy trans-fats and free radicals are generated).

Caution

Protein-rich foods should be eaten at least once a day with the timing of taking L-dopa calculated according to the recommended scheme (**see the part "L-dopa (Levodopa) - 'Sinemet', 'Madopar' or equivalent with Protein" in this chapter**). Protein is needed for anabolic function and provides the "building blocks" of the body. Dopamine is metabolised from dietary protein.

The list of foods compatible with L-dopa are overpage.

Popular Foods which are not Protein-rich
(more compatible with L-dopa)

Grains

Corn, rice, millet, buckwheat
Rice crackers
Gluten free breads: "EnerG" Rice or
Tapioca Bread (toasted), Corn breads

Grains may be taken as cereals,
used in confectionery and in
general cooking as well
as in bread

Comment
Gluten, a constituent of some grains (wheat, rye, oats, barley, spelt) has a high
protein content but the above grains are gluten-free

Vegetables

Potatoes *(sweet and other types)*	Cauliflower	Aubergines
Plantains	Cabbage	Courgettes
Pumpkins	Brussels Sprouts	Tomatoes
Squash	Dark green leafy vegetables	Celery
Carrots		Onions
		Leeks

Fruit

All fruit may be enjoyed. However, grapefruit should be avoided as it contains
naringenin, which slows the Phase1 liver detoxification pathway. Biochemical
testing will demonstrate whether grapefruit is an individual problem or not (see
the section "Biochemical Tests" in this chapter).

Dairy Substitute

Rice milk ("Rice Dream")

Comment
Dairy milk has a high protein content

Fats

Butter may be used sparingly. It is saturated fat and does not contain the
competing amino acids which are in milk. It may be used for cooking or
spreading.

Cold pressed olive oil, a mono-unsaturated oil, may be used for cooking
and dressings.

L-DOPA (LEVODOPA) "MADOPAR" AND "SINEMET" WITH VITAMIN B6

With the original version of the drug L-dopa, the co-enzyme vitamin B6 caused L-dopa's conversion to dopamine before it crossed the blood brain barrier. This was not effective.

Recommendations

Modern L-dopa drugs contain a decarboxylase inhibitor which inhibits premature decarboxylation of L-dopa before it crosses the blood brain barrier. In Sinemet this substance is carbidopa and in Madopar it is benserazide. As such, Vitamin B6 can be used together with "Sinemet"[24] and "Madopar"[25]. It is biochemically essential to the metabolic step between L-dopa and dopamine[26, 27] and if found to be deficient, should therefore be supplemented.

MONOAMINE OXIDASE INHIBITORS AND TYRAMINE-RICH FOODS[28]

Patients who are taking drugs containing monoamine oxidase (MAO) inhibitors run the risk of hypertension (high blood pressure) if eating tyramine rich foods in conjunction with them.

Recommendation

Selegiline is also used for Parkinson's disease. In higher doses (over 30 milligrams) the selectivity of Selegilene diminishes resulting in increased inhibition of MAO-A. There is, however, variability in patient reaction according to individual metabolic rate. Usually Parkinson's disease patients are on a daily dose closer to 10 milligrams and at this level, tyramine is not a problem. With all other drugs, however, drug-nutrient interactions should be monitored.

Foods Rich in Tyramine include

| cheddar, brie and other strong cheese | ripe avocado overripe bananas overripe or canned figs broad beans miso soup soy sauce | old liver pate fish (pickled, salted, smoked) caviar pepperoni salami summer-sausage meat concentrate in gravy or soup | yeast extract (marmite etc.) brewer's and other yeast-supplements | Chianti Vermouth and Drambuie | chocolate - (large quantities) caffeine - (large quantities) |

WHEN TO TAKE DRUGS - WITH OR WITHOUT FOOD?

All drugs used in treatment for Parkinson's disease need to be taken at optimum times in relation to food in order to be most efficacious. For drugs other than those listed below, it is recommended to consult the technical advisors of the drug manufacturers concerned in order to obtain information about drug-nutrient interactions and optimal times of taking drugs in relation to food and other drugs.

Cabergoline ("Cabaser")
Take as a single dose daily, with food[29]. If patients are nauseous it might be better to take the medication at the end of the meal (**see the chapter "Pharmaceutical Treatment" by Professor Aroldo Rossi**).

Pergolide Mesylate ("Celance")
The manufacturers do not give any guide as to whether this should be taken with or without food. However, it is recommend that agonists be taken after meals if patients tend to be nauseous.

Ropinerole Hydrochloride ("Requip")
Take three times daily with meals[30]. If patients are nauseous it might be better to take the medication at the end of the meal.

The manufacturers state, that as with other centrally active medication, patients should be cautioned against taking Ropinerole with alcohol[31].

Selegiline Hydrochloride ("Eldepryl", "Zelepar")
Take at breakfast in single dose or in two divided doses at breakfast and lunch[32]. It can also be taken together with L-dopa.

Entacapone ("Comtess")
Take together with L-dopa ("Sinemet", "Madopar" or equivalent). If supplementing iron, wait two or three hours before taking the drug as it forms chelates with iron, impairing its absorption[33].

ANTIBIOTICS AND GUT FLORA

Antibiotics are necessary for the elimination of certain pathogens. A side effect of their use, however, is the destruction of the friendly intestinal bacteria necessary for immunity in the gut.

Recommendations
A course of probiotics[34] needs to be supplemented if patients have taken antibiotics. "Friendly" cultures of intestinal bacteria which enhance gut immunity include bifidobacterium bifidum, lactobacillus acidophilus and lactobacillus bulgaricus.

DETOXIFICATION AND PARKINSON'S DISEASE

Parkinson's disease patients have been found to have compromised liver detoxification[35, 36, 37].

Recommendations
Patients and relatives can have biochemical tests to evaluate liver detoxification potential. If the results indicate, appropriate nutritional management may be instituted (see the section "Liver Detoxification and Optimal Liver Function - A Nutritional Approach" by Helen Kimber in this chapter). The effects of therapeutic and anaesthetic drugs should be noted by healthcare professionals.

As environmental factors may influence genetic expression, it would be prudent for people with Parkinson's disease and their blood relatives to reduce unnecessary exposure to chemical and other pollutants including organophosphates and organochlorines. Junk foods with harmful chemical colourings and additives as well as alcohol should be avoided or at least reduced to lessen the load on the liver. Mineral or purified water is preferable to tap water.

FOOD INTOLERANCE AND SYMPTOMS

It is important to identify any food allergy / intolerance as it has been clinically observed that eating problem foods may exacerbate symptoms.

Recommendations

- Biochemical tests - IgE identifies food allergy and IgG4 identifies food intolerance.

- Elimination or rotation of offending foods with delicious and nutritious substitutes.

- Digestive enzyme function should be assessed as incompletely digested food molecules, particularly protein molecules, may cause immune reactions. Patients may need to take digestive enzymes[38] for a limited period.

- Assessment of gut permeability: hyperpermeability of the intestinal mucosa ("leaky gut")[39] may also contribute to immune reactions. This is because the damaged intestinal lining allows incompletely digested larger food molecules to enter the blood stream. It may be necessary for patients to take nutrients, which stimulate repair of the gut mucosa. These include butyric acid, vitamin A, n-acetyl glucosamine and magnesium. The herb slippery elm[40] may be helpful and is also anti-inflammatory. Its use should be closely monitored in case it impedes the absorption of drugs.

- Clinical observation using a daily diary to identify possible reactions to food (see the chapter "The Patient's Diary").

Note

Common food intolerances noted in clinical practice are the gluten-containing grains wheat, rye, oats, barley and spelt as well as dairy foods (with the exception of butter).

MONOSODIUM GLUTAMATE (MSG), ASPARTAME AND FOOD ADDITIVES

Food with added glutamate such as in monosodium glutamate (MSG) and the sweetener aspartame[41], are best avoided. These are excito-toxins, which are contra-indicated in people with Parkinson's disease. Research has demonstrated in animals that MSG is implicated in the death of neurones[42].

Recommendations

- MSG is added to enhance the flavour of the food. Replacing MSG with fresh herbs produces a delicious result and can sometimes stimulate appetite. Peppers also improve flavour.

- Aspartame is used to sweeten food. A little honey, molasses or fructose can be used instead for sweetening. Fruit juice can also be used as a sweetener.

- Food containing artificial colours and non-essential preservatives should be avoided where possible, and substituted with healthier options.

BLOOD SUGAR LEVELS INFLUENCING ENERGY, MOOD AND NEURONES

The concentration of glucose in the plasma is dependent on nutritional and hormonal aspects which are carefully regulated by the body. Appropriate nutritional management helps in the control of blood sugar levels, in turn influencing energy production and mood. Patients with Parkinson's disease are often lacking in energy. Stress can also be a problem - it causes the hormone adrenaline (which is metabolised from dopamine) to be released. The concentration of blood glucose then increases, making for subsequent fluctuation in blood sugar levels.

It has been demonstrated that low blood sugar (hypoglycaemia) affects brain energy and can damage neurones[43, 44]. When blood sugar falls too low, for example, due to an inappropriate or irregular diet, mood swings and anxiety can often ensue. Insulin is complexed with zinc[45]. Chromium and vitamin B3 are implicated in glucose tolerance factor (GTF). Insulin and GTF are involved in blood sugar regulation.

Energy in body cells is produced by glucose metabolised primarily from carbohydrates such as grains, vegetables and fruit. If needed, glucose can also be metabolised from fat and protein. Specific vitamins and minerals, together with glucose, are co-factors in the production of energy in cells. These include B vitamins, NADH, Co-enzyme Q10, vitamin C, iron, copper, magnesium, manganese, and biotin.

Recommendations

It is essential for diabetics to have dietary supervision by their own personal physician, with attendant nutritionist or dietician. Otherwise general guidelines are as follows:

- Eat regular small snacks, every two hours, or between main meals. These snacks should contain small portions of complex carbohydrates (whole grains/apple) with a little raw salad.

- Avoid sweets and sugary foods, refined carbohydrates, alcohol and caffeine. Substitute these with whole grains, herb drinks and other natural foods.

- Fruit juices should be well diluted with still mineral water. Herb teas may be used.

- Oils, such as cold pressed olive oil or unrefined, unheated polyunsaturated oils may slightly slow down glucose release.

- Almonds and other nuts (not peanuts or cashews which may contain mycotoxins), together with fruit, are a good combination. Users of L-dopa need to be aware of the protein - L-dopa interaction and can only use this combination during a "protein window".

- If indicated medically, glucomannan fibre[46] can be taken as a supplement. This is a complex carbohydrate fibre, which is effective in stabilising blood sugar levels. However, the effects of this fibre on L-dopa ("Sinemet", "Madopar" or equivalent drug) should be assessed individually as the protein portion, although small, may compete at the absorption sites with L-dopa and undermine its effects.

- Nutritional biochemical testing assesses the status of vitamins and minerals involved in the regulation of blood sugar.

- Deficiencies need supplementing.

- Regular glucose monitoring, if indicated, may be necessary.

WEIGHT CONTROL[47]

It is important to monitor weight in patients.

Underweight or Weight Loss

There could be many reasons for this:

1. Insufficient daily intake of food.

2. Chewing and swallowing may be a problem.

3. Difficulty in controlling cutlery, crockery and cooking equipment.

4. Inability to buy, prepare, cook and store food hygienically.

5. Patients removing offending foods from their normal diet and not replacing these with other nutritious substances. This is a very common cause of weight loss in Parkinson's disease patients who embark upon a new diet without professional supervision.

6. Parasites or infection.

7. Loss of appetite.

8. Malabsorption and chronic diarrhoea.

9. "Leaky gut" (increased permeability of the intestinal mucosa).

10. Inadequate digestive enzyme function.

Recommendations for Underweight

■ Foods removed from the diet must be replaced with others of equivalent or better nutritional value.

■ Tests for parasites could be indicated.

■ Test permeability of the gut mucosa. If indicated, nutrients for the healing of the gut wall should be supplemented including butyric acid. Glutamine, although effective, is contra-indicated in Parkinson's disease because, in higher doses, it can function as an excito-toxin.

■ Occupational therapists may need to help patients find specialised utensils with which to eat and prepare food.

■ Health professionals should check that patients can buy, prepare and store food, hygienically. If there is a problem, the GP should be contacted with a view to organising home help.

■ It is essential for adults to have minimally 1,500 calories daily to sustain health. However, it is the quality of the food that is most important. If a patient is unable to achieve an adequate calorific intake due to inability to chew, nutritious foods can be liquidised. These can be supplemented with pre-digested elemental feeds such as Peptamen (Nestlé Clinical Nutrition). If swallowing is a problem, the nutritionist must advise the GP and discuss the possibility of naso-gastric or duodenal tube feeding. This is absolutely essential for the effective nutritional management of patients who have problems with swallowing.

■ In recommending a diet, it is helpful to assess the digestive enzyme potential in patients. This is possible non-invasively by stool examination[48] or by gastrogram (see section on Biochemical Tests). If there is a deficiency of hydrochloric acid or reduced pancreatic exocrine function, supplements of digestive enzymes may be necessary until the condition is corrected.

Overweight

Overweight does not seem to be a general problem in patients with Parkinson's disease. However, the following aspects, amongst others, can be considered if this is the case.

1. General medical differential diagnosis

2. Insufficient Exercise

3. Inappropriate Diet

4. Food Intolerance / Allergy

5. Fluid Retention

6. Sluggish Metabolism. Thyroid function may be implicated

Recommendations for Overweight

■ If exercise is a problem, the patient's doctor would be able to arrange a referral to a physiotherapist or remedial exercise therapist.

■ The diet should be checked for appropriate food and calorie content.

■ There may be different medical reasons for fluid retention. Food intolerance should also be considered. Biochemical tests IgG4 are useful. Allergy is identified by IgE.

■ Glucose handling should be checked.

■ Thyroid function should be checked. Tyrosine is the precursor of L-dopa, as well as of thyroxine. If deficient, inadequate thyroid metabolism might be considered.

PARASITES

Some patients suffer from chronic low weight and lack of energy. Although constipation is the more common problem, there are also patients who suffer from chronic or intermittent diarrhoea. They may have contracted intestinal parasites from contaminated foods or drinking water, both at home and abroad.

Recommendations

■ Stool samples for parasite detection (at least three samples).

■ Blood tests for parasites.

■ A breath test is also available, as well as blood and stool, for helicobacter.

■ Dark-field microscope assessment of blood.

■ Chemical or herbal therapy as medically indicated.

■ Food hygiene in the home should be checked. Washing of hands may also be difficult without help and pose a threat to hygiene.

■ Chilling or "holding temperatures" for heated foods, which may be left out to eat at a later time, should also be checked.

CONSTIPATION

Constipation is a problem for many patients who have Parkinson's disease. This can impair the optimum absorption of drugs and nutrients. The stress associated with this problem can exacerbate the symptoms of Parkinson's disease and affect wellbeing. Nutritional management is essential and helpful in regulating bowel function.

In acute cases, medical supervision may be necessary in the recommendation of an occasional enema or colonic. It is vital, however, for patients and carers to recognise when there is bowel obstruction (pain, abdominal distention, no bowel sounds) as this needs immediate medical intervention.

Otherwise, the following recommendations can often be helpful:

Recommendations

1. 10 glasses of still mineral water, at room temperature, should be drunk throughout the day.

2. Capsules of psyllium husks, always under professional healthcare supervision, should be taken between meals with at least two glasses of still mineral water. Start with two psyllium husks with two glasses of water on each ocassion, mid-morning and mid-afternoon. Increase the number of psyllium husks to the ideal amount as needed, no more than five per session and never have less than two glasses of water with the capsules.

3. Aloe Vera juice, as directed by a healthcare professional, can sometimes be helpful.

4. 6 to 8 prunes / apricots once or twice daily, seem to have the best laxative effect. Other helpful fruits with a slight laxative effect are strawberries / watermelon[49]. Fruit is best eaten or between meals to reduce bloating / flatulence.

5. Insoluble fibre: At each meal there should be sufficient complex carbohydrates containing insoluble fibre. Wholegrains such as brown rice with its bran is suitable in Parkinson's disease as it is gluten free. As such it does not have a high protein content, which is suitable, if L-dopa medication is needed. Raw salads, (finely processed or liquidised, if necessary) are helpful, especially when accompanying starchy meals. Laxative reactions appear to pre-dominate with insoluble fibre. For example rice bran has a greater laxative effect than guar[50].

6. Cabbage, celery, lettuce, carrots, radishes are beneficial as these readily absorb moisture[51].

7. Regular exercise and abdominal massage.

8. Osteopathic or chiropractic asssessment and gentle manipulation may sometimes be indicated.

9. Patients should sit regularly on the toilet, 10 to 20 minutes after each meal, even if there is no urge to defecate. They should sit and relax for at least 10 minutes without straining or pushing. It is hoped that eventually a rhythm for bowel emptying will establish itself[52].

10. Patients should not delay going to the toilet at any time when they do feel the urge to defecate.

Note
Blood or mucus accompanying bowel movement should be reported immediately to the medical practitioner.

FOOD SOURCE OF L-DOPA

Some foods, including the pods of broad beans (vicia faba[53]), do contain reasonable levels of L-dopa but the L-dopa content is variable. The author is not aware of any "standardised" formulations although these may well exist. Patients using food sources of L-dopa should do so under supervision as self-treatment can lead to problems of overdose. Broad beans may interact with monoamine oxidase inhibitors and are then contraindicated[54].

Serotonin, Dopamine and Acetylcholine

The correct balance between these neuro-transmitters is essential, otherwise their interaction could cause over or under-stimulation of neurons which may result in impaired motor control[54a]. They are normally metabolised from dietary sources. Serotonin is derived from tryptophane, for example in milk and pumpkin. Dopamine is derived from dietary protein containing the amino acids phenylalanine and tyrosine. Acetylcholine is derived from choline, for example in fish and soy lecithin.

The precursors of serotonin, dopamine and acetylcholine are available as nutritional supplements, but must only be taken when indicated and under strict professional supervision. In Parkinson's Disease, however, not all people are able to metabolise these.

EXAMPLE OF A DAY'S DIET FOR PATIENTS TAKING L-DOPA ("SINEMET", "MADOPAR" OR EQUIVALENT)

Before Breakfast

L-Dopa: wait 45 minutes to an hour before a carbohydrate breakfast.

Prunes: eat 6 to 8 prunes which have been simmered in a little still mineral or purified water, for a few minutes. Ideally wait 15 minutes before continuing with breakfast.

Breakfast

Should be gluten and dairy free (gluten and dairy products are highly proteinous). Ideally avoid or reduce caffeine (tea, coffee) as well as refined white sugars and artificial sweeteners.

Gluten foods to avoid	Substitute with
Wheat	Rice
Rye	Corn
Oats	Buckwheat
Barley	Millet
Spelt	
Dairy foods to avoid	**Substitute with**
Animal milk	Rice milk
Cheese	Home made vegetable spreads without yeast.
Yoghurt	Butter and single cream may be used sparingly.
Refined Sugars and artificial sweeteners to avoid	**Substitute with**
White table sugar	Manuka and organic Honey
Refined sugars	Fructose
Icing sugar	Fruit juices
Aspartame	Molasses
	Fruit spreads and jams
	Sweetened naturally
	Sugar cane
Caffeine drinks to avoid / reduce	**Substitutes for caffeine**
Tea	Herb teas
Coffee	Chicory
Chocolate	Carob

An Example of a Good Breakfast (compatible with L-dopa)

Fruit

Cornflakes (without added wheat) and "Rice Dream" rice milk

EnerG toast, butter and jam

Herb tea (peppermint, camomile, lemon verbena)

An Example of a Good Lunch (compatible with L-dopa)

- Fruit salad (no grapefruit)

  Jacket potato (sweet or ordinary type) with butter

  Vegetable sauce made from cold pressed olive oil, onions, tomatoes, sweet peppers, aubergine and courgettes, tomato passata or

  Heinz Tomato Ketchup.

  Salad including cabbage, carrot, lettuce, tomato, celery

  Salad dressing made with cold pressed olive oil, tomato juice, pepper and garlic

Or

- Fruit salad (no grapefruit)

  Vegetable soup including: sweet potato, broccoli, cauliflower, cabbage, leeks, turnip, swede, parsnips, plantains (boil gently in a little purified or still mineral water).

  Rice, corn or buckwheat pasta with tomato-vegetable sauce

  Salad with dressing

An Example of a Good Dinner including Complete Protein (not compatible with L-dopa)

Note about Drugs

- It is essential that this meal should be consumed at least one hour after your last L-dopa dose (tablet or dispersible which is absorbed more quickly than the tablet)

- L-dopa medication may be resumed 2 hours after the meal, if needed. However, if L-dopa medication is required before 2 hours, you may need to substitute protein with pre-digested amino acid drinks. Experience will be your teacher. For details see "L-dopa (Levodopa) - "Sinemet", "Madopar" or equivalent with Protein" in this section of the book.

Prunes: fifteen minutes before dinner 6-8 prunes should be taken if constipated

(Dinner continued overpage)

- Fish or chicken soup
  Fish or chicken or turkey or tofu (soy) or egg
  Dark green leafy vegetables (steamed)
  Yellow vegetables (pumpkin, squash, sweet potato, carrot, plantain)
  Salad
  Coconut pudding (coconut milk blended with bananas and pears)
  Readymade desserts can be eaten but the ingredients should not include carageenen (it can cause inflammation) or artificial sweeteners such as Aspartame, and the flavour enhancer MSG.

Note

At the evening meal avoid rice, pasta and ordinary potatoes if badly constipated. Eat extra yellow vegetables such as pumpkin and squash as substitutes.

During the "protein window", if patients are allergic to or intolerant of animal milk, soy, coconut, nut and seed milks can be substituted (blend almonds / sesame seeds with still mineral water in a liquidiser).

Optional Drinks at any Time
Still mineral water
Fruit juice diluted 50% with still water
Herbal drinks such as "Aqualibra" and "Ame" are excellent substitutes for alcohol, served chilled in wine glasses

Mid-Meal Snacks to Maintain Energy
Choices include
Brown rice cracker with salad and herb tea
Vegetable soup including sweet potato
1/2 a glass of Ultrafuel (Twinlab) diluted with 1/2 a glass of still mineral water

Bowel Function
The importance of regular fluid intake throughout the day cannot be stressed enough - minimally 10 cups. To assist with bowel function, take two cups of liquid with each meal and at least one in-between. High fibre fruits may be helpful such as figs and prunes, cabbage and celery.

DIETARY CONSIDERATIONS FOR THOSE WHO DO NOT TAKE L-DOPA

Food intolerances need to be identified biochemically or by clinical observation. The most common noted in clinical practice seem to be the gluten containing grains wheat, rye, oats, barley and dairy products (except for butter and cream).

It is important to have a well balanced diet throughout the day with choices, such as:

- deep-sea fish.

- chicken (white part).

- turkey.

- vegetables (including sweet potatoes, plantains, green leafy vegetables, courgettes, cabbage, celery, aubergine).

- fruit - 5 items including fruit and vegetables should be eaten daily - excluding grapefruit, if contra indicated (see section on Biochemical Tests).

- whole grains such as brown rice.

- plenty of fluids including herb teas, herbal drinks, chicory drinks and still mineral water. Fruit juices should be diluted with still mineral water and herb teas and soft drinks are preferable to tea and coffee, which contain caffeine.

- Cold pressed olive oil and limited butter should be used for cooking (no hydrogenated fats or oils or heated polyunsaturated oils such as sunflower and corn oils.) Unrefined polyunsaturated oils such as sunflower, corn and pumpkin seed oils can be used cold for food dressings.

- Food can be steamed or roasted on a low temperature. Use the water from boiling or steaming food for stock.

Notes

1. All oils, once opened, should be kept in the fridge. Olive oil will solidify. It needs to be removed from the fridge in time to become liquid again prior to use. Otherwise food can be steamed or roasted on a low temperature.

2. Organic food is preferable, if available. Non organic fruit and vegetables should be peeled. It has been demonstrated that Parkinson's disease patients have compromised detoxification[55, 56] processes. Alcohol could present problems.

3. Prunes are helpful if constipation is a problem as well as at least 10 glasses of still mineral or purified water, drunk daily.

References

1. *Biochemical Assessment of Nutritional Status of Zinc, Magnesium, Chromium, Copper, Manganese, Vitamins B1, B2, Niacin, Vitamin B6, Biotin, Essential Fatty Acids (Omega 6 and Omega 3) in patients with Parkinson's Disease*, Dr Geoffrey Leader MB ChB FRCA and Lucille Leader Dip ION, The London Pain Relief and Nutritional Support Clinic, London, UK: 2001: Tests performed at Biolab Medical Unit, London, UK.

1a. Diet and Parkinson's Disease I: *A Possible Role for the Past Intake of Specific Foods and Food Groups*: 1996: W Hellenbrand: A Seidler: H Boeing: B P Robra, P Vieregge, P Nischan, W H Oertel, E Schneider, G Ulm: Neurology 47: pps. 636 - 643:

2. *Parkinson's Disease and Brain Levels of Organocholorine Pesticides*: Ann Neural 36: pps. 100 - 103: 1994: L Flemming, JB Mann, J Bean, et al

3. *Ecogenetics of Parkinson's Disease: Prevalence and Environmental Aspects in Rural Areas*: Can J Neurol Sci 14: pps. 36 - 40: 1987

4. *Environmental Antecedents of Young-onset Parkinson's Disease*: J Amer Acad Neurol 43: pps. 1150 - 1158: 1993

5. *Herbicide (1-methyl-4-phenyl-1,2.3.6-tetrahydropyrinine is Implicated in Both Stiffness and Weakness in Parkinson's disease*: pps. 189, 266 (ref. 649) Save the Children and Yourself - A Guide to a Future Healthier Generation by Avoiding Toxins in Today's Food and Water: Nikolaus J Smeh, MS: 1996: Alliance Publishing Company, Garrisonville, USA

6. *Water Contaminants (hexachlorobenzene) has been shown to have nervous system effects* pps. 212, 276 (Environmental Protection Agency, Office of Water: EPA Health Advisory for Hexachlorobenzene. EPA HA d-438)

7. *Herbicide - nervous system effects including tremor*, pps. 225, 277 (ref. 935 - Environmental Protection Agency, Office of Water: EPA Health Advisory for simazine (Herbicide). EPA HA d-250

8. Biochemistry: pps. 303-6: Victor L Davidson, Donald B Sittman: Lippincott: 1999: Williams and Wilkins, Baltimore, Maryland, USA

9. Optimum Nutrition Workbook: pps. 33-5: Patrick Holford BSc Dip ION: 1992: ION Press: London, UK

10a. *Carbidopa/levodopa and selegiline do not affect platelet mitochondrial function in early Parkinsonism* - Neurology 45 (2): pps 344-8: 1995

10b. *Mitochondrial respiratory chain function in multiple system atrophy*: M Gu, M T Gash, J M Cooper, G K Wenning, S E Daniel, N P Quinn, C D Marsden, A H Schapira: May 1997: Movement Disorders 12 (3): pps. 418 - 422

11. *Chronic levodopa administration alters cerebal mitochondrial respiratory chain activity*. Ann Neurol 34 (5): 715-23: S Predborski, V Jackson-Lewis, U Muthane: 1993

12. *Dose related decrease of serum co-enzyme Q10 during treatment with HMG-CoA reductase inhibitors* - Mol Aspects of Med 18 (Suppl) S137-44: S A Mortensen, A Leth, E Agner: 1997

13. *Absorption tolerability and effects on mitochondrial activity of oral coenzyme Q10 in Parkinsonian patients*, Neurology 50: 793-795: CW Schults, MF Beal, K Fontaine, et al: 1998

14. BrainRecovery.Com: pps. 24-28, 30: Dr David Perlmutter MD: 2000: Perlmutter Health Center, Naples, Fl, USA

15. *Impaired oxidation of pyruvate in human embryonic fibroblasts after exposure to L-dopa*: European Journal of Pharmacology 263 (1-2): pps. 157 - 62: 1994 September 22

16. op. cit. n. 15

17. BrainRecovery.Com: p. 26: Dr David Perlmutter MD: 2000: Perlmutter Health Center, Naples, Fl, USA

18. Perales Y Herrero: *Mercury: Chronic Poisoning*: Encyclopaedia of Occ. Health and Safety: 3rd Edition, Vol. 2: 1983: Ed L Parmeggiani: Int. Labour Office, Geneva: pps. 1334 - 1335

19. *Epidemiological Study on Association between Body Burden Mercury Level and Ideopathic Parkinson's Disease: CH* Ngim, G Pevathasan: Neuroepidemiology: 1989 8: pps. 128 - 141

20. *Parkinson's Disease Mortality and the Industrial use of Heavy Metals in Michigan: RA* Rybick, CC Johnson, J Oman, JM Gorell: Movement Disorder: 8(1): 1993: pps. 87 - 92

21. *Parkinson's Disease and Occupational Exposure to Organic Solvents, Agricultural Chemicals and Mercury - A Case Reference Study*: CG Ohlson, C Hogstead: J Scand: Work Environmental Health 7L: 1981: p. 252

22. *British Society for Mercury Free Dentistry*, 225 Old Brompton Road, London, SW5 0EA, UK (telephone: +44 (20) 7373 3655).

23. *Dietary factors in the management of Parkinson's Disease*: P A Kempster MD MRCP FRACP, M C Wahlqvist MD FRACP: Nutrition Reviews Vol 52, No. 2: 1994

24. *ABPI Compendium of Data Sheets and Summaries of Product Characteristics (1999-2000)*: p. 371: Datapharm Publications Limited, London, UK

25. *ABPI Compendium of Data Sheets and Summaries of Product Characteristics* (1999-2000): p. 1334: Datapharm Publications Limited, London, UK

26. *Parkinson's Disease - The New Nutritional Handbook*: p. 6: Dr Geoffrey Leader MB ChB FRCA and Lucille Leader Dip ION: 1996: Denor Press, London, UK

27. *Wills' Biochemical Basis of Medicine*: p. 417: J Hywel Thomas PhD FIBiol and B Gillham PhD: 1989: Butterworth Heinemann: Oxford, UK

28. *The People's Guide to Deadly Drug-Interactions*: 1995: Joe Graedon & Teresa Graedon: pps. 45 - 48 St Martin's Press, New York

29. *ABPI Compendium of Data Sheets and Summaries of Product Characteristics (1999-2000)*, p.1169: Datapharm Publications Limited, London, UK

30. *ABPI Compendium of Data Sheets and Summaries of Product Characteristics (1999-2000)*, p.1609: Datapharm Publications Limited, London, UK

31. *ABPI Compendium of Data Sheets and Summaries of Product Characteristics (1999-2000)*, p. 1610: Datapharm Publications Limited, London, UK

32. *ABPI Compendium of Data Sheets and Summaries of Product Characteristics (1999-2000)*, p. 1105: Datapharm Publications Limited, London, UK

33. *ABPI Compendium of Data Sheets and Summaries of Product Characteristics (1999-2000)*, p.1104: Datapharm Publications Limited, London, UK

34. *Probiotics*: pps. 24-25, : Leon Chaitow ND DO and Natasha Trenev: 1990: Thorsons An Imprint of HarperCollins Publishers, London, UK

35. *Abnormal Liver Enzyme-mediated Metabolism in Parkinson's Disease - A Second Look - Neurology* 41(5 suppl 2): pps. 89 - 91: Discussion p. 92: C M Tanner: May 1991

36. *Metabolic Biomarkers of Parkinson's Disease* - Actor Neurologica Scandinavica - Supplementum 136: pps. 19 - 23: A Williams, S Sturman, G Steventon, R Waring: 1991

37. *Liver Enzyme Abnormalities in Parkinson's Disease*: Geriatrics 46 Suppl 1: pps. 60 - 63: August 1991:

38. *The Complete book of Enzyme Therapy*: pps. 38-41: Dr Anthony J Cichoke MD: 1999: Avery Publishing Group, Garden City Park, NY, USA

39. *The Complete book of Enzyme Therapy*: pps. 288-290: Dr Anthony J Cichoke MD: 1999: Avery Publishing Group, Garden City Park, NY, USA

40. *Prescription for Nutritional Healing* (2nd edition): p. 77: James F Balch MD, Phyllis A Balch CNC: 1997: Avery Publishing Group, New York, USA

41. *Excito Toxins - The Taste that Kills*: pps. 39 - 43: Russell Blaylock MD: 1997: Health Press, Santa Fe, USA

42. *Glutamate Neuroxtoxicity / A three-stage process / Neurotoxicity of Excitatory Amino Acids*: D W Choi: 1990: FIDA Research Foundation, Symposium Series (Vol. 4): Raven Press, New York, USA

43. *Hypoglycaemia-Induced Neuronal Damage Prevented by N-methyl-D-aspartate Antagonist*: Sci. 230 (1985): pps. 681 - 683

44. Excitotoxins: pps. 139, 156 - 158: Russell L Blaylock MD: 1997: Health Press, Santa Fe, New Mexico, USA

45. Nutritional Biochemistry: Second Edition: p. 808: Tom Brody: 1999: Academic Press, New York, USA

46. Optimum Nutrition Workbook: p. 148: Patric Holford BSc Dip ION: 1992: ION Press, London, UK

47. *Weight Change and Body Composition in patients with Parkinson's Disease*: Journal of the American Dieteic Association 95(9): pps. 979 - 983: September 1995: P L Beyer, M Y Palarino: D Michalek, K Busenbark, W C Koller

48. Comprehensive Digestive Stool Analysis (CDSA), Great Smokies Laboratory, Great Smokies, US Gastrogram, Biolab Medical Unit, London, UK

49. New Facts About Fibre: p.15: Betty Kaman PhD: 1991: Nutrition Encounter Inc.: Novato, California, USA

50. Fibre and Bulk Preparations, Extract from Gastrointestinal Transit (Pathophyisology and Pharmacology): pps. 212 & 213: K W Heaton: 1991: Wrightson Biomedical Publishing Ltd, Petersfield, Hampshire, UK

51. New Facts About Fibre: pps.19 & 59: Betty Kaman PhD: 1991: Nutrition Encounter Inc.: Novato, California, USA

52. Better Health through Natural Healing: p. 191: Ross Trattler ND DO: 1987: Thorsons Publishers Limited: London, UK

53. *Motor Effects of Broad Beans (vicia faba) in Parkinson's Disease*: PA Kempster MD et al: 1993:Asia pacific Journal of Clinical Nutrition:2: pps 85-89

54. The People's Guide to Deadly Drug-Interactions: 1995: Joe Graedon & Teresa Graedon: p. 47: St Martin's Press, New York

54a. Parkinson's Disease: Balance of Transmitters: p.35: Dr Abraham Lieberman and Frank Williams: Thorsons, London, UK

55. op. cit. n. 35

56. op. cit. n. 36

Bibliography

Nutritional Biochemistry: Second Edition: Tom Brody: 1999: Academic Press, New York, USA

Biochemistry: Victor L Davidson, Donald B Sittman: Lippincott: 1999: Williams and Wilkins, Baltimore, Maryland, USA

Wills' Biochemical Basis of Medicine: J Hywel Thomas PhD and Brian Gillham PhD: 1989

Environmental Medicine in Clinical Practice:Honour Anthony, Sybil Birtwistle, Keith Eaton, Johnathan Maberley: 1997: BSAENM Publications, Southampton, UK

Complete Guide to Food Allergy and Intolerance: Dr Jonathan Brostoff and Linda Gamlin: 1998: Bloomsbury, London, UK

Excitotoxins: The Taste that Kills: Russell L Blaylock MD: 1997: Health Press, Santa Fe, New Mexico, USA

BrainRecovery.Com: Powerful Therapy for Challenging Brain Disorders: David Perlmutter MD: 2000: Perlmutter Health Center, Naples, Fl, USA

Fats that Heal, Fats that Kill: Udo Erasmus: 1993: Alive Books, Burnaby BC, Canada

Nutrition Nutrition Almanac 4th edition: Gayla J Kirschmann, John D Kirschmann: 1996: McGraw-Hill: New York, USA

Save the Children and Yourself - A Guide to a Future Healthier Generation by Avoiding Toxins in Today's Food and Water: Nikolaus J Smeh, MS: 1996: Alliance Publishing Company, Garrisonville, USA

Food for Life - Preventing Cancer through Healthy Diet: Oliver Gillie (World Cancer Research Fund): 1998: Hodder & Stoughton, London, UK

Menace in the Mouth? Your mercury fillings may be affecting your health: Dr Jack Levenson: 2000: Brompton Health, London, UK

The Food Doctor: Vicki Edgson & Ian Marber: 1999: Collins & Brown Limited, London, UK

CHAPTER 9.2

Nutrients in Food

by Lucille Leader Dip ION

Calories, Quantity and Quality of Food

An adult usually needs minimally 1,500 calories daily in order to sustain health. However, in this book the emphasis is on the frequency of ingesting quality foods, which include the macronutrients carbohydrates, fats and proteins together with vitamins, minerals and essential fatty acids.

It is to be hoped that this approach will automatically provide a balanced diet with adequate calories. However, should weight control remain a problem - either too much or too little weight - it would be advisable to check the calorie intake daily, the absorption potential, as well as the physical exercise pattern with the relevant specialist. Even if there is no weight problem, exercise is an essential dimension to maintaining a healthy metabolism. Advice should be sought as to which type of exercise is suitable for the individual.

Some Good Food Sources of Nutrients

Not all the foods are suitable for everyone, eg citrus, dairy or gluten grains might have to be excluded, if these are a problem. However, there are always choices available.

Carbohydrates
Whole grains
Honey
Fruit
Vegetables

Fats
Butter
Vegetable oils (cold pressed only)
Nuts and seeds

Protein
Fish and poultry
Soybean
Eggs
Whole grains and Pulses

Water
Mineral water
Purified water
Beverages
Fruits
Vegetables

Vitamin A and beta-carotene
Liver (provided organic)
Eggs
Yellow fruits and vegetables
Dark-green fruits and vegetables
Whole milk and milk products

Vitamin B1
Brewer's Yeast
Whole grains
Blackstrap molasses
Brown rice
Fish
Poultry
Egg yolks
Legumes
Nuts (not peanuts, cashews or brazils)

Vitamin B2
Brewer's yeast
Whole grains
Blackstrap molasses
Egg yolks
Legumes
Nuts

Vitamin B3 (Niacin)
Brewer's yeast
Poultry
Fish
Whole grains
Milk products
Rice Bran

Vitamin B5 (Pantothenic Acid)
Brewer's yeast
Egg yolks
Legumes
Whole grains
Salmon

Vitamin B6
Whole grains
Brewer's yeast
Blackstrap molasses
Legumes
Green leafy vegetables

Vitamin B12
Fish
Eggs
Cheese
Milk and Milk Products
Unprocessed spirulina
B12 supplements advised for vegetarians

Biotin
Egg yolks
Brewer's yeast
Whole grains
Sardines
Legumes
Egg yolks
Soy Beans
Fish
Legumes

Folic Acid
Dark green leafy vegetables
Brewer's yeast
Root vegetables
Whole grains
Oysters, Salmon, Milk

Inositol
Whole grains
Citrus fruits
Brewer's yeast
Molasses
Milk
Nuts (no peanuts, cashews and brazils)
Vegetables

Para-Aminobenzoic Acid (PABA)
Yoghurt
Molasses
Green leafy vegetables

Pantothenic Acid
Brewer's yeast
Egg yolks
Legumes
Whole grains
Salmon

Vitamin C
Citrus fruits
Rose hips
Acerola cherries
Cantaloupe
Strawberries
Broccoli
Tomatoes
Green peppers

Vitamin D
Salmon
Sardines
Herring
Egg yolks
Vitamin E
Cold pressed oils
Eggs
Molasses
Sweet potatoes, leafy vegetables

Vitamin K
Cauliflower
Green leafy vegetables
Egg yolks
Safflower oil
Blackstrap molasses
Cauliflower
Soy beans

Bioflavonoids
Citrus fruits
Fruits
Blackcurrants
Buckwheat

Unsaturated Fatty Acids
Sunflower oil
Corriander oil
(unrefined, unheated)

Monounsatured oil
Cold pressed olive oil

Calcium
Milk
Sesame seeds (Tahini) - extremely
high content comparable with milk
Green leafy vegetables
Shellfish
Molasses
Sesame seeds (Tahini) - extremely
high content comparable with milk
Seafood
Ripe olives

Choline
Fish
Soy lecithin

Chromium
Honey
Grapes
Raisins
Corn oil (cold pressed)
Clams
Whole grain cereals
Brewer's yeast

Cobalt
Oysters
Clams
Poultry
Milk
Green leafy vegetables
Fruits

Copper
Seafood
Nuts
Legumes
Molasses
Raisins

Cruciferous Vegetables
Broccoli
Cauliflower
Brussels sprouts
Cabbage

Fluoride
Iodine
Seafood
Kelp

Iodine
Kelp
Seafood

Iron
Eggs
Fish
Poultry
Blackstrap molasses
Cherry juice
Green leafy vegetables
Dried fruits
Liver (organic)

Magnesium
Seafood
Whole grains
Dark green vegetables
Molasses
Nuts and seeds

Manganese
Whole grains
Green leafy vegetables
Legumes
Nuts
Pineapples
Egg yolks

L-Methionine
Eggs
Poultry

Molybdenum
Legumes
Whole-grain cereals
Dark green vegetables

PABA
Molasses
Green leafy vegetables

Phosphorous
Fish
Poultry
Eggs
Legumes
Milk and Milk Products
Nuts
Whole grain cereals

Polyphenols
Yams
Onions
Tea (green)
Apples
Nuts

Potassium
Whole grains
Vegetables
Dried fruits
Bananas
Legumes
Sunflower seeds

Selenium
Tuna
Herring
Brewer's yeast
Whole grains
Sesame seeds

L-Tryptophane
Pumpkin
Kelp
Spirulina
Milk
Jacket Potato

Sodium
Seafood
Celery

Sulphur
Fish
Garlic
Onions
Eggs
Cabbage
Brussels Sprouts
Horseradish

L-Taurine
Eggs
Fish

Vanadium
Fish

Zinc
Pumpkin seeds
Sunflower seeds
Sesame seeds
Seafood
Oysters
Mushrooms
Brewer's yeast
Herring
Eggs

Bibliography:

Nutrition Almanac 4th edition:
Gayla J Kirschmann, John D Kirschmann:
1996: McGraw-Hill: New York, USA

Some Approximate Food Values of Popular Carbohydrates, Proteins & Fats

*by **Lucille Leader** Dip ION*

Carbohydrates

Brown Rice

Measure	1 cup
Weight	196 grams
Calories	704
Carbohydrate	152
Protein	14.8
Total Lipids	3.6

Rice Flour

Measure	1 cup
Weight	125 grams
Calories	479
Carbohydrate	107
Protein	7.5
Total Lipids	0.4

Millet Flour

Measure	1 cup
Weight	30 grams
Calories	100
Carbohydrate	21
Protein	3
Total lipids	1

Millet Flakes

Measure	1 cup
Weight	30 grams
Calories	100
Carbohydrate	21
Protein	3
Total lipids	1

Buckwheat Flour

Measure 1 cup	
Weight	100 grams
Calories	333
Carbohydrate	72
Protein	11.7
Total lipids	2.5

Carob Flour

Weight	8 grams
Calories	14
Carbohydrates	6.5
Protein	0.4
Total lipids	0.1

Quinoa

Measure	1 cup
Weight	100 grams
Calories	335
Carbohydrates	59.9
Protein	14.9
Total lipids	5.8

Pumpkin

Measure	1 cup
Weight	245 grams
Calories	49
Carbohydrates	12

Protein	1.76
Total lipids	.17

Yams

Measure	1 cup
Weight	200
Calories	210
Carbohydrates	48.2
Protein	4.8
Total lipids	.4

Plantain

Weight	100 grams
Calories	112
Carbohydrates	28.5
Protein	0.8
Total lipids	0.2

Sweet Potato

Weight	100 grams
Calories	87
Carbohydrates	21.3
Protein	1.2
Total Lipids	0.3

Proteins

Soy Beans (cooked)

Measure	1 cup
Weight	180 grams
Calories	234
Carbohydrates	19.4
Protein	19.8
Total lipids	10.3
Total unsaturated	7.68
Cholesterol	Nil

Raw Green Peas

Measure	100 grams
Carbohydrate	10
Protein	6
Total lipids	1.6

Chicken (light meat)

Measure	4 ozs
Weight	116 grams
Calories	216
Carbohydrate	Nil
Protein	23.5
Total lipids	12.8
Total unsaturated	7.96
Cholesterol	78

Turkey (light meat)

Measure	6.4 ozs
Weight	180 grams
Calories	286
Carbohydrate	Nil
Protein	39
Total lipids	13.2
Total unsaturated	8.18
Cholesterol	117

Fish (cod)

Measure	3 ozs
Weight	85 grams
Calories	70
Carbohydrate	Nil
Protein	15
Total lipids	.57
Total unsaturates	.276
Cholesterol	37

Eggs (whole)

Measure	1 large
Weight	50 grams
Calories	79
Carbohydrates	.6
Protein	6.07
Total lipids	5.58
Total unsaturates	2.97
Cholesterol	274

Baker's Yeast (dried)

Weight	100 grams
Calories	169
Carbohydrates	3.5

Protein	35.6
Total Lipids	1.5

Fats

Almonds

Measure	1 cup
Weight	142 grams
Calories	849
Carbohydrates	27.7
Protein	26.4
Total lipids	77
Total unsaturated	67
Cholesterol	Nil

Sesame Seeds

Measure	1 cup
Weight	150 grams
Calories	873
Carbohydrates	26.4
Protein	27.3
Total lipids	80
Total unsaturated	64
Cholesterol	Nil

Coconut - Desiccated

Weight	100 grams
Calories	604
Carbohydrates	6.4
Protein	5.6
Total lipids	62
Total unsaturated	1.5
Saturated	4.7
Monounsaturated	50
Cholesterol	Nil
Olive Oil	
Measure	1 tablespoon
Weight	13.5 grams
Calories	119
Carbohydrates	Nil
Protein	Nil
Total lipids	13.5
Total Unsaturated	11
Cholesterol	Nil

Butter

Measure	1 tablespoon
Weight	14.1
Calories	101
Carbohydrates	.008
Protein	.12
Total lipids	11.5
Total Unsaturated	3.74
Cholesterol	31

Light Whipping Cream

Measure	1 cup
Weight 239 grams	
Calories	699
Protein	5.15
Carbohydrates	7.07
Total lipids	73.8
Total unsaturated	23.8
Cholesterol 265	

Bibliography:

Nutrition Almanac 4th edition:
Gayla J Kirschmann, John D
Kirschmann: 1996: McGraw-Hill: New
York, USA

Recipes

by Lucille Leader *Dip ION*

These delicious and simple recipes are suitable for use whether people are on L-dopa medication or not. If you wish to eat around the time of taking L-dopa (Sinemet or Madopar), choose recipes which do not contain a relatively large amount of protein (these include meat, poultry, fish, eggs, dairy, soy, the gluten containing grains wheat including couscous and bulgar, rye, oats, barley, spelt, sago, coconut, nuts, seeds, avocado, asparagus and pulses). The timing for eating protein in relation to your Sinemet or Madopar is explained in the section "L-dopa (Levodopa - Sinemet, Madopar or equivalent) and protein" on page 82. Remember, however, to eat good sources of protein at least once a day as they are the body's building blocks.

If not using L-dopa, you can substitute egg for lecithin wherever listed. However, egg may be included in the recipes by users of L-dopa when not needing the effects of the medication.

It is important to chew food as well as possible. If this is a problem however, a food processor or liquidiser can be used. It is, however, important to let your doctor know if swallowing and chewing are a problem. You may need more specialised nutritional support, which includes the use of pre-digested complete liquid meal formulas. These are also suitable for tube feeding if swallowing is not possible.

A special note about cooking soy beans: It is important to soak them over night then throw away the water and boil three times vigorously, each time in fresh water for 15 minutes.

Safety in the kitchen requires a fire blanket or fire extinguisher to hand. For those who do not have help and movement is difficult, a microwave oven may be the only solution. However, for optimal health, it would be best to use conventional methods of cooking if at all possible. Remember to wash your hands well before preparing/eating food. Ensure adequate heating through or chilling of foods. If you are on your own and food preparation is difficult, do enquire whether your general practitioner is able to direct you to an organisation, which could help with providing meals. Supermarkets and shops can also be helpful in delivery of foods. An occupational therapist can direct you to specialised utensils and cups, if holding them is a problem. **Bon Appetit!**

SOUPS

Important Note:
If using a food processor or chopping food is a problem, keep the vegetables whole.

Satisfying Winter Soup
- 3 potatoes, cut into medium-size hunks
- 1 medium onion
- Pumpkin pieces (peeled), quantity as desired
- 1 celery stick, cut in large pieces
- 1 carrot
- 1 bunch parsley
- 1 courgette
- 2 tomatoes, chopped
- 1 leek (cut in two)
- 1 litre of water

1. *Boil all the ingredients in 1 litre of purified or still mineral water. Cover and simmer on low heat.*

2. *As soon as vegetables are soft, remove from the water and liquidise in a food processor or mash with potato masher.*

3. *Return blended mixture and purified or still mineral water to pan, heat and serve.*

Gazpacho Soup   (Serves 5)
- 5 large tomatoes, chopped
- 1 clove garlic, crushed
- $\frac{1}{2}$ cup celery, diced
- 1 cup cucumber, grated
- $\frac{1}{2}$ cup green pepper, diced
- $\frac{1}{2}$ cup sweet red pepper, diced
- 1 cup tomato juice
- $\frac{1}{2}$ cup fresh parsley, chopped
- 2 Tbsp olive oil (cold-pressed)
- 2 tsp basil, chopped
- Black pepper (optional)

1. *Combine all ingredients in a large bowl or food processor. Mix well and chill in refrigerator. Serve cold.*

Vichyssoise (Serves 4)
- 4 large potatoes
- 1 large leek
- 1 onion
- 1 pt water (purified or still mineral)
- Black pepper to taste

1. *Put all the ingredients into a pot and cook until soft.*

2. *Blend the vegetables to a smooth liquid in a food processor and then add back to the water.*

3. *Serve hot or chilled with fresh chopped parsley to decorate.*

For Special Occasions:
Add a drop of single cream just before serving

SALAD DRESSING

Mediterranean Olive Oil Dressing
- 6 tbs cold pressed olive oil (remove from the fridge 10 minutes before use)
- 2 tbs lemon juice or tomato juice
- 1 pressed garlic clove (to taste - optional)
- Ground Black pepper

SALADS

Potato Salad (Serves 2)
- 4 potatoes (in skins) (if organic)
- 1 celery stick (chopped)
- 1 apple (chopped)
- 2 spring onions (chopped)
- A sprinkling of chives (chopped)
- Dressing made with 3 Tbsp cold pressed olive oil and 1 Tbsp lemon juice (or tomato juice) crushed garlic and black pepper

1. *Mix the ingredients together in a bowl and toss with the Mediterranean Dressing.*

Fresh Mixed Salad (Serves 2)
- Pepper (red, green or yellow)
- Tomatoes (finely sliced)
- Lettuce
- Finely grated carrot
- Cucumber

1. *Dressing made with 3 Tbsp cold pressed olive oil and 1 Tbsp lemon juice (or tomato juice), crushed garlic and black pepper to taste.*

Carrot Salad
Grate as many carrots as desired and serve either mixed through with soaked sultanas, orange or pineapple juice, or on their own.

GRAIN RECIPES (GLUTEN FREE AND LOW PROTEIN)

Simple Rice Recipes
- 1 cup white rice
- $2\frac{1}{2}$ cups water (purified or still mineral water)

1. *Wash rice 3 times in cold water.*

2. *Put rice and water together in a pot.*

3. *Bring to boil.*

4. *Stir once.*

5. *Put lid on and simmer on a low heat for 20 minutes.*

6. *If rice is still moist, leave to simmer a few minutes longer. However, if the rice is still hard, add a little more water and simmer on a low heat for a further few minutes with the lid on until rice is tender.*

For Special Occasions:
Add sultanas to the rice when cooking. Sauté sliced bananas in a cold pressed olive oil and stir through the rice when cooked.

For Brown Rice
Use the same recipe as for white rice, (2 cups of water to 1 cup of rice) but add an extra cup of water. It will take longer to cook - about 40-50 minutes. A

delicious variation when cooking rice is to put some handfuls of sultanas into the water, and a little tomato sauce. In a separate pan you could sauté some chopped up bananas, spring onions and dried ginger flakes in a little olive oil. When these are turning golden, pour them with the oil into the already cooked rice and mix through.

For Special Occasions:
Add sultanas to the rice when cooking. Sauté sliced bananas in a cold pressed olive oil and stir through the rice when cooked.

Vegetable Risotto (Serves 6)
- 8 oz. brown rice
- 1 celery stick, diced
- 1 medium onion, chopped
- 1 courgette, diced
- 8 oz. beansprouts
- 4 oz. sweetcorn kernels
- 8 oz. broccoli florets
- 2 tomatoes, diced
- 1 Tbsp olive oil (cold-pressed)

Note: You can use any vegetable of your choice.

1. *Cook rice as package directs.*

2. *Blanch vegetables for a few seconds in boiling water.*

3. *Heat olive oil in wok or large pan and stir-fry all vegetables until tender.*

4. *Add cooked rice to the wok or pan, mix well and heat through. Serve.*

Countryside Peppers   (Serves 6)
- 6 medium red/yellow/orange peppers
- 3 cups water (purified or still mineral water)
- 1 cup millet
- 1 $1/2$ cups onion, chopped
- 1 clove garlic, crushed
- $1/2$ cup mushrooms, diced
- 1 Tbsp olive oil (cold-pressed)
- Crushed black pepper (optional)

1. *Blanch peppers in boiling water. Allow to cool slightly.*

2. *Bring water and millet to a boil. Reduce heat. Cover and simmer on a low heat for 30 minutes.*

3. *In a pan heat oil and sauté garlic, onion and mushrooms. Season to taste.*

4. *Combine cooked millet, and add to onion mixture.*

5. *Fill peppers with millet mixture. Cover with a little Cold pressed olive oil Bake at 180oC for 30 minutes, then serve.*

Polenta Aux Tomates   (Serves 6)
- 2 pints purified or still mineral water
- 8 oz yellow cornmeal (Polenta)
- 1-2 oz. Butter
- 1 tsp fresh basil
- Sauce
- 1 tsp fennel seed
- 2 Tbsps. olive oil (cold-pressed)
- 1 clove garlic, crushed
- 1 medium onion, chopped
- $^1/_2$tsp. fructose (health food shop)
- 1 lb. chopped tomatoes
- 3 Tbsps. tomato puree
- 1 tsp fresh oregano
- Crushed black pepper (optional)

1. *Bring the water to a boil in a large saucepan. Gradually add it to the cornmeal, continually stirring to avoid lumps. Add butter, continuing to cook over a low flame for 20 minutes. The mixture should have a creamy consistency. If not, it may be necessary to add more butter/water.*

2. *Pour into a 13 x 9 inch baking tin, level and set aside to cool.*

3. *Meanwhile, prepare sauce by heating oil in a saucepan, sauté garlic and onion till tender, then add oregano, basil, fennel seeds and black pepper. Stir in chopped tomatoes and puree, add fructose, cover and simmer for 20-30 minutes or until sauce thickens.*

4. *Slice polenta into squares, cover with sauce and serve.*

Note:
Polenta may be bought "ready made" at Delicatessen Shops. If using it, re-heat or grill the polenta, make the sauce and cover thin slices of polenta with it.

POTATO DELIGHTS

Mouth-watering Potato Cakes (Serves 4)

- 4 medium potatoes (2 sweet and 2 plain
- 1 dessertspoonful of lecithin granules or 1 egg
- 2 onions
- 2 Tbsp. brown rice flour
- 2 Tbsp. olive oil (cold-pressed)

1. *First chop the potatoes and onions into quarters. Place in a food processor together with the flour, lecithin granules or egg and 2 Tbsp. of olive oil. Chop to a fine, coarse mixture but do not allow to become a liquid. If watery, add a little more rice flour, so that the consistency does not fall apart, but is still soft.*

2. *Heat a frying pan or griddle with a dash of olive oil, sufficient so that the cakes will not stick to the bottom. Keep heat at medium setting.*

3. *Drop the mixture by the dessert spoon onto a pan or onto griddle (mixture should form a mini pattie), cover but keep checking to make sure cakes don't burn or stick. Flip over when lightly browned and cook underside. Total cooking time for each should be about 20 minutes or until the potatoes are cooked through.*

Alternative Method

The cakes may be grilled or baked. Lightly grease an oven dish or baking tin with cold pressed olive oil. Drop spoonfuls of potato mixture into the dish and pour a little olive oil over each one. Cover with tin foil, not touching the food. Keep under the grill or very hot oven until the potato is cooked through. Take off the tin foil about 10 minutes before serving in order to crisp.

Jacket Potatoes with Butter (Serves 4)

- Potatoes (organic preferably sweet or also plain)
- Butter

1. *Scrub clean the skins of sweet or ordinary potatoes and prick the potatoes with a fork.*

2. *Brush the with a little olive oil and wrap first in greaseproof paper and then in aluminium foil. Make sure that the aluminium foil completely covers the greaseproof paper or it will catch alight in the oven.*

3. *Bake in the oven 160oC - 190oC for an hour and a half or until soft.*

4. *Serve with butter and a salad or vegetables.*

Roast Potatoes   (Serves 6)

- 6 potatoes in jackets, (sweet or usual). (Pumpkin can also be used)
- Olive oil

1. *Steam potatoes until soft.*

2. *Coat potatoes with cold-pressed olive oil.*

3. *Roast in the oven at 190oC in an open dish. Turn potatoes intermittently and eat when crisp.*

Mediterranean Potatoes

- 4 potatoes
- 1 Tbsp olive oil
- 2 oz/50g unsalted butter
- 1 clove garlic, crushed
- 1 medium onion
- Freshly ground black pepper
- 1 green pepper, seeded and sliced
- 1 tsp mixed herbs
- 14oz/400g tin tomatoes

1. *Peel and cut into halves or quarters. Steam in a covered dish till the potatoes are done. Put aside.*

2. *Meanwhile, heat the oil and butter in a frying pan, add garlic, onion and pepper and cook for 5 minutes.*

3. *Add tomatoes and their juice, breaking up the tomatoes, then add the herbs and seasoning. Cook for 10 minutes.*

4. *Pour the sauce over the potatoes and serve hot.*

Alternatively:
Put all your ingredients, uncooked, into an oven casserole with a cup of water. Cover the dish with tin foil and cook at 180oC for about a 1 or 2 hours or until cooked.

PASTAS

Tomato Delight
- Rice Noodles / Buckwheat Noodles / Corn Noodles
- Readymade pasta sauce without wheatflour

1. *Cover noodles generously with water.*

2. *Boil gently with the lid off, stirring regularly*

3. *Heat the pasta sauce on a low heat and stir it into the noodles after they have been cooked.*

Tuna Surprise a la Ray   (contains Protein) (Serves 3)
- Half a packet of Rice Noodles / Buckwheat Noodles / Corn Noodles
- 2 small tins of tuna fish in spring water or olive oil
- 1 Tbsp. Cold pressed olive oil (if not using tinned tuna with olive oil)
- Juice of half a lemon

1. *Cover noodles generously with water.*

2. *Boil gently with the lid off, stirring regularly*

3. *Flake the tuna and mix into the cooked noodles.*

The Dressing
Mix a little cold pressed olive oil and lemon through the noodles
or use 1 Tbs. organic mayonnaise and 2 Tbs. Heinz Tomato Ketchup (mixed to taste) or just serve the noodles with the plain flaked tuna and a little cold pressed olive oil stirred through them.

DESSERTS

Exotic Coconut Pudding (contains Protein) (Serves 2)
- 1 tin coconut milk
- 4 bananas
- 1 large tin of pears naturally sweetened and drain off liquid
- 1 passion fruit (optional)

1. *Blend all the ingredients in the food processor until a creamy consistency is reached. If a thicker consistency is required, use less coconut milk.*

2. *Serve chilled in dessert dishes. The mixture may be festively decorated with other fruit, if desired.*

3. *This recipe can also be turned into ice cream in an ice-cream maker.*

Fruit Salad with or without Cream

1. *Chop fruit of your liking to bite size, using fruits of the season. This can include berry fruits. Passion fruit gives an exotic taste as do papayas, lychees, mangoes and red grapes.*

2. *Serve with or without cream.*

Luxury Noodle Pudding a la Ray   (Serves 6)

- $^1/_2$ packet of Chinese rice noodles
- 1 tablespoon of lecithin granules or an egg
- 1 jar of jam, naturally sweetened
- 2 handfuls raisins or sultanas (unsulphured or organic)
- 4 apples, cored, peeled and grated
- Knob of butter

1. *Preheat oven to 100oC*

2. *In a small bowl, soak raisins or sultanas in boiling water to soften.*

3. *Meanwhile boil noodles as package directs. Drain.*

4. *In a mixing bowl, mix jam, lecithin or egg, grated apples, raisins and noodles together. Add the drained noodles and mix through.*

5. *Lightly grease a square baking dish with olive oil and place noodle mixture in the dish.*

6. *Bake for 35 minutes, covered by foil (which does not touch the food). Remove the foil for the last ten minutes.*

Apple Crumble   (Serves 2)

- 4 chopped sweet eating apples, steamed with a little water (sufficient to cover apple puree) until tender
- Manuka honey or fructose to taste
- Crumbs made from soft butter and rice flour blended together
- Butter to grease dish
- Cinnamon to taste

1. *Grease baking dish with butter.*

2. *Pour the pureed apple into the dish, mixed with sweetener and cinnamon. Sprinkle with the crumbs and bake for 1/2 hour or until the crumbs are brown, at 180°C.*

Baked Apples (Allow one apple per person)

- Cored sweet cooking apples
- Cinnamon
- Manuka honey
- Soaked sultanas or raisins
- Butter
- Cloves

1. *Grease baking dish with butter.*

2. *Stuff the apples with the sultanas, honey and stick a few cloves round the top of the apple.*

3. *Cover the dish with foil and bake at the bottom of the oven for approximately 1-hour at 180°C or until soft.*

Fruit Whirl

- Apple
- Banana
- Mango
- Passion fruit
- or fruits of your choice

No melon or plums, as these ferment when together or with other foods. Whirl in a blender or food processor and serve in a festive glass decorated with a sprig of mint. If eating during the "protein window period", sprinkle with chopped nuts and seeds (which have been blended in a food processor.) Remember to keep the nuts and seeds in the refrigerator.

FISH, POULTRY AND SOY

Tomato Chicken (Serves 4)

- 4 breasts of chicken/turkey or whole chicken
- Heinz tomato sauce
- Onions

- Leeks
- Potato and sweet potato
- Green pepper
- 1 cup purified or still mineral water
- A few basil leaves
- 4 - 6 dessertspoonful cold pressed olive oil
- 2 Apples, quartered (optional)

1. *Chop onions, leeks, pepper, apples and basil leaves. Sauté in olive oil together with the Heinz Tomato Sauce (enough sauce to make gravy), for a few minutes, until a golden colour. Stir in one cup of mineral water. Pour this sauce over the chicken and whole potatoes and bake in a tightly covered oven dish. If you do not have enough gravy to cover the chicken and potatoes, add tomato sauce and a little water.*

2. *Bake in the oven, in a tightly covered dish for about 1 to 1_ hours, or until the chicken is soft.*

Note:
This dish can also be cooked on top of the stove, in a covered pot, at a low temperature for 1 to $1^1/_2$ hours or until the chicken and vegetables are tender. Check sauce level frequently. Stir intermittently.

Indonesian Plaice   (Serves 1)
- 1 Fillet of Plaice/Cod or other fish
- Black pepper
- Grated ginger root or ginger powder
- Pressed fresh garlic
- Chopped spring onions or leeks
- Cold pressed olive oil

1. *Lace the frying pan or dish with cold pressed olive oil.*

2. *Place all the vegetables in the dish / pan and gently sauté, whilst stirring.*

3. *When beginning to cook, place fish on top of the vegetables.*

4. *Put the lid on the pan and allow to cook through on a very low heat, adding a little water if food is sticking to the pan.*

5. *Check continuously that the mixture is not drying out and turn the fish, if necessary.*

6. *Cook for 15 minutes or until the fish is properly cooked through.*

Note:

This dish could also be baked in an oven in a tightly covered dish for 1 hour or until cooked through.

Cooking soy beans: It is important to soak them over night before boiling three times vigorously, each time in fresh water for 15 minutes.

Tofu (soy) a la Alison   (Serves 2)

- Tofu pieces (not genetically modified)
- Peppers (green, red, yellow, orange)
- Onion
- Chopped fresh tomatoes (or tinned)
- Cold pressed olive oil
- 1 cup of mineral or purified water
- Paprika (optional)
- Salt (optional)
- Pepper (optional)
- Heinz Tomato Ketchup (optional)

1. *Chop onion and peppers and place in a large frying pan or casserole dish laced with cold pressed olive oil.*

2. *Sauté the vegetables and as soon as they are slightly softened, lower the heat and add the tofu pieces.*

3. *Stir in a cup of water and add spices and ketchup, if desired.*

4. *Place a tightly fitting lid on the pot. Gently cook on a low heat, stirring regularly, until the ingredients are cooked through (approximately 30 minutes).*

5. *Serve with rice (see rice recipe in the above section)*

Soy Mince a la Ray

- Soy mince (not genetically modified)
- Onions
- Fresh tomatoes
- Cold pressed olive oil
- Organic soy sauce (wheat free)
- Heinz Tomato Ketchup, to taste
- Black pepper

1. *Sauté the onion with tomatoes in a large frying pan or casserole dish laced with cold pressed olive oil.*

2. As soon as the vegetables are slightly softened, lower the heat and stir in the soy mince.

3. Add stirring, boiled mineral or purified water to just cover the mixture, adding spices and ketchup, to taste.

4. Place a tightly fitting lid on the pot. Gently cook on a low heat, stirring intermittently, until the ingredients are cooked through (approximately 30 minutes).

5. Serve with rice (see rice recipe in the above section)

CAKES BISCUITS AND PASTRY

Fruit-Chip Biscuits (Gluten Free)
- 200 grams butter
- $1^1/_2$ cups brown sugar or $^1/_2$ cup fructose (fruit sugar)
- 2 Tbs lecithin granules or 1 egg
- 2 tsp vanilla essence
- $1^1/_2$ cups rice flour
- $^1/_2$ cup buckwheat flour
- $^1/_2$ cup millet flakes
- 1 tsp baking soda - bicarb.
- 1 cup chopped fruit

1. Cream butter, sugar, lecithin or egg, vanilla.

2. Add the dry ingredients and mix thoroughly.

3. Add fruit and mix.

4. Form into cookies and bake on a greased baking tray for about 10 minutes at 190°C

Pastry (Gluten Free)
- 5 oz brown rice flour
- 3 oz millet or buckwheat flour
- 5 oz butter
- 2 large sheets of grease-proof paper

1. *Preheat oven to 190ºC*

2. *Combine dry ingredients, mixing in oil with a fork.*

3. *Add water to mixture to form a dough.*

4. *This pastry is tricky to roll so you might like to do it between greaseproof paper.*

5. *Sprinkle the lower piece with rice flour, place dough on it, then lay sheet of greaseproof paper on top and flatten with a rolling pin. When it is rolled remove top piece of paper and carry dough to dish on bottom piece of paper. Invert dish onto it, and then turn dish right way up, allowing pastry to fall into it. Push into shape. Alternatively, you can roll it out carefully, using plenty of rice flour.*

6. *Prick well all over then bake blind* for about 25 minutes until set but not hard.*

7. *Use with your favourite filling or vegetables in tomato puree with a little fresh garlic and spring onion, or pureed fruit.*

Alternatively: Process an equal amount of butter and rice flour in a food processor. Roll out as desired. Example: 6 ozs rice flour and 6 ozs butter.

*   To bake blind, line the oven dish with pastry, cover with grease-proof paper and weight this down with a small quantify of rice grains to hold the paper down and absorb moisture. This seems to make the pastry crunchier.

"Special Treat" Birthday Cake ala Karen
(Gluten Free) (contains Nuts - walnuts)
- 10 eggs separated and at room temperature
- 10 Tbsps (about 2/3 cup) fructose
- 6 ozs bittersweet or semi-sweet chocolate melted over hot water and cooled or preferably use plain chocolate sweetened with fructose available from health shops or delicatessens
- 2 cups finely chopped walnuts (not ground)

1. *Preheat oven to 180ºC.*

2. *Beat the egg yolks and sugar until very thick and lemon coloured. Stir in the chocolate and fold in the chopped nuts.*

3. *Beat the egg whites until stiff but not dry and fold into the chocolate-nut mixture. Put into a greased 10-inch spring form pan and bake for 1 hour or until the centre springs back when lightly touched with the fingertips. Cool in the pan.*

4. *A variant could be to use finely grated carrots in place of chocolate.*

Mouthwatering Chocolate-Chip Cookies (Gluten Free)

- 200 grams butter
- $1^1/_2$ cups brown sugar or $^1/_2$ cup fructose
- 2 eggs
- 2 tsps vanilla essence
- $1^1/_2$ cups rice flour
- $^1/_2$ cup buckwheat flour
- $^1/_2$ cup millet flakes
- 2 cups chocolate chips
- 1 cup chopped almonds (optional)
- 1 cup desiccated coconut
- 1 tsp baking soda-bicarb. (optional)

1. *Cream butter, sugar, vanilla, eggs.*

2. *Add the dry ingredients and mix thoroughly.*

3. *Add chocolate chips, almonds, coconut and mix.*

4. *Form into cookies and bake on a greased baking tray for about 10 minutes at 190ºC.*

Note:
Experiment baking these biscuits without the soda-bicarb. If absolutely necessary, use the minimum amount.

Biochemical Tests

by Lucille Leader Dip ION and Dr Geoffrey Leader MB ChB FRCA
with a contribution by Dr John McLaren-Howard DSc FACN

Assessing patients on a cellular level enables healthcare professionals to plan patient management based on biochemical individuality. Some of the following tests may be useful in the assessment of metabolic, nutritional and general health status, as a confirmation of clinical judgement.

Haematology and Biochemistry - *(Blood)*
General screen investigating immune function and response to infection, electrolytes, kidney function, liver function and iron status.

Thyroid Function - *(Blood)*
General thyroid assessments may be indicated. Tyrosine is synthesised from the essential amino acid phenylalanine. Tyrosine metabolises three ways - to form melanins, L-dopa and thyroxine.

Liver Detoxification Test (Phase 1 and Phase 2) - *(Saliva, Urine)*
(see Note 1 on page 132)
Phase 1 (Cytochrome P450) liver detoxification in patients with Parkinson's disease has been shown to be sub-optimal[1]. It is important to assess both Phase 1 and Phase 2 detoxification pathways in order to optimise nutritional management.

Toxic Metals and Pesticides Screen - *(Sweat / Blood)*
(see Note 2 on page 132)
Patients may have been excessively exposed to organophosphates and toxic metals.

Mercury Toxicity Tests - *(Blood, Sweat, Stool, Electrical Measurements)*

Minerals - *(Sweat or other methods)*
(see Note 3 on page 132 and Table of Results in the section Nutritional Supplementation)
Minerals are essential as co-enzymes. Some examples: *zinc* plays a role in protein metabolism and may be deficient in Parkinson's disease patients. *Magnesium*, together with calcium, controls contraction and relaxation of muscles. *Chromium* is essential to glucose tolerance factor. *Manganese* is a co-enzyme to delta-6-desaturase, the enzyme necessary in the metabolism of essential fatty acids.

Red Cell Magnesium - *(Blood)*
Deficiency of magnesium may contribute to the degree of muscle spasm.

Myothermogram (see Note 4 on page 132)
Magnesium plays an important part in enabling muscle relaxation in Parkinson's disease and similar conditions. In some patients, it can be quite difficult to correct intra-cellular magnesium deficiency. In these, and when the label "Parkinson's disease" may have been inappropriately applied, the Myothermogram can be used to assess the magnesium-related components of tremor. The Myothermogram indirectly monitors the intra-cellular changes of muscle action using sensitive detectors of the changes in heat output from a muscle during simple muscle movements. It is a remarkably effective way of investigating biochemical causes of tremor.

Dr John McLaren-Howard DSc FACN

Functional Tests
- **Biotin - *(Blood)***
  (see Note 5 on page 132 and Table of Results in the section "Nutritional Supplementation")
  This contributes to mitochondrial energy production.

- **B Vitamins 1,2,3,6 - *(Blood)***
  (see Note 6 on page 132 and Table of Results in the section "Nutritional Supplementation")
  These are essential to the Krebs Cycle and the making of cellular energy (adenosine triphosphate, ATP.) Vitamin B6 is essential in the metabolic step from L-dopa to dopamine.

Vitamin B12 - MMA *(Urine)*
(see Note 7 on page 132)
This is essential for nervous/muscular function.

Digestive Enzymes - *(Gastrogram/Stool)*
(Comprehensive Digestive Stool Analysis) (see Notes 8 & 9 on page 132)
Patients with Parkinson's disease may demonstrate deficiencies in the production of hydrochloric acid and/or pancreatic exocrine function. As dopamine is metabolised from protein it is essential that protein be adequately digested to initiate this metabolic pathway. The digestion and absorption of carbohydrates and fats are essential to metabolism. Incompletely digested food molecules can contribute to food allergy or intolerance, which might aggravate symptoms in some patients with Parkinson's disease. Large incompletely digested protein molecules can also contribute to increased permeability of the gut mucosa.

Gut Permeability - *(Urine)* (see Note 10 on page 132)

The integrity of the intestinal mucosa is essential for nutritional absorption and protection against potential allergens. Permeability could be affected by disease, drugs, surgery and radiation. Patients with increased gut permeability are often very fatigued.

Food Allergy (IgE) and Food Intolerance (IgG4) - *(Blood)*

It has been observed clinically that certain foods and chemicals may aggravate symptoms in patients with Parkinson's disease.

Antioxidant Profile - *(Blood)* (see Note 11 on page 132)

It is thought that free radical damage may play a role in the destruction of neurones in Parkinson's disease. Antioxidant therapy may be indicated.

Amino Acid Profile - *(Blood / Urine)* (see Note 12 on page 132)

L-dopa is derived from the amino acid tyrosine. It is useful to assess the amino acid status of Parkinson's disease patients in the interest of all anabolic functions. Amino acid supplements may be indicated.

Essential Fatty Acids - *(Red blood cells)*
(see Note 13 below and Table of Results in the section Nutritional Supplementation)

These are essential to the integrity of cell membranes. They play a role in the control of inflammation (forming prostaglandins), and contribute to immune system function.

Parasites - *(Stool, Blood, Breath for Helicobacter, Dark-Field Microscope)*
(see Note 14 on page 132)

Parasites may be a problem for patients who present with malabsorption, chronic diarrhoea, fatigue or anal irritation.

Adrenal Stress Index - *(Saliva)* (see Note 15 on page 132)

This test is a measure of cortisol and DHEA levels and is used as a biochemical marker of stress. Manipulation of the levels of these hormones may have beneficial therapeutic effects.

Male and Female Hormone Profiles - *(Saliva)* (see Note 16 on page 132)

Patients often present with sexual, fertility, menstrual and menopausal problems.

Agglutination Tests

These include Coombs tests, Complement Fixation and ELISA. They may sometimes be indicated in special circumstances if pregnancy is contemplated.

Reference

1. *Metabolic Biomarkers of Parkinson's Disease* - Actor Neurologica Scandinavica - Supplementum 136: pps. 19 - 23: A Williams, S Sturman, G Steventon, R Waring: 1991

Notes

1. Great Smokies Diagnostic Laboratory, Ashville, North Carolina, USA:
   UK representation: Nutri Limited: 0800 212 742 *or* Health Interlink: 01582 794091
2. BioLab Medical Unit, 9 Weymouth Street, London, W1, UK
   Telephone: 020 7636 5959
3. BioLab Medical Unit, 9 Weymouth Street, London, W1, UK
   Telephone: 020 7636 5959
4. BioLab Medical Unit, 9 Weymouth Street, London, W1
   Telephone: 020 7636 5959
   Dr John McLaren-Howard
5. BioLab Medical Unit, 9 Weymouth Street, London, W1, UK
   Telephone: 020 7636 5959
6. BioLab Medical Unit, 9 Weymouth Street, London, W1, UK
   Telephone: 020 7636 5959
7. The Doctors Laboratory, 55 Wimpole Street, London, W1, UK
   Telephone: 020 7460 4800
   BioLab Medical Unit, 9 Weymouth Street, London, W1, UK
   Telephone: 020 7636 5959
8. Gastrogram (capsule): BioLab Medical Unit, 9 Weymouth Street, London, W1, UK
   Telephone: 020 7636 5959
9. Great Smokies Diagnostic Laboratory (stool samples), Ashville, North Carolina, USA:
   UK representation: Nutri Limited: 0800 212 742 or Health Interlink: 01582 794091
10. Great Smokies Diagnostic Laboratory, Ashville, North Carolina, USA:
    UK representation: Nutri Limited: 0800 212 742 or Health Interlink: 01582 794091
11. BioLab Medical Unit, 9 Weymouth Street, London, W1, UK
    Telephone: 020 7636 5959
12. The Doctors Laboratory, 55 Wimpole Street, London, W1, UK
    Telephone: 020 7460 4800
13. BioLab Medical Unit, 9 Weymouth Street, London, W1, UK
    Telephone: 020 7636 5959
14. Great Smokies Diagnostic Laboratory, Ashville, North Carolina, USA:
    UK representation: Nutri Limited: 0800 212 742 or Health Interlink: 01582 794091
    Parascope: A joint project between Nutrition Associates, York, UK: 01904 691591 and
    Department of Microbiology, Leeds Infirmary, Leeds, UK: 0113 3924657:
    UK representative: BioLab Medical Unit, 9 Weymouth Street, London, W1, UK
    Telephone: 020 7636 5959
15. Great Smokies Diagnostic Laboratory, Ashville, North Carolina, USA:
    UK representation: Nutri Limited: 0800 212 742 or Health Interlink: 01582 794091
16. Great Smokies Diagnostic Laboratory, Ashville, North Carolina, USA:
    UK representation: Nutri Limited: 0800 212 742 or Health Interlink: 01582 794091

CHAPTER 9.4

Oral Nutritional Supplementation

by Lucille Leader Dip ION

In every patient (100%) with Parkinson's disease seen at The London Pain Relief and Nutritional Support Clinic at The London Welbeck Hospital in London (aged between 16 and 75 years, males and females, some on L-dopa and others not), there has been evidence of nutritional deficiencies of various nutrients. These were measured by blood, sweat and urine and included vitamins, minerals and essential fatty acids (see Table 1 on page 136). Deficiencies of hydrochloric acid and pancreatic enzymes as measured by gastrogram, as well as increase in gut permeability, were also often demonstrated.

In addition to the use of regular *oral* supplements, *sublinguals* (designed to be absorbed under the tongue), *transdermals* (designed to be rubbed in and absorbed through the skin) and *intravenously administered* nutrients are recommended if available, as absorption appears to be a general problem. Sublingual nutrients avoid the gut and enter the blood stream directly through the oral mucosa. Some sublingual nutritional products are available but in their absence, capsules, powders, liquids and tablets will have to suffice. The essential fatty acids (Omega 6 and Omega 3) can also be administered by massaging them into thin-skinned areas of the body. Fat soluble vitamins A and E can also be transdermally absorbed.

Nutritional supplementation should always be based on the biochemical individuality of each patient and be supervised by a nutritionist, dietician or physician conversant with nutritional medicine. Biochemical tests are available to assess nutritional status (see the section "Biochemical Tests"). A typical oral nutritional supplement programme tends to include the following:

■ Vitamin B complex:

B vitamins play a role in mitochondrial energy production. Modern L-dopa drugs contain a decarboxylase inhibitor, which has the desired effect of inhibiting premature decarboxylation of L-dopa before it goes through the blood brain barrier. As such, Vitamin B6 can be used together with "Sinemet"[1] and "Madopar"[2]. Vitamin B6 is a biochemically essential co-enzyme in the metabolic step between L-dopa and dopamine[3,4]. Vitamins B6 and B12 with folate are also recommended if homocysteine levels are increased.

Vitamin B12: This is implicated in neuromuscular function.

■ General vitamin and mineral complex:

In addition to this -

Vitamin C: This is a coenzyme with dopamine B hydroxylase.

Vitamin D3:   Deficiencies have been detected in Parkinson's Disease[5].

Zinc: Zinc is implicated in many enzyme functions and protein metabolism.

Magnesium: Deficiency can exacerbate muscle spasm and is a co-enzyme in fatty acid metabolism.

Manganese: This is an important delta 6-desaturase co-enzyme in fatty acid metabolism.

Chromium: This is implicated in blood sugar control.

NADH: This is a derivative of vitamin B3 and forms an essential part of the electron transport chain in the metabolisation of cellular energy. Although some practitioners prescribe this as an oral supplement for Parkinson's disease, the authors have not found it to be efficacious by this route in their patients. However intravenous administration has been found to be of benefit[6].

- **Broad-spectrum amino acids:** This form of pre-digested protein is for anabolic function. Protein may need to be supplemented if patients are on a reduced protein diet because of L-dopa medication. Pre-digested amino acids are quickly absorbed, which makes them eminently suitable for those who need L-dopa medication frequently.

- **Phosphatydil serine:** This is for membrane stability[7].

- **Gingko biloba:** This is an anti-oxidant which dilates capillaries.

- **Anti-oxidants:** These are implicated in control of free-radials and include alpha lipoic[8] acid and other anti-oxidants such as vitamins A, C, E and selenium. The immune enzyme glutathione peroxidase is selenium dependent.

- **N-acetyl-cysteine**[9]. This stimulates the body's own production of glutathione and is an antioxidant.

- **Acetyl-L-carnitine**[10]. This is an important antioxidant.

- **Alpha-lipoic acid**. This is a powerful antiantioxidant.

- **Healing agents for increased gut permeability.** These include butyric acid, biotin and micellised vitamin A. *Glutamine is contra indicated, as it is an excito-toxin.*

- **Digestive enzymes as indicated.**

- **Bifidobacterium bifidum, Lactobacillus acidophilus, Lactobacillus bulgaricus and other cultures of intestinal bacteria**[11]. These friendly cultures of intestinal bacteria enhance gut immunity. Probiotics need to be supplemented if patients have taken antibiotics.

- **Valerian.** This much documented herb aids sleep.

- **Essential fatty acids** (Omega 6 and Omega 3). Omega 6 is found in primrose and borage oils and Omega 3 in fish oils. These enhance cellular membrane integrity, upregulate the immune system and are involved in the metabolisation of anti-inflammatory prostaglandins series 1 and 3.

Table 1.
Table of Nutritional Deficiencies

A small sample of Parkinson's Disease patients at The London Pain Relief and Nutritional Support Clinic, London

The sample below does not represent a controlled trial but is only a report of some nutritional deficiencies encountered in Parkinson's disease patients. It is not intended to draw any conclusions as regards the relationship of these with Parkinson's disease but merely to demonstrate the necessity for nutritional supplementation as part of a management programme to optimise the functional health of these patients. It is interesting to note the significant zinc deficiency (75%) in patients whether they take L-dopa or not. Significant zinc deficiency in the cerebrospinal fluid of Parkinson's disease patients has been demonstrated in a controlled trial[12]. Zinc was also deficient in another controlled study assessing the nutritional status of patients with Parkinson's disease[13].

The table below involves males and females with Parkinson's disease, ages ranging from 31 to 75 years.

Minerals		Number of Patients	Zinc	Manganese	Magnesium	Chromium
tested by sweat	On L-dopa	28	21 (75%)	8 (29%)	19 (67.8%)	9 (32%)
	Not on L-dopa	12	9 (75%)	4 (33%)	7 (58%)	1 (8%)

Essential Fatty Acids		Number of Patients	GLA	DGLA	EPA	DHA
tested by blood	On L-dopa	28	7 (24%)	7 (24%)	15 (16%)	16 (55%)
red blood cells	Not on L-dopa	12	1 (8%)	7 (24%)	7 (58%)	8 (67%)

Functional B Vitamins		Number of Patients	Vit B1	Vit B2	Vit B6
tested by blood	On L-dopa	25	5 (20%)	7 (28%)	6 (24%)
	Not on L-dopa	12	6 (50%	6 (50%)	1 (8%)

Niacin		Number of Patients	Vit B3
tested by blood	On L-dopa	23	12 (52%)
	Not on L-dopa	11	1 (9%)

Biotin		Number of Patients	Biotin
tested by blood	On L-dopa	18	13 (72%)
	Not on L-dopa	11	6 (55%)

References:

1. *ABPI Compendium of Data Sheets and Summaries of Product Characteristics* (1999-2000): p. 371: Datapharm Publications Limited, London, UK

2. *ABPI Compendium of Data Sheets and Summaries of Product Characteristics* (1999-2000): p. 1334: Datapharm Publications Limited, London, UK

3. *Parkinson's Disease - The New Nutritional Handbook*: p.6: Dr Geoffrey Leader MB ChB FRCA and Lucille Leader DipION: 1996: Denor Press, London, UK

4. *Wills' Biochemical Basis of Medicine*: p.417: J Hywel Thomas PhD FIBiol and B Gillham PhD: 1989: Butterworth Heinemann: Oxford, UK

5. *High Prevalance of Vitamin D deficiency and reduced bone mass in Parkinson's Disease -Neurology* 49(5): pps. 1273-79: Y Sato, M Kikyuama, K Oizumi

6. *NADH - A new therapeutic approach to Parkinson's Disease. Comparison of oral and parenteral application*: D Volc, J G Birkmayer: C Vrecki, W Birkmayer: 1993: Acta Neurologica Scandinavica Suppl. 146: pps. 32-35:

7. *BrainRecovery.Com*: pps. 23-24: Dr David Perlmutter MD: 2000: Perlmutter Health Center, Naples, Fl, USA

8. *BrainRecovery.Com*: p. 25: Dr David Perlmutter MD: 2000: Perlmutter Health Center, Naples, Fl, USA

9. *BrainRecovery.Com*: p. 26: Dr David Perlmutter MD: 2000: Perlmutter Health Center, Naples, Fl, USA

10. *Effect of intraventricular injection of l-methyl-4-phenylpyridinium protection by acetyl-L-carnitine*: V Steffen, M Santiago, C P de la Cruz, et al: 1995: Human Exp Toxicol 14:865-871

11. *Probiotics*: pps. 24-25, : Leon Chaitow ND DO and Natasha Trenev: 1990: Thorsons An Imprint of HarperCollins Publishers, London, UK

12. *Trace Element Status of Cerebrospinal Fluid of Individuals with Neurological Diseases by ICP-MS*: N I Ward, N Walker A E Ward: 1988 Trace Element Analysis in Diagnosis and Pathological States: Vol 5, pps 513-550: proceedings of the 5th International Workshop in Nuremburg, Rep of Germany: Trace Element Analytical Chemistry in Medicine and Biology ISBN 31101111113406: Walter de Gruyter & Co, Berlin, Germany & New York, USA

13. *Diet, Body Size and Micronutrient Status in PD*: Abbott RA, Cox M, Markus H, Tomkins A: 1992: European Journal of Clinical Nutrition 46(12): pps. 879 - 884:

Bibliography

Clinical Nutrition - A Functional Approach, Geoffrey S Bland PhD et al, 1999, The Institute for Functional Medicine Inc, Gig Harbor, WA, USA

Biochemistry: The National Medical Series for independent Study, Victor L Davidson, PhD, Donald B Sittman, PhD, 1994, Harwal Publishing. A Waverly Company, Baltimore, USA.

Wills' Biochemical Basis of Medicine: Second Edition, J Hywel Thomas, PhD, FIBiol & Brian Gillham PhD, 1993, Butterworth Heinemann Limited, Oxford, England

Antioxidant Adaptation - Its Role in Free Radical Pathology, Stephen A Levine PhD & Parris M Kidd PhD, 1994, Allergy Research Group, California, USA

Fats that Heal, Fats that Kill, Udo Erasmus, 1993, Alive Books, Burnaby BC, Canada

Nutritional Influences on Illness, Melvyn R Werbach MD, 1989, Thorsons Publishers Limited, London, UK

The Lactic Acid Bacteria - Their Role in Human Health, Nigel Plumber BSc PhD, 1992, Biomed Publications Limited, Shirley, UK

Probiotics, Leon Chaitow ND DO & Natasha Trenev, 1990, Thorsons, London, UK

Parkinson's Disease - The New Nutritional Handbook, Geoffrey Leader MB ChB FRCA & Lucille Leader DipION, 1997, Denor Press, London, UK

Encyclopaedia of Natural Medicine, Michael Murray ND and Joseph Pizzorno ND, 1991, Prima Publishing, Rocklin, CA, USA

Intravenous Nutritional Support in Parkinson's Disease

by Dr Geoffrey Leader MB ChB FRCA
Dr Dieter Volc MD and Dr David Perlmutter MD

I ntravenous administration of vitamins and minerals, NADH and glutathione, have been found to be useful for some patients as part of the nutritional management of Parkinson's disease. It has been noted that this form of nutritional administration can be more effective than oral supplementation. Vitamins, minerals and NADH are often helpful in improving energy and wellbeing. Glutathione administration has also been shown to improve patients' symptoms. To optimise functional health, physicians are able to combine these techniques. Protocols for their administration are presented below.

Nicotinamide Adenine Dinucleotide (NADH)[1]

NADH supplementation was pioneered by Professor Walter Birkmayer and Dr George Birkmayer in Vienna, Austria. It is used as part of Parkinson's disease management by Dr Dieter Volc who joined, and later succeeded the late Professor Walter Birkmayer in his clinic in Vienna. NADH is available in Vienna (see Note 1 on page 143).

Protocol for Intravenous NADH

by Dr Dieter Volc MD

10mgs of NADH powder is dissolved in 100ml of normal saline. It is administered slowly, via an antecubital vein, over a period of twenty minutes. This administration is usually repeated daily for 10 days. After a number of weeks or months, when the observed feeling of wellbeing starts to wane, a booster series may be given. If patients are unable to have daily sessions, twice weekly may still be of benefit. Due to metabolic individuality, some patients may benefit from NADH and others may not.

Vitamins and Minerals

VITAMINS AND MINERALS which play a role in energy metabolism (the Kreb's Cycle) as well as any deficient nutrients, are administered by Dr Geoffrey Leader in London, UK. This type of nutritional support is useful in patients who have cellular deficiencies and who are suffering from malabsorption. The nutrients are easily obtainable by the medical profession. (see Note 2 on page 143).

Protocol for Intravenous Vitamins and Minerals

by Dr Geoffrey Leader MB ChB FRCA

The patient is required to sign informed consent as the effect of administration cannot be predicted with certainty and must be regarded as "nutritional support" and in no way therapeutic. Thereafter, the "cocktail" is dripped slowly into the vein over a period of half an hour, with the patient either in the lying or sitting position, whichever is more comfortable. However, for the first administration, the lying position is always used together with pulse rate and blood pressure monitoring, before, during and after, so as to assess the patient's reactions. Up until the present time, no side effects and especially no allergic reactions have been encountered in a series of 100 administrations.

A typical protocol follows in which vitamins and minerals are added to 200ml of sterile water together with heparin 100iu and lignocaine 20mg to prevent any discomfort.

Ideally the mixture is given twice a week via alternating arm veins. If this is not possible, then it may be given at least once a week, up to a total of eight administrations. After the initial course a maintenance infusion is usually necessary once a month in order to maintain an increased feeling of wellbeing. Due to metabolic individuality, some patients may benefit and others not.

Sterile water	200ml	Lignocaine 1%	2ml
Heparin	100iu	Vits B1, B2, B3	50mg, 25mg, 50mg
Cyanocobalamine	1000mcg	Dexpanthenol	500mg
Folic Acid	5mg	Magnesium Sulphate	500mg - 1000mg
Manganese	0.1mg	Molybdenum	50mcg
Pyridoxine	50-100mg	Copper	0.4mg
Zinc	5mg - 10mg	Selenium	80mcg
Chromium	4mcg	Ascorbic acid	2gm

Glutathione

Intravenous glutathione administration has also been shown to alleviate patients' symptoms whilst reducing oxidative stress. This technique is used as part of nutritional management in Parkinson's disease by Dr David Perlmutter in Naples, Florida, USA.

Protocol for Intravenous Glutathione

by Dr David Perlmutter MD

There are several factors that explain why glutathione is so beneficial in Parkinson's disease. Glutathione has the unique ability to make certain areas of the brain more sensitive to dopamine[2], so that even though dopamine is decreased, it nevertheless becomes more effective. The concept of enhancing cellular receptor sensitivity has become quite familiar in medicine today. In diabetes for example, before actually administering insulin, physicians often begin therapy by prescribing the drug metformin, which acts by enhancing the sensitivity of cells to whatever insulin is still being produced.

Our protocol for using glutathione is relatively simple. Glutathione is inexpensive and easily obtained (see Note 3 on page 143). We use liquid glutathione, not reconstituted powder. It should be administered by a qualified healthcare practitioner as follows:

1. Dilute the appropriate dosage of glutathione liquid in 10cc of sterile normal saline. Usually vials contain 200mg.

2. This solution is then injected through a 21-gauge butterfly catheter intravenously over a 15 to 20 minute period of time.

3. Alternatively, many patients choose to have an intravenous access port inserted. This allows frequent glutathione administration without repeated intravenous injections.

Treatment begins at 1000mg glutathione 3 times a week and may be increased to injections every other day of up to 1200mg, depending on results.

The Importance of Glutathione

With so much emphasis placed on L-dopa therapy, it is important to recognise that another vital brain chemical is also profoundly deficient in Parkinson's disease. This chemical, glutathione, is substantially reduced, virtually across the board, in Parkinson's patients. And yet, this deficiency seems to receive precious little attention[3].

Glutathione is a critically important brain chemical. It is clearly one of the most important brain antioxidants. That is, glutathione helps to preserve brain tissue by preventing damage from free radicals[4] - destructive chemicals formed by the normal processes of metabolism, toxic elements in the environment, and as a normal response of the body to challenges by infectious agents or other stresses. In addition to quenching dangerous free radicals, glutathione also acts to recycle vitamin C and vitamin E, which, because of their antioxidant activity, also reduce free radicals in the brain.

So, with the understanding that glutathione is important for brain protection, and that this protection may be lacking in the brains of Parkinson's patients because of their glutathione deficiency, wouldn't it make sense to give glutathione to Parkinson's patients experimentally and observe their outcome? That's exactly what was done in a landmark study from the Department of Neurology, University of Sassari, Italy. In this research protocol Parkinson's patients received intravenous glutathione twice daily for 30 days. The subjects were then evaluated at one month intervals for up to six months. The published results indicated "all patients improved significantly after glutathione therapy, with a 42% decline in disability. Once glutathione was stopped, the therapeutic effect lasted 2-4 months." Further, the researchers indicated "...glutathione has symptomatic efficacy and possibly retards the progression of the disease"[5].

It is unclear exactly why this study has remained almost completely unrecognised. In the United States, the use of L-dopa, or other drugs designed to mimic it, remains the standard of care. And yet, this Italian study demonstrated that providing glutathione, a substance naturally occurring in the brain, provided Parkinson's patients substantial benefit. Quite simply, we know that the brains of Parkinson's patients are profoundly deficient in this important chemical, with clinical research supporting its incredible effectiveness.

In my clinic, we began administering intravenous glutathione in late 1998. The effectiveness of this brain antioxidant in Parkinson's disease is nothing short of miraculous. Certainly, its administration is more complicated than simply "taking a pill", but on the other hand, there are essentially no reported side effects. In addition, while our Parkinson's patients are now realising profound improvements with respect to reduction of rigidity, increased mobility, improved ability to speak, less depression, and decreased tremor, glutathione has the added benefit of protecting the brain from free radical damage, thus slowing the progression of the underlying illness. This contrasts so vividly with the simplistic approach of only treating symptoms.

Following even a single dosage of intravenous glutathione, many of the symptoms of Parkinson's disease are rapidly improved, often, in as little as

15 minutes. Injections are typically repeated from 3 times a week to as often as daily.

Here is an example of a typical response to glutathione therapy in a patient with moderately advanced Parkinson's disease:

Dear Dr Perlmutter

This letter is to advise you of the progress of my husband's response to the glutathione therapy started two weeks ago.

As you know (HS), now 72 years old, had been diagnosed with Parkinson's disease five years ago, starting with a tremor in his right hand. The disease progressed rapidly, impairing his walking ability, balance, and reducing his voice volume and clarity. Most recently, his inability to walk had made it necessary for him to use a wheelchair when leaving the house. At home, he has used a walker for the past two years.

His prescribed medications have included Sinemet®, Mirapex®, and Tasmar® over the past years, the effects of which have diminished.

Almost immediately after your first treatment of glutathione IV two weeks ago, there was a marked improvement in his facial expression, his voice volume, and ability to walk and turn. He started with 400 mg., 3 times a week. The effective period of time after injection has increased from one hour to almost the whole day. When we visited your office last he received 600 mg., and his ability to walk almost normally lasted the full day and part of the next.

He also reports that he has a general feeling of wellbeing after each treatment. He is now taking 400 units of glutathione IV once a day, together with the supplements you have prescribed.

References

1. *NADH - A new therapeutic approach to Parkinson's Disease. Comparison of oral and parenteral application*: D Volc, J G Birkmayer: C Vrecki, W Birkmayer: Acta Neurologica Scandinavica Suppl. 146: pps. 32-35: 1993

2. *Modulation of Glutamate Receptor Functions by Glutathione*: SS Oja, R Jankay, V Varga, P Saransaari: Neurochem Int Aug-Sept 37 (2-3): pps. 299-306: 2000

3. *Parkinson's Disease: A disorder due to nigral glutathione deficiency?*: T L Perry, D V Godin, S Hansen: Neurosci Lett 33: pps. 305-310: 1982

4. *Review of oxidative stress in brain and spinal cord injury: Suggestions for pharmacological and nutritional management strategies*: B H Juurlin, P G Paterson: J Spinal Cord Med Oct: 21 (4): pps. 309-334: 1998

5. *Reduced Glutathione in the treatment of early Parkinson's Disease*: G Sechi, M G Deledda, G Bua, et al: Prog Neuropsychopharmacol Biol Psychiatry 20(7): pps. 1159-70: 1996:

Notes

1. *Intravenous NADH is available from:*
   Dr Dieter Volc, Schottenfeldgasse 45, A-1070 Vienna, Austria
   Email: Prosenex@abacus.at

2. *Intravenous Vitamins and Minerals are available from:*
   McGuff Company, 3524 West Lake Center Drive, Santa Ana, CA 92704
   Telephone: 714 545 2491   Facsimile: 714 540 5614

   College Pharmacy, 3505 Austin Bluffs Pkwy,
   Ste 101, Colorado Springs, CO 80918
   Telephone: +1 719 262 0022   Facsimile: +1 719 262 0035

3. *Injectable Glutathione (non powder form) is available from:*
   Wellness Health and Pharmaceuticals
   2800 South 18th Street, Birmingham, Alabama 35209, USA
   Telephone: (800) 227-2627   Facsimile: (800) 369-0302

Liver Detoxification & Optimal Liver Function
A Nutritional Approach

by Helen Kimber BSc

The liver is the hardest working organ in the human body. It performs many functions that are vital to life. It plays an important role in digestion (breaking down nutrients) and assimilation (building up body tissues). It is the storage site for many essential vitamins and minerals - iron, copper, B12, vitamins A, D, E and K. Red blood cells, which are responsible for carrying oxygen around the body, are also produced in the liver and Kupffer cells help to devour harmful micro-organisms in the blood so helping to fight infection.

Amongst its many functions the most important role of the liver is that of Detoxification. The liver detoxifies harmful substances by a complex series of chemical reactions. The role of these various enzyme activities in the liver is to convert fat-soluble toxins into water- soluble substances that can be excreted in the urine or the bile depending on the particular characteristics of the end product.

Detoxification

Toxins

↓

Liver — See Phase I & Phase II detoxification

Blood   Bile

↓   ↓

Kidneys   GI Tract

↓   ↓

Urine   Faeces

Every day our bodies are bombarded with toxins from both outside (exotoxins) as well as toxins from within the body (endotoxins). Exotoxins include the polluted environment, medications, alcohol, cigarette smoke, car exhaust emissions. Endotoxins include the by-products of nutrient breakdown, hormones and bacterial waste products from the intestines. All produce harmful substances. It is the role of the liver to render these potentially harmful products into less harmful compounds.

The effect of exposure to toxins varies from individual to individual. Some people are highly sensitive to different endo and exotoxins. Others, because their livers can detoxify more efficiently, are not so sensitive and are therefore more resilient. In 1994, it was suggested that Parkinson's disease could be a form of accelerated ageing associated with environmental toxins.[1]

Researchers are exploring the environmental agents and possible defects in the liver's detoxification ability, which may predispose an individual to Parkinson's disease. A study carried out at the University of Birmingham Medical School in 1991 demonstrated that individuals who have compromised liver detoxification are more prone to developing either Parkinson's Disease or Alzheimer's disease.[2] A build up of potentially toxic products can cause free radical damage and oxidative stress, which could be attributed to the destruction of cells in the substantia nigra. The use of nutrition to ensure optimal liver detoxification and adequate antioxidant nutrients to quench free radicals is therefore essential in supporting the Parkinson patient.

The rate at which the liver can eliminate toxins can determine an individual's susceptibility to toxic overload which in turn can lead to symptoms of ill health. When the liver becomes so overloaded with harmful toxins that the enzymes that break them down can no longer cope, the toxins build up and this then manifests itself in a specific disease state.

Parkinson's disease is more prevalent in individuals who have been exposed to occupational toxins. And although not everyone exposed to toxins will develop the disease, those unfortunate enough to have an inherited flaw in their detoxification ability are at a far greater risk to the brain damaging effects of a wide variety of toxins.

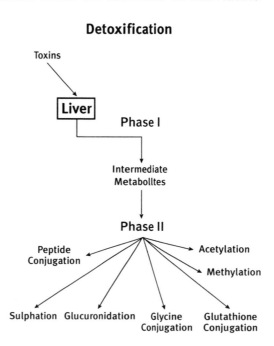

Detoxification

Detoxification - Phase I

There are two stages of liver detoxification, Phase I and Phase II.

Phase I is carried out by the cytochrome P450 enzyme system and consists of oxidation and reduction reactions. Various nutrients are required in order for the phase I detoxification system to be carried out efficiently. There are many substances, which can induce P450. Cytochrome P450 reactions generate free radicals and this can cause secondary damage to cells. An adequate supply of key antioxidants and free radical quenchers is therefore essential to prevent tissue damage.[3]

Phase I Nutritional Support

Antioxidants

Reduced glutathione is a critically important brain chemical. It acts as an antioxidant, protecting against free radical damage. Furthermore, it helps to recycle two other antioxidants, vitamin E and vitamin C. Glutathione has also been found to be lacking in patients suffering from Parkinson's disease.[4] A study in Italy using intravenous glutathione twice daily for 30 days showed some remarkable results. All patients improved significantly after glutathione therapy, with a 42% decline in disability. The researchers also noted that once the glutathione therapy was stopped the therapeutic effect lasted for 2-4 months.[5]

N-Acetyl-L-Cysteine (NAC) is an effective sulfhydryl donor and precursor to Growth Stimulating Hormone (GSH) synthesis. It enhances glutathione-S-transferase activity, promotes detoxification, and directly quenches free radicals.[6] The detoxifying properties of NAC make it an ideal nutritional agent to help eliminate intestinal endotoxins and xenobiotics. (See Phase II Nutritional Support)

Coenzyme Q10 (CoQ10) is ubiquitous in biological systems. It is found in all tissues of the body, but is concentrated in the adrenals, kidneys, lungs, spleen and especially the heart. The primary role of CoQ10 is in oxidative phosphorylation, as an integral component of the mitochondrial energy-transducing assembly. As an antioxidant, CoQ10 is especially active in cell membranes. It protects low-density lipoproteins (LDL) from oxidative damage and enhances the antioxidant function of vitamin E.[7] Because of its global use in the body, CoQ10 plays a significant role in the recovery from many health problems.

Vitamin C is a well-known antioxidant. Depletion of vitamin C is associated with oxidative stress throughout the body. Vitamin C is required for the activity of the Mixed-Function Oxygenase System. This xenobiotic-metabolizing system operates in the microsomes and reticuloendothelial tissues of the liver. Depletion of vitamin C also destabilises the integrity of cytochrome P450 electron transport. Lastly, breakdown of cholesterol by hydroxylation occurs in the liver microsomes, and vitamin C is required for this process.[8]

Vitamin E is a powerful free radical scavenger, halting the chain reaction of lipid peroxidation in biological membranes. Despite the presence of glutathione peroxidase and other antioxidant systems, vitamin E deficiency in membranes will lead to insufficient protection against damage by hydroxyl radicals produced during cellular respiration. Conversely, if other antioxidant enzyme systems are impaired (e.g. lower glutathione peroxidase activity associated with selenium deficiency), the requirement for vitamin E's free radical scavenging activity increases proportionally.[9]

Selenium is used as a cofactor for glutathione peroxidase, the enzyme that catalyses GSH reduction reactions.

Phase I Herbal Support

Bioflavonoids are ubiquitous in photosynthesising cells. They are in the highest concentration in fruits and vegetables, especially citrus fruits, where they may represent as much as 1% of the fresh material. Over 4000 bioflavonoids have been identified from both higher and lower plants, and the list is constantly expanding. Plant flavonoids are powerful antioxidants and detoxicants. They inhibit lipid peroxidation, and provide direct scavenging activity. As therapeutic agents, several important flavonoids have been studied, including quercetin, green tea catechin, silymarin from Milk Thistle, flavonoid glycosides from Ginkgo biloba, and anthocyanins.

Quercetin is a bioflavonoid with antioxidant properties. After oral supplementation, quercetin is conjugated in vivo, yielding metabolites that exhibit antioxidant properties.[10] Reactive oxygen species contribute to many diseases. Flavonoids, such as quercetin and silibinin, can effectively protect cells and tissues against the injurious effects of reactive oxygen species.

Green Tea has been shown to increase antioxidant enzyme activity. The condensed tannins from Camellia sinensis have a free radical scavenging activity that is significantly greater than vitamin E.[11]

Milk Thistle (Silybum marianum) contains several therapeutic phytochemicals, including silymarin, silybin and silibinin. These constituents make Milk Thistle a unique hepatoprotective agent. Silymarin has been shown to protect liver cells from several toxic agents, including Amanita mushroom.[12]

Ginkgo (Ginkgo biloba) is an antioxidant and inhibits membrane lipid peroxidation.[13] The benefits of Ginkgo as an antioxidant have been studied primarily in the cardiovascular and neurological systems.

Anthocyanins were compared to other flavonoids in a study by Galvez et al to determine their capacity for flavonoid inhibition of membrane lipid peroxidation. The authors compared anthocyanins with catechins, flavonoids, flavones, and flavonones. Anthocyanins were found to be the most efficient at inhibiting lipid peroxidation. They were 2.5 times more effective than epicatechin and 40 times more effective than quercetin.[14]

Other nutrient cofactors required for cytochrome P450 reactions include riboflavin, niacin, magnesium, and iron.

The metabolites from phase I detoxification are often potentially more harmful than their original toxic compounds and it is important for health that they are not allowed to build up. This is where **Phase II detoxification** comes in. In phase II, glutathione conjugation is the primary pathway for these intermediate metabolites. Increased exposure to toxins as well as poor dietary supply of glutathione can soon lead to glutathione depletion and increased damage from these highly reactive intermediates. Oral supplementation with reduced glutathione or N-acetyl-cysteine may help to increase glutathione levels.

Detoxification - Phase II

Phase II Conjugation Reactions
Phase II reactions are biosynthetic reactions in which a xenobiotic or a Phase I-derived metabolite is linked to a molecule that makes it more water-soluble and less toxic. Excretion of conjugated toxins is dependent on their capacity to participate in transport mechanisms located in the liver, kidney and intestinal membranes.

Phase II Nutritional Support

Conjugating Agents
Glucuronidation is the most important Phase II conjugation reaction.

Glucuronidation pathways in Phase II can be reversed by beta glucuronidase enzymes produced by pathological bacteria, which causes toxins to be reabsorbed, increasing toxicity. Studies have shown that Calcium D-Glucarate, a natural ingredient found in certain vegetables and fruits can inhibit beta glucuronidase activity resulting in increased elimination of toxins. Supplements of Calcium D-

Glucarate may also be taken to enhance the glucuronidation pathway. [15]

By inhibiting beta-glucuronidase activity, the net elimination of carcinogens, toxins and steroid hormones via glucuronidation is increased.

Glutathione conjugation with glutathione S-transferase enzymes is critical to protect vital cellular components. These enzymes catalyse reactions that conjugate and detoxify a diverse group of xenobiotics. The cofactor for reactions catalysed by glutathione S-transferase enzymes is **reduced glutathione** (GSH), a tripeptide composed of glycine, cysteine and glutamic acid. The glutathione S-transferase enzymes protect cells from electrophilic xenobiotic compounds. These compounds, and their reactive intermediates produced by cytochrome P-450 metabolism, bind with GSH instead of covalently binding with cellular constituents and damaging cells.

Sulphation is another important conjugation reaction, and represents an effective means to decrease the activity of pharmacologic and toxicologic agents. In addition to detoxifying drugs, sulphation is important in the metabolism of endogenous compounds, such as catecholamines, some steroids and bile acids. By supporting Phase II sulphation and GSH conjugation, N-Acetylcysteine (NAC) is another protective agent against the toxic effects of many chemicals. It is the treatment of choice for acetaminophen overdose.[16] In animal studies, NAC had a protective effect against alcohol-induced ulcers. As an immune stimulant, NAC specifically supports the function of the Gut-Associated Lymphoid Tissue (GALT) by mediating communication between macrophages and lymphocytes and stimulating cytotoxic T-cells.

Methylation is a common conjugation reaction. Methyl groups are added to many exogenous and endogenous compounds to reduce their toxicity. Important examples include the O-methylation of catechol oestrogens and the biotransformation of homocysteine to methionine. Methylation is supported by methyl donors, such as betaine, folic acid and adenosylcobalamin.

Ornithine is an endogenous amino acid conjugator in birds and reptiles. However, L-ornithine-L-aspartate has clinical applications in humans. Clinical trials of ornithine aspartate have shown that it reduces ammonia levels, improves mental status, reduces the risk of coma and improves other clinical parameters in patients with hepatic encephalopathy and hyperammonemia.[17]

Other nutrients which play vital roles in Phase II pathway include the amino acids - cysteine, methionine, glutamic acid and aspartic acid.

In some people the detoxification pathways (Phase I and II) are out of balance.

For example, if Phase I is more active than Phase II, a build up of reactive intermediate metabolites can occur which in turn can lead to tissue damage and disease. These people are referred to as **Pathological Detoxifiers**.

Pathological detoxifiers can be identified as those individuals who are highly sensitive to fumes e.g. paints and perfumes, react adversely to various pharmaceutical drugs and they may have a reaction to drinking caffeine. Alternatively a liver detoxification test, available from Great Smokies Diagnostic Laboratory, can pinpoint exactly how efficiently one's liver is carrying out the detoxification process and if you are indeed a pathological detoxifier.

There is now an extensive body of evidence indicating that diet plays a crucial role in modifying the body's detoxification pathways. Even in allopathic medicine, grapefruit juice is used as a phytochemical for transplant patients because grapefruit contains naringenin which slows down Phase I enzyme activity. This enables such drugs as cyclosporin, which is given to these patients to prevent organ rejection, to stay in the system for longer, prior to the drug being detoxified. Pathological detoxifiers may also find it very useful to include grapefruit juice in their diet.

Vitamins and minerals - particularly the B vitamins - play a major role acting as cofactors for many enzyme systems including those of liver detoxification. Ensuring a plentiful supply of the B complex group of vitamins is of prime importance for optimum detoxification. Therefore, including plenty of whole grains containing dietary B vitamins, as well as taking a good B complex supplement, will aid the liver in this crucial role.

Depletion of vitamin C may also impair the detoxification process. Vitamin C also prevents free radical formation and is found in citrus fruits and green leafy vegetables. However, in order to obtain optimum amounts, supplementation is required. At least 1000mg a day is recommended.

Some individuals are unable to tolerate high doses of vitamin C in the form of ascorbic acid due to the acidity. Therefore pH buffered vitamin C, obtained from the Sago Palm, is an alkaline form of vitamin C, which can be tolerated by most individuals.

Vitamin E and selenium are cofactors for glutathione peroxidase activity as well as being powerful antioxidants. Vitamin E is a well-documented, free radical scavenger. It terminates free radical propagation reactions in the cellular membrane, thus helping to protect the membrane from lipid peroxidation. Vitamin E also works synergistically with Vitamin C.

Today, our diets are very low in selenium due to the depletion of this vital mineral in the soil. Supplementation is therefore imperative. Brazil nuts are one of the best food sources of selenium.

Cruciferous[18] vegetables such as broccoli, cauliflower, brussels sprouts and cabbage in the diet have been shown to enhance Phase I activities. It is thought that the indoles, which are the active ingredients in these foods, are the major contributors to this activity.

Zinc is another essential nutrient and acts as a cofactor for many enzyme systems. Zinc deficiency can cause a whole range of consequences. One important role that zinc plays is in the functioning of the enzyme alcohol dehydrogenase involved in the conversion of alcohols to aldehydes in Phase I detoxification.

Dietary Guidelines For Optimum Detoxification

The diet should include plenty of organic, unrefined, unprocessed foods, as fresh as possible in their natural state. Fresh vegetables, fruits, whole grains and unrefined carbohydrates should make up the majority of the diet. Red meats, animal fats, sugars and refined foods should be avoided, as should caffeine, alcohol and other stimulants.

Drink plenty of bottled water or diluted juice, at least two litres per day. Try to omit tea and coffee from the diet and instead drink herbal teas. A minimum of one serving daily of cruciferous vegetables and at least five servings of fresh fruit should be included in the daily diet. Protein sources can be obtained from lentils, soy, beans, nuts, seeds, fish, organic chicken, turkey and eggs.

In summary, therefore, it can be said that an efficient liver detoxification system is vital to health. In order to support this process it is essential that many key nutrients are included in the diet.

CAUTION: It is vital that a qualified healthcare practitioner supervise any diet. There are many specialised detoxification regimes but none of these may be advisable for Parkinson's disease patients. In Parkinson's disease, the ability of the liver to detoxify efficiently may be impaired making a detoxification programme completely inappropriate. When toxins are released too quickly, this can lead to ill health. However, just simple avoidance and removal of toxins from the diet could give many positive health benefits - increased energy, clear skin, more vitality and a general better feeling of wellbeing.

References

1. *Journal of Neural Transmission - Parkinson's disease and dementia section* 1994: 7(2): 83-100.

2. Williams, Steventon, Sturmann, Waring. *"Heredity variation involved with detoxification and neurodegenerative disease" Journal of Inherited Metabolic Disorders*: 1991: Vol 14 no. 4

3. *Casarett and Doull's Toxicology*: 1991: pps 88-126.

4. Perry et. al. *Neurosciences* lett. 33 1982.

5. Sechi, G et. al. *Prog Neuropsychopharmacol Biol Psychiatry* 20(7) 1996.

6. J Cell *Biochem* 1993:17F:S270-S277.

7. Mol *Aspects Med* 1994: 15 Suppl:S97-102.

8. *Modern Nutrition in Health and Disease* 8th ed.: 432 - 448.

9. *Modern Nutrition in Health and Disease* 8th ed.; 326-341.

10. Am J *Physiol* 1998; 275(1 Pt 2): R212-9.

11. *Plant Flavonoids in Biology and Medicine II*. Alan R. Lis Inc. 1988:135-38.

12. *Hum Toxicol* 1983:2:183-195.

13. *Presse Med* 1986:15:1475-1479

14. *Pharmacology* 1995:51(2):127-33.

15. *Biochem Med Metabol Biol* 1990;43(2):83-92, *Cancer Detect Prev* 1997;21(2):178-90.

16. J Pharm *Exp Ther* 1986: 238: pps54-61.

17. J Hepatol 1998; 28(5):856-64.

18. Zhang Y, *Tallalay P*, Cho GG. Posner GM.

    "A Major Inducer of Anticarcinogenic Protective Enzymes from Broccoli: Isolation and Elucidation of Structure: 1992: *Proceedings of the National Academy of Sciences* Vol 89 pps 2399-2403

Bibliography

BrainRecovery.com: David Perlmutter M.D: The Perlmutter Health Center, Naples Fl, USA.

Phytonutrients and Detoxification: Dr Mark Percival 1997: Clinical Nutrition Insight: Vol 5 No 2:

The 20 Day Rejuvenation Diet: Dr Jeff Bland: 1997: Keats Publishing, New Canaan, USA

Standard Detoxification Profile: Application Guide: 1997: Great Smokies Diagnostic Laboratory, Ashville, N Carolina USA

Innovative Clinical Approaches to the Cascade of Chronic Illness: 1997: Nutri Ltd, Buxton, UK

The Detoxification Process Simplified, HeathComm International: 1997: Gig Harbour, Washington USA

Functional Medicine Symposium - Course Notes: The Gut Liver Connection: Mitchell Kaminski M.D: 1998: Functional Medicine Institute, Gig Harbour, Washington, USA

Appleton J: *Phytonutrition for Hormonal Health* Vol 2 No 2 May 1999: Tyler Encapsulations Oregon USA

CHAPTER 9.7

Pregnancy

by Professor Lia Rossi Prosperi and Lucille Leader Dip ION

The following chapter is of potential interest to young people who have Parkinson's disease and are considering a pregnancy. We can currently only present guidelines, as there is not much scientific information on this subject available for people with Parkinson's disease. Both men and women must consult their neurologists and gynaecologists before embarking upon any pre-conceptual regime. There is much to be considered including genes, cellular status, general health, pharmaceutical treatment, social and care implications. As such, the authors cannot be held responsible for any individual nutritional programme followed and patients need the guidance of their own medical team.

Development of the Foetal Brain and Nutritional Aspects of Pregnancy

Malnutrition during pregnancy

The foetus grows and develops because of the nourishing substances (nutrients) and oxygen in the placenta[1].

A well-developed placenta is fundamental for the optimal development of the nervous system whereas a small placenta leads to the formation of fewer neurones[2].

During gestation the development of the nervous system begins very early on: the neural plate appears on the 18th day and head processes appear on the 20th day.

During foetal development, the localisation of neurones is organised. Their axons are developed and finally the nerve connections are established, starting from an immature pattern that will be perfected and completed in the adult.

In the foetus the process of cerebral development is programmed with perfect precision: every specific cerebral structure has to be constructed and completed in a very precise, genetically pre-arranged period of time.

In order to complete each of these stages it is necessary for adequate quantities of the essential nourishing substances to be available during this time; if these are lacking, the development of the nervous system will be impaired. Serious nutritional deficiencies cause serious damage, but even slight deficiencies even though of minimal entity may lead to sub-optimal development of the brain[3].

A slight nutritional deficiency can lead to reduced proliferation of neurones, to fewer dendritic branches and synapses and as a result, to insufficient cognitive and intellectual development[4].

Critical Periods in which the growth of the nervous system is particularly rapid.

First Criticial Period

This is from the 15th to 20th week[5] of gestation, during which neurones multiply and with optimal nourishment and oxygen supplies reach their maximum number.

If the mother is deficient in protein, vitamins and minerals, this can lead to a lower weight of the foetal brain at brain as a result of fewer neurones[6].

Nutritional deficiencies in the first critical period diminish the total number of neurones[7] and in particular the auxiliary neurones, which start working when those designed to carry out certain functions are damaged.

Nutritional supplementation at a later stage will not be able to compensate for the damage suffered[8]. As stated previously, the development of the nervous system follows very precise chronological steps and if nutritional deficiencies set in at these particular moments in time, the development of the nervous system will often be impaired.

Second Critical Period

This begins during the 25th week[9] of gestation and continues until the 2nd year after birth.

This second period is characterised by the process of "myelogenesis" during which the glial (neuroglia) cells produce a substance called myelin.

Myelin consists of 21.3% of protein and 78.7% of lipids; this substance covers the nerve fibres like a sheath and enables transmission of nervous impulses[10].

Insufficient quantities of myelin considerably diminish the speed with which the nervous impulse is transmitted.

Nutritional deficiencies of essential amino acids (lysin, methionine, threonine, leucine, isoleucine, valine, phenylalanine, tryptophan, histidine) and essential fatty acids (alpha linoleic acid and gamma linolenic acid) impair the process of "myelogenesis"[11].

During the last three months of pregnancy there is progressive transport of polyunsaturated fatty acids from the maternal to the foetal circulation[12].

During pregnancy serious or slight nutritional deficiencies may lead to cells being unable to synthesise vital enzymes for cell multiplication and maturity[13].

Folic acid deficiency and possible foetal damage

Research has demonstrated the close relationship between folic acid deficiency during gestation and subsequent defects in the nervous system of the new-born child. Folic acid is an important co-factor during the development of the foetal central nervous system when cells are dividing rapidly[14].

A varied, balanced diet will not always ensure adequate quantities of folic acid and for this reason women trying to conceive and those in the first trimester are advised to supplement with 0.4 mg of folic acid per day[15] in order to lower the risk of malformations in the baby's nervous system. Neural tube defects have been associated with folic acid deficiency.[16] It is recommended, however, to have the folate status of patients assessed and corrected during pre-conceptual preparation.

Iodine deficiency

Maternal iodine deficiency can cause irreversible damage to the child's brain and these effects can be avoided by correcting maternal iodine deficiency before pregnancy[17]. Prolonged iodine deficiency may cause cretinism characterised by mental deficiency and spastic diplegia[18]. Professional nutritional advice must be taken.

Lead, Methyl-mercury and Cadmium

There are heavy metals, which damage the foetal brain[19]. During pregnancy lead and methyl-mercury may pass through the placental barrier and reach the foetus. As the blood-brain barrier is not completely developed, heavy metals can accumulate inside the brain of the foetus.

An accumulation of methyl-mercury can cause serious motor, cognitive and intellectual deficiencies in the newborn baby and in the developing child[20].

Cadmium is a metal, which indirectly damages the nervous system of the foetus[21]. This metal does not pass from the mother to the foetus, but accumulates in the placenta and competes with the absorption of two fundamental minerals, zinc and copper, which are important for the development of the nervous system[22].

Nutritional Recommendations for Women and Men who are Contemplating a Pregnancy

It has been scientifically shown there is a close link between nutrition and foetal development of the nervous system. The nutritional status of both parents should be assessed before conception (at least 6 months beforehand).

Dental Treatment Considerations

It would be prudent to check dental health before embarking on pregnancy. Exposure to mercury presents a hazard to the developing foetus.

Some Practical Nutritional Advice for Future Parents

- Follow a varied and balanced diet including good sources of protein such as fish, eggs, soy, nuts (not cashews or peanuts) and seeds.

- Choose organic food, if possible, and food which is GMO free (Genetically Modified Organisms[23])

- Choose cooking methods such as steaming, using the residual water for stock. Grilling or roasting should be on lower temperatures. Boiling should be avoided as nutrients are lost by this method. When oil is heated during frying, free radicals are formed. This process is increased when temperatures soar above 180°C. It is ideal to use cooking or frying pans with a thermostat, if frying is unavoidable.

- Avoid cooking methods that lead to the formation of poisonous substances such as polycyclic hydrocarbons and benzopyrene. Barbecued food especially if the flames come into contact with it can cause the formation of benzopyrene and polycyclic hydrocarbons. Blackened food from pizza ovens, toasting and grilling should be avoided.

- Avoid cooking methods that excessively decrease the nutritional value of food such as boiling.

- Do not use aluminium or enamel pots and pans

- Do not heat or cook with polyunsaturated fats, margarine and oils. Only use unrefined polyunsaturated oils cold for salad dressings. Cook with cold pressed olive oil or a little butter

- Avoid alcoholic drinks and reduce caffeine consumption

- Regularly exercise gently, under professional supervision.

- Insure a well-functioning bowel without the use of harsh laxatives. Plenty of still mineral water, fruit and vegetables can be helpful. Prunes and apricots may also benefit.

- Try to get enough sleep - nine to ten hours, if possible, during a 24-hour period

- Eat smaller meals and snacks every couple of hours to help balance blood sugar and give energy

- Have your weight checked, regularly, by a health professional. Do not embark on any calorie restrictive diets on your own, as these are may not be appropriate during pregnancy. It is essential that all diets must be supervised

- Cows milk and gluten containing grains seem to be common sources of food intolerances. These should be checked. If indicated, these foods should be substituted.

- Do not smoke.

Dental Treatment Considerations

It would be prudent to check dental health before embarking on pregnancy. Exposure to mercury presents a hazard to the developing foetus (see the chapter *Mercury in Dentistry,* by Dr Jack Levenson).

Useful Biochemical Profiles (pre-conceptual assessment)

We recommend that the ideal time to have nutritional assessment is at least six months before conception. This allows adequate time for any nutritional deficiency to be corrected. Further assessments can be made during pregnancy, if indicated. Any nutritional therapy must be under the joint supervision of a doctor and a nutritionist.

Recommended nutritional tests are to be found on page 158.

NUTRITIONAL TESTS
Vitamins
B12 - (MMA Urine)
B1 - blood
B2 - blood
B3 - blood

B6 - blood
Biotin - blood
Folate - blood/urine

Minerals - sweat/blood/hair
Zinc
Magnesium
Manganese
Chromium
Selenium

Lead
Cadmium
Aluminium
Mercury

Essential Fatty Acids
Omega 6- red blood cells
Omega 3- red blood cells

Amino Acid Profile - blood/urine
Allergy/Food Intolerance - blood

GENERAL BIOCHEMICAL TESTS
Haematology and Biochemistry - blood
(to include Hb, Iron status and Ferritin)
Glucose monitoring - urine/blood
Hormone profiles (male and female) - saliva/blood
Genito-urinary tests to exclude infection
Parasites - stool/blood

Drugs and Pregnancy[24, 25, 26, 27, 28]
There is not much research data available about drugs and their effects on pregnancy in people with Parkinson's disease. However, the same recommendations would surely be prudent for people whether they have Parkinson's disease or not. It is always advisable to avoid the use of any potentially harmful drug[29] during pregnancy and even for a few months before as there is the risk that some chemicals may be harmful to the developing foetus. However, all cases are different and require careful consideration by the neurologist, gynaecologist and patient, well in advance of a pregnancy being contemplated.

Contraception
Methods of contraception should be discussed with the patient's gynaecologist or general practitioner. Patients with tremor and stiffness may find the use of

barrier methods difficult. Although practical, the contraceptive pill has associated risks and side effects which need to be taken into account[30]. It is essential that the pros and cons of all methods should be carefully assessed for each individual patient.

If patients are taking L-dopa or other drugs, they must discuss the possibility of temporary withdrawal of these from the therapeutic programme for some months before conception and during the pregnancy with their medical advisors. If a patient is able to have adequate movement without drugs, this might well be an option.

L-dopa should not be given to pregnant women or women of childbearing potential in the absence of adequate contraception. If pregnancy occurs in a woman taking "Madopar" the drug must be discontinued[31]. There is evidence of harmful effects in studies in pregnant rabbits and the benserazide component has been found to be associated with skeletal malformations in the rat[32].

Breast Feeding

Certain drugs taken by the mother are found in breast milk and may be harmful to the baby[33]. Patients taking L-dopa "Madopar" (Roche Products Limited) should not breast-feed their infants. The manufactures of L-dopa "Sinemet" also state that "Sinemet" (DuPont Pharmaceuticals Limited) should not be given to women during pregnancy or to nursing mothers[34]. It has appeared harmful in animal trials (visceral and skeletal malformations in rabbits). The safety of other drugs used needs to be assessed. Organophospates (pesticides) have been detected in breast milk. As organophosphates are thought to be implicated in the pathogenesis of Parkinson's disease, it would be advisable for the nursing mother to eat organic food, if available and also not have mercury fillings put in the mouth. Mercury has been found in breast milk and is highly toxic.

In strict collaboration with her gynaecologist, neurologist, paediatrician and nutritionist, she will either need to

a) Remain off drugs until the baby is weaned off the breast

OR

b) Resume the Parkinson's drug regime after the birth and feed the baby by bottled formula.

If it is possible for the mother to cope physically with the baby without the use of drugs, it is preferable for her to breast-feed. The nutritional formula offered by breast milk from a mother, providing she has an adequate nutritional status, is best for the baby as it contains valuable ingredients which are not always found in bottled formulas. These are essential to vital immune processes including at intestinal level.

Infertility

Some general considerations

Assessment by the appropriate medical specialist is recommended. Medical conditions other than Parkinson's disease may affect fertility.

Genito-urinary infections can affect fertility.

Physical difficulties experienced during intercourse may need remedial measures. In-vitro fertilisation (IVF) may be necessary.

The status of male and female hormones and nutrients is relevant to fertility and should be assessed.

Stress management and counselling may be necessary.

References

1. Malnutrizione E Sviluppo Cognitivo, Estratto Da *"Trattato Enciclopedico Di Psicologia Dell'eta' Evolutiva"* Volume Ii – Tomo Ii: P. 762: E. Caracciolo: Ed.Piccin: Italia

2. Malnutrizione E Sviluppo Cognitivo, Estratto Da *"Trattato Enciclopedico Di Psicologia Dell'eta' Evolutiva"* Volume II – Tomo II: pps. 763, 764, 765: E. Caracciolo: Ed.Piccin: Italia

3. Malnutrizione E Sviluppo Cognitivo, Estratto Da *"Trattato Enciclopedico Di Psicologia Dell'eta' Evolutiva"* Volume II – Tomo II: P. 764: E. Caracciolo: Ed.Piccin: Italia

4. Malnutrizione E Sviluppo Cognitivo, Estratto Da *"Trattato Enciclopedico Di Psicologia Dell'eta' Evolutiva"* Volume II – Tomo II: pps. 763, 764: E. Caracciolo: Ed.Piccin: Italia

5. Malnutrizione E Sviluppo Cognitivo, Estratto Da *"Trattato Enciclopedico Di Psicologia Dell'eta' Evolutiva"* Volume II – Tomo II: P. 754: E. Caracciolo: Ed.Piccin: Italia

6. Malnutrizione E Sviluppo Cognitivo, Estratto Da *"Trattato Enciclopedico Di Psicologia Dell'eta' Evolutiva"* Volume II – Tomo II: pps. 765,767,769: E. Caracciolo: Ed.Piccin: Italia

7. Malnutrizione E Sviluppo Cognitivo, Estratto Da *"Trattato Enciclopedico Di Psicologia Dell'eta' Evolutiva"* Volume II – Tomo II: pps. 753, 766: E. Caracciolo: Ed.Piccin: Italia

8. Malnutrizione E Sviluppo Cognitivo, Estratto Da *"Trattato Enciclopedico Di Psicologia Dell'eta' Evolutiva"* Volume II – Tomo II: P. 773: E. Caracciolo: Ed.Piccin: Italia

9. Malnutrizione E Sviluppo Cognitivo, Estratto Da *"Trattato Enciclopedico Di Psicologia*

Dell'eta' Evolutiva" Volume II – Tomo II: P. 754: E. Caracciolo: Ed.Piccin: Italia

10. Malnutrizione E Sviluppo Cognitivo, Estratto Da *"Trattato Enciclopedico Di Psicologia Dell'eta' Evolutiva"* Volume II – Tomo II: pps. 753, 756, 766: E. Caracciolo: Ed.Piccin: Italia

11. Malnutrizione E Sviluppo Cognitivo, Estratto Da *"Trattato Enciclopedico Di Psicologia Dell'eta' Evolutiva"* Volume II – Tomo II: pps. 758, 766, 767, 776: E. Caracciolo: Ed.Piccin: Italia

12. Nutrizione E Cervello Cap.VI: pps 217 - 218: M.Giovannini, C.Agostoni: Pytagora Press-Milano: Italia

13. Malnutrizione E Sviluppo Cognitivo, Estratto Da *"Trattato Enciclopedico Di Psicologia Dell'eta' Evolutiva"* Volume II – Tomo II: P. 773: E. Caracciolo: Ed.Piccin: Italia

14. Le Vitamine: A Fidanza: Cap.VII: P. 95: 1990: Ed.Agnesotti-Roma: Italia

15. ASM Associazione Studio Malformazioni :P.1

16. *Prevention Of Neural- Tube Defects With Folic Acid In China*: R.I. Berry,Z. Li, J.D. Erickson Et Al: New England J Of Med 1999:341:pps 1485-90

17. Gli Oligoelementi Nella Nutrizione E Nella *Salute Dell'uomo-Schede Informative* N°3-4: P 46: 1996: Istituto Scotti Bassani (In Collaborazione Con World Organization-Geneva)–Milano: Italia

18. Gli Oligoelementi Nella Nutrizione E Nella *Salute Dell'uomo-Schede Informative* N°3-4: P 46: 1996: Istituto Scotti Bassani (In Collaborazione Con World Organization-Geneva)–Milano: Italia

19. Gli Oligoelementi Nella Nutrizione E Nella *Salute Dell'uomo-Schede Informative* N°3-4: P 141: 1996: Istituto Scotti Bassani (In Collaborazione Con World Organization-Geneva)–Milano: Italia

20. Nutrizione E Cervello Cap.XIII:P. 413: A Giacobazzi, C Truzzi, R Avallone, A. Ventura E M. Baraldi: Pytagora Press-Milano: Italia

21. Gli Oligoelementi Nella Nutrizione E Nella *Salute Dell'uomo-Schede Informative* N°3-4: P 141: 1996: Istituto Scotti Bassani (In Collaborazione Con World Organization-Geneva)–Milano: Italia

22. Gli Oligoelementi Nella Nutrizione E Nella *Salute Dell'uomo- Schede Informative* N°3-4: P 141: 1996: Istituto Scotti Bassani Milano: Italia (In Collaborazione Con World Organization, Geneva, Switzerland)

23. *Effects Of Diets Containing Genetically Modified Potatoes Expressing Galanthus Nivalis Lectin On Rat Small Intestine* (Lett): S.W. Ewen, A. Pusztai : 1999: The Lancet: 354 (9187) (Letter): pps. 1353 -1354

24. *Parkinson's Disease And Pregnancy*: L I Golbe: 1987 July: Neurology 37 (7): pps. 1245 - 1249

25. *Pregnancy And Parkinsonism: A Case Report Without Problem*: H Allain, D Bentue-Ferrer, D Milon, P Moran, F Jacquemard, G Defawe: 1989 June: Clinical Neuropharmacology, 12 (3): pps. 217 - 219

26. *Pregnancy And Parkinson's Disease: A Review Of The Literature And A Case Report*: 1998 January: Movement Disorders 13(1): pps. 34 - 38

27. *Selegiline, Pregnancy And Parkinson's Disease*: A Kupsch And W H Oertel: 1998 January: Movement Disorders 13(1): pps. 175 - 176

28. *The Effect Of Pregnancy In Parkinson's Disease*: L M Shulman, A Minagar, W J Weiner: 2000 January: Movement Disorders 15(1): pps. 132 - 135

29. *Folic Acid Antagonists During Pregnancy And The Risk Of Birth Defects*: New England J Med:2000: 343: Pps1608-14

30. *The Bitter Pill*: pps. 77 - 102, 115 - 151, 61 - 67, 203 - 225, 26 - 40, 41 - 60, 200, 106: Dr Ellen Grant: 1986: Corgi Books (Transworld Publishers Limited): London, UK

31. *ABPI Compendium Of Data Sheets And Summaries Of Product Characteristics*: P. 1332: 1999/2000: Datapharm Publications Limited, London, UK.

32. *ABPI Compendium Of Data Sheets And Summaries Of Product Characteristics*: P. 1333: 1999/2000: Datapharm Publications Limited, London, UK.

33. *ABPI Compendium Of Data Sheets And Summaries Of Product Characteristics*: P. 1333: 1999/2000: Datapharm Publications Limited, London, UK.

34. *ABPI Compendium Of Data Sheets And Summaries Of Product Characteristics*: P. 372:1999/2000: Datapharm Publications Limited, London, UK.

Bibliography

Nutritional Biochemistry:Tom Brody:1999:Academic Press (Harcourt Brace& Co):San Diego Ca, USA, London, UK

Sex, Health And Nutrition:Robert Erdmann Phd And Meirion Jones:1992:Thorsons:London, UK

Planning For A Healthy Baby:Belinda Barnes And Suzanne Gail Bradley:1990:Vermilion An Imprint Of Ebury Press, Random House UK Ltd, London, UK

The Bitter Pill: Ellen Grant MB Ch BD Obst RCOG:1986:Corgi Books (Transworld Publishers Limited): London, UK

CHAPTER 10

Sexuality and Parkinson's Disease

by Dr Michael Perring MA MB BChir FCP(SA) DPM

Introduction

The study by health professionals of the sexual lives of patients with chronic disease is relatively recent, focusing principally during the past 20 years on multiple sclerosis, diabetes, post-coronary care, stroke, spinal injuries and cancer.[1]

- Parkinson's disease has received greater attention as more young people have been affected. Quality of life issues, including the maintenance of sexual function for Parkinson's disease patients and their partners, are now recognised as being, for them, a primary concern.[2]

- Sexual problems arise from the cumulative effects of the disease process itself, from the effects of medication, and from the stress of social and psychological factors.

This article reviews the nature of sexual problems amongst Parkinson's disease sufferers and the management of the individual with Parkinson's disease to optimise sexual function.

Definition - What is Parkinson's Disease?

Parkinson's disease is a chronic, progressive disease of the central nervous system. The classic symptoms are tremor at rest, rigidity (stiffness), bradykinesia (slowness of movement) and hypokinesia (reduced body movement). There is postural instability (unsteadiness) with difficulty in stopping, starting and turning when walking. Typically tremor and stiffness develop on one side of the body, later becoming bilateral. Involvement of the autonomic nervous system may lead to difficulty in controlling the bladder, constipation, disturbed sleep, excessive sweating, intolerance to extremes of heat and cold, postural hypotension, and sexual problems. The disease is progressive but clinical symptoms do not follow a regular pattern. Most people are diagnosed over the age of 60, but one in 20 are under 40 years of age at the time of diagnosis.

Prevalence - how common is Parkinson's disease?

165/100,000 of the general population will develop Parkinson's disease[3]. This increases to one person in 200 over the age of 65, and one in 50 over the age of 80. Approximately 120,000 people in the UK have Parkinson's at the present time.

Pathogenesis - how does the disease process develop?

The hallmark of Parkinson's disease is degeneration in the mid-brain of the dopaminergic nigrostriatal pathway. These are pigmented nerve cells located in the substantia nigra producing dopamine. Recently adjacent neurones in the locus coeruleus and ventral tegmental areas have been implicated along with the neurotransmittors nor-adrenaline and serotonin.

The principle function at these mid-brain sites is the control of muscle movement. When 80% of the dopamine producing cells are destroyed symptoms of Parkinson's disease appear and the severity of Parkinson's disease thereafter is proportional to a further loss of cells.

The underlying cause of the condition in certain families may be genetic with involvement of a site on chromosome 4[4]. A genetic precipitant would also require an environmental trigger - contaminated well water and pesticides have been described as risk factors. An infective cause was clear in the epidemic of cephalotis lethargica in the 1920's.

Sexual Function

- Sexual function in humans is varied and complex! In its expression it may be limited to the imagination, or sublimated in other ways, for instance, in the arts or at work.

- Sexual activity, on the other hand, involves the body as well as the mind, and requires structural integrity of the endocrine, neurological, and musculo-skeletal systems. Furthermore sexual activity occurs within a supportive social setting and depends, amongst other things, on the availability of a partner and the opportunity for sexual activity. Functionally sexual activity involves anticipation, arousal, and orgasm, and is followed in men, but not in women, by a refractory period when no sexual activity can take place. Sexual interest, or libido, provides the drive which leads to sexual activity being sought out. A psychosexual response cycle has been described by Masters and Johnson[5] for the phases of sexual arousal:

Physiology of the Sexual Response in Men

In men, penile tumescence is an early sign of sexual excitement and arousal. Erection results from dilatation of the arterial vasculature of the penis, so that more blood flows into the penis, and closure of the venous valves so that less blood flows out[6]. The size of the non-erect penis does not relate to its size when erect and in the obese it appears smaller than it is as a prepubic pad of fat makes it less visible.

In later stages of arousal (Master and Johnson's Plateau phase of the cycle) increased excitement is accompanied by further engorgement of the tip of the penis (the glans). Secretions from the paraurethral glands lubricate the urethral opening. The duration of this phase is under voluntary control, but is brief if the individual is anxious and may lead to premature ejaculation.

The Orgasmic phase of the cycle is preceded by a moment of 'ejaculatory inevitability' (the point of no return) after which voluntary control is lost. This moment is marked by the contraction of 'smooth' muscle fibres in the prostate gland and seminal vesicles (supplied by the autonomic nervous system) The second phase of ejaculation involves rhythmic contractions of smooth muscle in the perineum and urethra. During this phase closure of the internal sphincter of the bladder prevents retrograde flow of ejaculate into the bladder.

Immediately following ejaculation there is a refractory period when further ejaculation is impossible.

Sensation in the male genitalia is derived via the pudendal nerve which arises from the spinal cord at the level of the sacrum (S2-4). The functions of erection and orgasm are controlled by the autonomic nervous system, parasympathetic activity (S2-4) predominating during erection and sympathetic activity (T11-L3) during ejaculation. While erection can occur as a spinally mediated event (reflex spinal erection) fibres from the autonomic nervous system are relayed via the spinal cord to higher centres in the brain (the limbic system). Animal studies have shown that erection and ejaculation may occur by electrical stimulation of the preoptic area, lateral hypothalamus, tegmentum, and anterior cingulate gyrus[7]. Both excitation and inhibition of erection may be induced by stimulation of different cortical centres. An overall inhibitory effect of the cortex on erection is suggested by the lowered threshold to erection which follows spinal cord transection.

Male Sex Hormones

Male hormones, or androgens, include testosterone, dihydrotestosterone, androstenedione, and Dihydroepiandrosterone (DHEA). They are produced in the testis and adrenal glands under the control of stimulating hormones (FSH and LH) from the pituitary gland. The pituitary in turn responds to stimuli from higher centres by producing more FSH and LH as androgen levels drop (a feedback loop mechanism). There is, thus, a sensitive means of maintaining androgens levels in the blood.

Androgens provide the sex-drive (libido) which motivates sexual behaviour and heightens sexual arousal (leading to an increase in spontaneous erections). There are widespread actions of androgens which serve to maintain secondary sex and other male characteristics (muscle bulk, bone density, cardiac blood flow, and mental alertness).

The Effects of Ageing on Male Sexuality

Hormone levels usually decline very gradually from a peak in late adolescence. In some men a more rapid decline in their late 50's leads to symptoms akin to the menopause in women (hot flushes, aches and pains in joints, loss of energy including libido, and a sense of slowing up mentally). Various elements of the sexual response cycle are effected: there is a reduction in the ease of erection, and in its firmness and sustainability; erection, once lost, is less easily recovered. Orgasms are less intense and rhythmic contractions of smooth muscle are of shorter duration. The volume of the ejaculate (seminal and prostatic fluid) is reduced and the refractory period following ejaculation is longer. While the need to ejaculate is experienced less intensely sexual satisfaction amongst older men (and women) is often reported to be good, and the ability to continue functioning sexually certainly remains an important element of the older male's self-image. The frequency of sexual activity decreases with age but is very variable. Men (and women) who commence sexual activity early in life are more likely, disability aside, to continue sexual activity till late in life. Frequency of sexual activity for men and women correlates positively with the availability of a partner and inversely with the duration of a relationship[8].

Physiology of the Sexual Response in Women

For women the choice of a sexual partner and courtship underline the importance of the social context in which female sexuality takes place. Emotional closeness for women is more often than for men a prerequisite for sexual activity.

- The stages of the sexual response cycle, as in men, are arousal, orgasm and resolution - arousal may be considered as having an initial excitement phase followed by a plateau phase. In the excitement phase an increase in the blood flow to the genitals leads to labial and vaginal engorgement, and lubrication. The speed and intensity of arousal varies greatly. The plateau phase describes a more or less steady state of high arousal, which is still not so intense as to trigger orgasm. In this phase there is retraction of the clitoral hood. The anatomy of the clitoris has recently been shown (in dissection studies of younger women) to be more extensive than previously thought[9].

- With further stimulation and vascular engorgement to the clitoris a sense of orgasmic inevitability (similar to the male experience of inevitability) occurs and is followed by orgasm. Orgasm is an intense pleasurable sensation in the genital region and is accompanied by rhythmic contractions of the vaginal wall, Fallopian tubes and pubo-coccygeus muscle (a 'sling' of muscle in the floor of the pelvis), and with widespread changes elsewhere. A skin flush from dilation of blood vessels occurs indicating involvement of the autonomic nervous system throughout the body. A difference from the male sexual response cycle is the absence in women of a refractory period after orgasm. This enables women to have several orgasms within a short period of time. The experience of orgasm by women is very variable and in a significant proportion of women is not regularly achieved except by self-stimulation. Female ejaculation from glands homologous to the male prostate occurs in a proportion of women at the time of orgasm.

- In the resolution phase of the sexual response cycle detumescence occurs. The more prolonged the arousal the more gradual is resolution. If sexual tension has been high but without an orgasm, then resolution is slower.

The neurological basis to sexual arousal in women is similar to that in men: pudendal and autonomic nerve supplies are responsible for tumescence, lubrication, and orgasm, corresponding to the functions of erection and ejaculation in men.

Female Sex Hormones
The ovary produces oestrogens - oestradiol, oestrone and oestriole - and progesterone, in amounts which wax and wane with the menstrual cycle. Their production is under the control of stimulating hormones (FSH and LH) from the anterior pituitary gland, and their action is to create in the womb a suitable milieu for the implantation of a fertilised ovum. Under the influence of oestrogens and later progesterone the endometrial lining of the womb proliferates in preparation for implantation. In the absence of a fertilised ovum it is subsequently shed at menstruation (the menstrual period).

Androgens (testosterone and DHEA) are secreted by the adrenal gland and assist in maintaining libido. They are sometimes prescribed for this purpose, in which case there are additional benefits to energy and wellbeing.

The Effects of Ageing on Female Sexuality
Women's capacity to respond sexually peaks in the 4th decade. Changes in hormone production (reduced oestrogen and increased FSH) and corresponding changes in body function occur when ovulation ceases. This is termed the menopause and may be accompanied by hot flushes, night sweats, aching in the joints, and a reduction in physical and mental energy and well being. Other ageing changes include diminished intensity to sensation and orgasm and a

general reduction in the bodies' sexual responsiveness. Oestrogen, however, continues to be produced in the bodies' fat stores and may moderate the effects of the menopause. Where loss of oestrogens is severe supplemental oestrogen and progesterone (or synthetic Progestogens) may be considered. Continuing sexual activity helps to maintain genital function such as vaginal lubrication, while reported sexual satisfaction remains high even when the physiological response of arousal is reduced.

Studies on Sexual Dissatisfaction, Sexual Dysfunction and Frequency of Sexual Activity.

- **How common is dissatisfaction with sex or specific sexual problems amongst the disabled?**
  Stewart[10] studied the frequency of sexual dissatisfaction amongst UK individuals living in the community with physical disability. In a sample of 212 disabled people, aged from 20-64 years, he found that most (77%) were married and over half (54%) were 'suffering some problem which served as an obstacle to satisfaction of their sexual need'.

- **How do the able-bodied compare?**
  Unfortunately there are few reports for comparison of sexual satisfaction amongst healthy couples in the 50 plus population. Frank[11], in the US, studied 100 'well-educated and happily married couples', with a mean age range of 35-37 years. 14% of the men and 15% of the women reported their sexual relationship to be 'not very', or 'not at all', satisfying.

  Osborn[12], in the UK, studying a sample of 436 healthy women of varying ages, found 10% of respondents 'believed they had a sexual problem'.

  Welsh et al reported in 1997 on 27 women with Parkinson's disease comparing them to a healthy control group. 50% of each group were sexually active but dissatisfaction with the quality of the sexual experience was more often expressed by the group with Parkinson's disease. This group had higher levels of anxiety, vaginal tightness (a symptom of anxiety), and problems with bladder control. The self-image of women was poor in this group and they had a higher incidence of depression. In this study, as in others, increasing age correlated with a reduction in sexual activity and satisfaction.

■ **How do patients with Parkinson's disease compare with the disabled?**

A study of a younger population with Parkinson's disease was undertaken by Brown (1990) in the UK. He found that amongst 34 couples 59% of the males and 36% of the females were moderately or severely dissatisfied sexually, whilst analysis of sexual dysfunction in this group showed 65% of the male patients and 52% of their partners had sexual problems. It was notable that moderate or severe sexual difficulty was reported more frequently in those couples where the male was the patient. However, couples who perceived themselves as having a sexual problem were not necessarily sexually dissatisfied. The authors suggest this may indicate that couples develop strategies to minimize the impact of Parkinson's disease on their sex life. In the same study sexual problems were commoner amongst individuals who were older, had more severe symptoms, and who were depressed.

The Frequency of Sexual Activity

The frequency of sexual activity is commonly reduced in Parkinson's disease in both sexes. This arises from a combination of factors, including disability due to Parkinson's disease itself, fatigue, side effects of medication, and psychological factors in patients and their partners.

Symptoms of Parkinson's disease interfere with the physical act of intercourse: muscle stiffness and rigidity with resistance to movement of the limbs, a reduction in spontaneous movement; difficulty in maintaining balance and tremor. Sometimes involvement of the autonomic nervous system may lead, for example, to difficulty in sexual arousal, control of the bladder or bowel, changes in postural blood pressure causing faintness or dizziness, and increased sweating.

Because of drug regimes motor function is best for many patients in the morning and worst at night. Consequently sexual activity may be preferred in the morning.

Psychological factors in the Parkinson's disease sufferer co-exist with physical disability. The Parkinson's disease patient and their partner need to think flexibly. For example, a less active role in lovemaking for a man who has reduced mobility requires a partner willing to initiate sexual activity. Change from an active role to one of greater dependency may effect how he or she feels about himself or herself. Loss of self-esteem may be compounded by social factors, such as financial dependence or job insecurity, and physical factors, such as fatigue. Depression often, and anxiety sometimes, reduce the frequency of lovemaking whether associated with Parkinson's disease or in a physically healthy population.

What sort of Sexual Dysfunction do patients with Parkinson's Disease have?

Male sexual dysfunction's are categorized as loss of desire, problems with arousal and/or maintaining an erection, premature ejaculation, and retarded ejaculation.

In women, sexual dysfunctions are loss of desire, problems with arousal (anorgasmia), and painful spasm of the vagina (vaginismus).

Physical and psychological reasons for sexual problems often overlap, and this certainly holds true for individuals with Parkinson's disease.

Brown (1990)[13] studied sexual function in 34 young patients and their partners. The commonest symptom amongst couples was reduced frequency of sexual activity. This may have reflected loss of desire due to psychological factors such as depression and anxiety; or it may have been secondary to a specific sexual problem such as impotence; or for social reasons, for instance a lack of opportunity for sexual activity. A common finding was difficulty in communicating between spouses, particularly where the Parkinson's disease sufferer was male.

Amongst younger male patients the commonest sexual problems were erectile dysfunction (60%) and premature ejaculation (65%). The women patients had problems with arousal (orgasm) and, less commonly, vaginismus. Both avoidance of sex and impaired sensation were reported in the spouses of both sexes indicating possible problems with attraction for their partner, and anxiety.

Singer et al (1990)[14] found a similar prevalence of erectile problems (62%) in a Parkinson's disease group as against a matched control group in whom 37% had erectile problems. While autonomic symptoms, duration of treatment with L-dopa, and age, did not correlate with the presence of erectile dysfunction, the authors thought erectile dysfunction might be directly attributable to the severity of Parkinson's disease. On the other hand other reports have implicated the autonomic nervous system in the development of erectile problems.

Psychological Factors

For the patient with Parkinson's disease and for their partner there are many reasons why sexual function may be effected by psychological issues. Sexual behaviour is often a barometer of general health and in Parkinson's disease may reflect the unhappiness and quiet desperation which clinically manifests itself as a depressive illness. A psychological reaction to the diagnosis of physical disease process, and to side-effects of the drugs used in its treatment, is inevitable.

As described below in the story of John Smith, shock as an initial reaction, with denial, anger and emotional lability, is common. In some respects it is similar to the process of mourning - after all, death has occurred to aspects of the self, and this loss needs to be grieved. A satisfactory outcome to this process, which may take 18 months to 3 years, is indicated by acceptance and adaptation, in which the patient has a realistic appreciation of his/her situation and can focus on effective outcomes within limits imposed by the disease. The pre-morbid personality of the patient indicates the likely extent to which adjustment may be achieved. Social issues include loss of perceived attractiveness, independence and self-esteem, uncertainty about the future, and financial difficulties.

What help can care-givers provide? In the first instance, clear information about the nature of the disease process, on-going counselling throughout the course of the disease, and practical help with aids and services to the Parkinson's disease patient and their household. The aims of helpers throughout the course of the illness should be to improve the quality of the patient's daily living and to maintain their independent lifestyle.

Effects of Medication on Sexual Function

It is difficult to distinguish sexual symptoms due to medication from those due to the direct involvement of Parkinson's disease in the autonomic nervous system, depression and other psychological issues.

In contrast to the hypokinesis that is typical of Parkinson's disease, dyskinesias related to anti-parkinsonian drugs involve hyperkinetic choreo-athetoid, lurching, and jerky movements. For many patients these abnormal involuntary movements are unsightly, exhausting, painful and disabling, They often occur at the same time as the effects of each levodopa dose decline.

The side-effects of levodopa may affect the timing of sexual activity: there is less fatigue and better control of movement in the morning. Fatigue is associated with loss of libido and reduced frequency of sexual activity. Fatigue also adds to the stress that a Parkinson's disease patient is experiencing and we may therefore expect them to have problems of arousal: erectile dysfunction and anorgasmia. Since wakefulness may occur as a consequence of taking levodopa, lack of sleep may lead to exhaustion. The distracting nature of these side-effects are associated with a poor self-image and with depression. This lack of self-confidence and alteration of mood are further reasons for sexual difficulties.

L-dopa is occasionally associated with increased sexual activity. This may be a problem when heightened sexual interest in the patient is not shared by their partner, or is present in a patient who has dementia, or is in an institution.

Optimizing Sexual Function in Parkinson's Disease

The problems for those suffering from Parkinson's disease, typically in their 60's at the onset of the disease, are superimposed on the other problems of a population of that age. Myocardial infarction, for example, has been shown to lead to an approximately 50% reduction in sexual activity after rehabilitation is completed.

In any case, there is by the age of 60 in a healthy population, a wide range in the level of sexual activity and interest. We know, for instance, that the frequency of sexual activity in couples relates inversely to the time they have lived together[15] and in a relationship of over 30 years duration many will have evolved into a companionate rather than sexually active lifestyle . On the other hand an individual who is sexually active from an early age is more likely to remain active sexually than someone whose first sexual experience occurred late. Brecher's survey of sexual lifestyles in the States showed continuing sexual activity into the 80's where there was no significant disease and while sexual activity was desired.

It follows that what we might consider to be 'normal' as regards frequency and interest in sexual activity is very variable. The guiding principle for carers is that the Parkinson's disease sufferer is to be supported in maintaining a sexual identity, while the means to sexual activity, should they so wish it, needs to be considered in the context of their personal and social situation.

Managing Sexual Problems in Men with Parkinson's Disease

Erectile Dysfunction

The commonest sexual problem in Parkinson's disease is erectile dysfunction (ED), or impotence. It is defined as a failure to achieve or maintain an erection sufficient for penetration to take place. It occurs most probably in Parkinson's disease as a result of the depression which so frequently complicates the illness. Conversely, depression may itself be a consequence of sexual difficulties. It should be remembered, though, that in healthy adults of this age erectile failure occurs in 30-40% of the population. In Parkinson's disease the incidence is about 60%. Difficulty in maintaining an erection after penetration occurs commonly in Parkinson's disease and progresses in parallel with the disability from the disease.

The approach to treatment advocated by Masters and Johnson in the 1970's emphasized psychological factors and the removal of 'performance anxiety' in a behavioural programme which structured sexual activity for the couple. They suggested that at the beginning of the programme physical contact should be non-genital only. Such an agreement allowed exploration of shared sensual pleasure by touching and stroking. A 'sensate focus' exercise was agreed as an assignment reported in a therapy session after a few sessions of practice at home. The essence of 'sensate focus' exercises is that the recipient focuses attention on the spot of their body which is being touched. There is increased awareness and sensation at that spot, and attention is diverted by this means from thoughts about overall sexual performance. Repeating the exercise, taking turns to be the receiver, leads to relaxation and heightened sensual pleasure. Later assignments with increasing body contact (from non-genital to genital touching) leads after 8-10 sessions to penetrative sex. In the course of sessions with the therapist there is opportunity to explore emotional issues that may be limiting arousal, for example undisclosed anger, feelings of shame, or loss of self-esteem. Initially the outcome to treatment was considered by Masters and Johnson to have been successful (in a highly selected group of patients) in as many as 75% of cases, but their success rate was not replicated in the modified behavioural programmes adopted in the UK. Subsequently there has been greater recognition of the role of physical factors in the causation of ED - diffuse arterial disease and the side-effects of drugs being common examples.

Current approaches to treatment in ED utilise relaxation techniques and focusing to counter performance anxiety, as well as psychotherapy to explore underlying issues. But a high proportion of adults who have an accompanying physical disease such as Parkinson's disease can now benefit from the advent of new drugs which enhance erection. There are several drugs on the market which increase the vascular supply to the penis: Sildenafil, which is taken orally, and Alprostadil taken as a pellet placed in the tip of the urethra or by injection directly into the penis (the corpus cavernosum). The use of these drugs is discussed below. I have placed them in an order which reflects their ease of use. Which one is preferred will depend on the individual's situation.

Sildenafil (Viagra)

Clinically available since 1998 this is the simplest to use of the new chemical aids to erection. Taking it is socially discrete, there are minimal side-effects, and, when it works, it is consistent in its action. A distinctive feature about Sildenafil is that erection only occurs when the individual is sexually excited. An initial dose of 25-50mg (subsequently increasing to a maximum of 100mg in a 24 hour period) may cause side-effects of facial flushing in about 15 minutes, and mild indigestion, coloured haloes around objects and a mild headache. These effects are dose-related and transient. If Sildenafil is taken before an evening meal an increased erectile response occurs with sexual excitement for up to 18 hours; the peak effect lasts about 4 hours starting about an hour after taking the tablet. There are no reported interactions with drugs (L-dopa and dopamine agonists) used in Parkinson's disease, though metabolism of Sildenafil by a cytochrome P450 isoform in the liver is shared with certain other drugs including Erythromycin and Cimetidine, so that concurrent use of either drug may be taken with a half dose of Sildenafil.

In one small study ten men with erectile dysfunction and Parkinson's disease were given 50 mg Sildenafil on 8 occasions of attempted intercourse. The average age of the men was 72.8 years with Parkinson's disease of 7.5 years duration. Significant improvement was found in sexual satisfaction, sexual desire, ability to achieve and maintain erection, and ability to achieve orgasm[16].

Alprostadil (Muse)

Alprostadil is structurally similar to the natural substance in the body called Prostaglandin E1. It acts by widening blood vessels so that blood can flow into the penis more easily. Marketed in the form of a pellet the size of a pin-head the drug is placed in the opening at the tip of the urethra using an applicator. The technique for doing this is easy and painless. To assist the drug's action, physical activity such as walking which mobilises blood flow to the pelvis, may be needed.

The initial dose of Alprostadil is 250 micrograms increasing to a maximum of 1000 micrograms as necessary. Erection occurs within 10 minutes and lasts between 30 to 60 minutes. Not more than two doses are recommended in any 24 hour period. Interaction with other medication is unlikely because of the low levels of alprostadil in the blood. Decongestants, appetite suppressants and some drugs used to control high blood pressure may diminish the response to Alprostadil.

Alprostadil (Caverject)

The first of the new drugs for erection Caverject remains for some men the most reliable way to get an erection. It is also the most invasive in that individuals need to learn the technique of self injection into the corpus cavernosum.

Doses vary between an initial dose of 1.25 micrograms and a maximum of 60 micrograms. Usually an effective dose is between 5 and 20 micrograms which gives an erection after a few minutes and lasts about an hour. If the erection with Alprostadil lasts more than four to six hours (priapism) blood needs to be drawn off the corpora cavernosa in order to detumesce the penis. Failure to do this may otherwise make subsequent erection more difficult. Bruising sometimes occurs at the site of injection, though this is less likely with a good injection technique.

Rarely a bend develops in the penis after repeated injections (Peyronie's disease).

There are prepared syringes of Alprostadil available for injection under the trade name of Viridal Duo and Caverject Dual Chamber. These may be easier to administer and their action is similar to Caverject.

Male Hormones

Male hormones or androgens, of which testosterone is an example, are indicated when the bodies' production of its own hormones has declined (hypogonadism). Androgens have numerous actions in the body which help to maintain mental and physical performance. They also increase libido, sexual fantasies and spontaneous erections. As a consequence they may be taken to enhance men's sexual experience. Some men have an 'andropause' in the mid-fifties akin to the female menopause. It is heralded by flushes, joint pains, fatigue, loss of libido, and a sense of ageing. Men may also have at the andropause an increased difficulty in maintaining an erection and flattening of affect. Blood levels of free testosterone (which measures testosterone activity) indicate whether testosterone replacement should be considered. A level of testosterone of less than 11.0 nmol/L or a free testosterone of less than 40% justify supplementation. Testosterone is taken most easily by mouth, as Testosterone Undecanoate, in a starting dose of 160 mg daily. Alternatively there are skin patches, injections and creams which are effective, and since absorption by these routes of administration occurs directly into the blood, any consequences of impaired bowel or liver function are avoided.

A caution about the use of male hormones: if there are symptoms of prostate gland overactivity (nocturia, a dribble at the end of passing urine, difficulty in starting to urinate and a poor stream) then testosterone should be administered with caution. Rectal examination and an ultrasound will show the degree of enlargement and possible tumours in the gland. Serial measurements of prostate specific antigen (PSA) enable prostate activity to be monitored (a total PSA of up to 4.0 nmol/L is normal).

Traditional Drugs

There are a number of other drugs which are effective in enhancing erection. Yohimbine, derived from the bark of a West Indian tree, has been used in the UK for at least 80 years[17]. A number of double-blind controlled studies have shown significant improvement in 'sustained erections' for men taking between 20 and 40 mg daily. The drug acts centrally in the brain to increase arousal and motivation[18]. It has also been taken on an 'as required' basis one hour before anticipated intercourse in a 5 mg dose, though Morales has suggested the drug needs to be taken for several weeks to be effective[19]. The drug is generally well tolerated but with high doses other drugs acting on alpha 2 adrenoreceptors may be blocked leading to increased blood pressure, agitation, and other central nervous symptoms.

Premature Ejaculation (PE)

Premature ejaculation is everyman's experience at certain times in their life, reflecting nervousness or a momentary lapse in technique. It is most often a feature of early sexual relationships. In Parkinson's disease it is more common at the onset of the disease and usually reflects anxiety about the disease process itself and the ability to maintain adequate sexual function.

The problem is variously defined but in essence is when ejaculation occurs too quickly and, if present to a severe extent, before penetration has been achieved. Once established it becomes a source of anxiety in its own right and may lead to avoidance of love-making or, in single people, of social contact.

Traditionally PE was thought to be due to 'performance anxiety' and identified as a problem of younger men. In these cases the problem usually settled down with time; or, otherwise, the 'stop-start' technique could be taught (see below). The symptom is aggravated in a relationship where the man feels (or actually is!) challenged by his partner, and sometimes it expresses a more deep-seated ambivalence to women, in which case psychotherapy may be indicated.

Usually the symptom is treated with a behavioural programme (the 'stop-start' technique described below), medication (with Clomipramine or Paroxetine), or counselling. Attempting to relax by taking alcohol, relaxing drugs such as diazepam and chlordiazepoxide, and ejaculating a second time do not usually help.

The 'Stop-start' technique: In this technique the man stimulates himself to just before the moment of inevitability (see physiology section) and at that point of 'pre-inevitability' he stops and waits for the urge to ejaculate to settle down. He then stimulates himself again to the same point and again stops. This can be repeated several times before allowing himself to ejaculate. The exercise now continues with the partner sitting alongside and then on top of him. The partner inserts the penis into the vagina and gives penile stimulation by her pelvic movements to the same point of pre-inevitability. The exercise continues until he has mastered the art of relaxation necessary to delay ejaculation. Practice of the technique requires the couple to talk clearly about his level of excitement during intercourse; sufficient lubrication of the penis to minimize friction which will accelerate ejaculation, and forbearance on the part of the woman to focus on his needs for the duration of the exercise.

Clomipramine is taken as a 25-50 mg tablet one hour before intercourse. The drug is one of a group, the tricyclics, which are used as antidepressants. There may be some dryness of the mouth, and blurring of vision, due to the acetyl choline-like action of the drug, which is a part of the bodies' response, including the delay to ejaculation.

Recently Paroxetine 40 mg/day, in a double blind control study, was shown to give a significant improvement in ejaculatory control[20].

Retarded Ejaculation

This refers to difficulty in achieving an ejaculation (or orgasm) despite an adequate erection. It is rarer than either of the preceding dysfunctions and it is also more difficult to cure. In Parkinson's disease it is likely that the best way to promote ejaculation is by increasing stimulation to the penis and by practicing a relaxation technique. If there is a long-standing fear of emotional closeness associated with the condition, as is sometimes the case, psychotherapy which addresses childhood issues may be required. There is no specific medication generally recommended for retarded ejaculation.

Managing Sexual Problems in Women with Parkinson's Disease

The commonest sexual dysfunctions in women with Parkinson's disease describe are loss of libido, difficulty with arousal, anorgasmia, and, rarely, vaginismus. Other parameters of sexual function that have been reported are the frequency of sexual activity, which is reduced, and problems in communication. It is often unclear whether these symptoms are primary, occurring due to the disease itself or arise as a consequence of the stress, anxiety and depression that so frequently accompany the disease.

Loss of Libido

In Parkinson's disease loss of libido is about three times as common in women as in men. It occurs typically after the onset of the disease[21]. As discussed above, loss of libido coexists with difficulty in arousal, fatigue, stress, lack of communication, and the 'on-off' symptoms of prolonged medication. It follows that an approach to management is required that is based on an assessment that is broad-ranging, inclusive of medical history, drugs taken, and psychological and social factors. It is helpful if the partner is also seen. Once physical health has been assessed counselling can help explore any underlying problems.

What can Counselling Offer?

Counselling helps people to make or adjust to changes in their life. In Parkinson's disease it may include practical recommendations such as adopting different routines for making love (changing the time or the position for intercourse); it may involve listening while an individual or couple talk about what is distressing them. Counselling helps with communication skills. For instance, the individual who has difficulty in identifying, or misidentifies, a feeling, and in communicating to others what they want.

If depression is present it should be treated; selective serotonin re-uptake inhibitors (SSRI's) such as fluoxetine or paroxetine are used but occasionally may aggravate sexual difficulties.

As regards general health HRT may have a place in promoting well-being and energy. Testosterone 2.5 mg as a tablet daily (or equivalent dose of a cream) may improve libido and is justified if blood levels are depleted. DHEA, a building block in the metabolism of the sex hormones in women, has also been shown recently to increase libido in women, but not men[22]. A recommended dose is 5-10 mg by mouth daily. The blood level of DHEA should be checked before treatment is started.

Anorgasmia

Failure to achieve an orgasm is present in about 15% of the normal population, and many more women probably require manual stimulation to be orgasmic[23]. In Parkinson's disease the frequency of anorgasmia described is similar. In this same group studied by Welsh it was noted that women's sexual satisfaction was reduced and they expressed concern over body appearance, incontinence, and vaginal tightness.

Medical assessment should precede counselling and a sensate focus programme (see section on managing erectile dysfunction) may be offered. This should help relaxation, and with increased stimulation to the clitoris and surrounding area may enable orgasm to be achieved.

Vaginismus

Involuntary tightening of the adductors (clasping muscles of the thigh) and tightening of the vaginal sphincter are a response to anxiety. As a consequence penetrative sex is difficult (and painful), or impossible. Women may be orgasmic, despite their fear of penetration, as a result of non-penetrative sex with clitoral stimulation. In Parkinson's disease the vaginismus is probably due to muscle spasm arising from the disease itself and treatment will require adjustments to medication. Vaginismus may also be secondary to poor lubrication leading to pain on penetration.

Breathing and relaxation may be used as part of a behavioural treatment programme. If necessary additional help, using progressively larger dilators, may be sought from a gynaecologist.

Considerations of general health which relate to good sexual function in both sexes

Sleep is often disturbed in Parkinson's disease and levodopa is reported as a cause of difficulty in getting to sleep. Anxiety and agitation may have a similar effect. There is in any case a common tendency for changes to the sleep pattern with ageing which leads to disturbed sleep at night and drowsiness during the day. This pattern is accentuated in Parkinson's disease. Typically depression leads to early morning waking. Rigidity of the Parkinson's disease itself may cause difficulty in turning over and repositioning in bed without waking. If the individual gets insufficient sleep, irritability and deteriorating mental function (alertness, memory impairment) may occur. Other disorders of sleep include sleep talking or walking, and vivid dreams or nightmares (possibly due to L-dopa).

The usual recommendations to assist sleep include a warm bath, a hot drink at bed-time with removal of noise and light sources. Exercise during the daytime, if possible, will help (see below). Satin sheets can make turning over in bed easier. If sleep continues to be disturbed a short-term course of hypnotics such as Chloral Hydrate, or a benzodiazepam such as Temazepam 10 mg, may help break the pattern of sleeplessness. Valerian root extract may also be helpful.

Physical exercise increases well-being, improves sleep, helps maintain a good circulation (including to heart, brain and genital region, is an aid to weight control, and prevents muscle wasting. About half the population take insufficient exercise. The minimum recommended for good health is half an hour of moderately intense exercise three times a week, and the population over 60 in the UK have responded positively to the chief medical officer's advice. For the Parkinson's disease patient the principle remains the same, but the sort of activity depends on the level of disability and has to remain within the lever of exercise tolerance.

Kegel's exercises are a specific way to strengthen the pelvic floor muscles. They were originally described for women who had problems with incontinence after childbirth; in men voluntary contraction during intercourse enhances the erection. The muscle forms a sling attached to the pubic bone at the front and the coccyx behind and has openings in the mid-line for the sphincters of the rectum, urethra, (and vagina in women). The exercise consists of alternate tightening and relaxing of the sphincter muscles, holding them in the constricted position for a second or so before relaxing. Repeating the exercise ten times whenever urine is passed strengthens the pelvic floor musculature significantly within three or four weeks.

Thoughts on Sexual Technique -
Having Sex and Making Love

Introduction

Curiosity and the pursuit of physical pleasure are expressed in acts of love for which descriptive prose is inadequate. Technique and positions for love-making are important, but less important than the mind-set with which we relate to one another. People with Parkinson's disease who are physically compromised, sex may require greater inventiveness and the ability, as a couple, to communicate well. Our experience of making-love, as opposed to having sex, may be limited by problems but reflects better our aspirations and the sort of person we are.

Foreplay

Massage: Perfumed massage oil provides a pleasant medium with which to caress and stroke one another; the combined effect of the perfume and massage leads to relaxation. Some oils, for instance baby oil, can be applied to the genitals if a couple decide to transform the massage into love-making.

Massage is given in long stroking movements which may extend over the trunk and down the limbs without breaking contact. Focusing on the person massaged allows attunement to their experience, sharing the rhythms and sense of relaxation achieved. Rocking the body lulls the senses.

The head, where much perception is localised, is also most sensitive to stroking - gentle massage of the muscles round the nose, gentle pulling of the ears or the hair on the crown of the head, or rhythmic rolling of the head from side to side. The neck holds tension (we are alerted to what's going on around us by movements of the head). Pressing with the thumbs from the nape of the neck to the points of the shoulders eases the tension held there.

Erogenous areas vary but include the side of the neck, areas adjacent to the genitals, the nipples (in both sexes), and over the buttocks - stroking or light scratching may give goose pimples as the hairs literally stand on end (autonomic arousal).

Breathing, particularly expiration, and relaxation go together - at the end of breathing out we can relax muscle tone by focusing on the part we want to relax, starting at the top of the body and working down to the tips of out toes. As we relax successfully we may feel waves of sensation or involuntary muscle contractions, especially in the low back region where tension is often held.

Many of the body's sexual movements were laid down originally as reflex responses, so that we can, for instance, initiate pelvic thrusting movements by relaxation rather than by deliberate thrusting. These involuntary movements are slower than those that may be adopted voluntarily and lead to tingling and movement of the limbs. Since we have all evolved these same reflex patterns, two people attuned to their own body rythms may move in unison with one another during intercourse and may more easily climax together. The emotional connection that precedes and accompanies' sexual contact is very important.

Initiation of sexual activity by either sex is equally of benefit for men and women. In Parkinson's disease initiation of the sexual act may be less easy but it need make little difference to foreplay involving eye contact creating emotional closeness, talking, kissing and touching, which heighten sexual arousal.

Intercourse
Positions
- Spooning describes a couple's position where one lies curled round the back of the other with the free arm looped around the others waist. The position offers good body contact and may be adopted as a position in which to fall asleep.

  Penetration may be easier from the rear. The vaginal opening is more accessible with a pillow between the legs.

- The active partner does best to be on top for intercourse. The active partner then may take some responsibility for the arousal of their partner as well as themselves. The 'non-active' partner can assist pelvic movements of the other by pushing with their hands on the iliac crests of the pelvis.

- If disability requires it alternate positions may be sought standing, kneeling or leaning with cushions or pillows. Don't be discouraged at the prospect of using sex-aids that may be recommended by your therapist.

Lubrication
After the menopause women may find that vaginal lubrication is less during sex irrespective of the level of arousal. Lubrication may be better if they are on HRT or using topical oestrogen gel. Alternatively Senselle or KY jelly may be used - Senselle is very slippery and KY a bit sticky as it dries.

Quality of Life - The Story of John Smith

John Smith is a professional man in his mid sixties who had been diagnosed as having Parkinson's disease some years before I met him. He asked me, as a physician, to help him with his general health, including his failing sex-life. He was at that time already receiving Sinemet and had been battling with the problem of fluctuating energy levels. What I report here is his own account of his experience which I have changed slightly to protect his anonymity, and to which I have added my own thoughts in retrospect.

The diagnosis of his condition at first was a shock to him. As he saw it, an illness such as cancer is well-known and dealing with it is clear - you can cut it out and, if you're lucky, you will be cured of it. Whereas Parkinson's disease, once you have it, is there for life, like a life sentence. And, what's more, with Parkinson's disease not being so common as a disease, John didn't know anyone amongst his colleagues or friends who had it, or to whom he felt he could talk about it.

His first response was blankness, then fear, and then anger. But he lived, to start with, as though it wasn't there. He busied himself with his career keeping to his normal heavy work schedule while continuing to undertake other activities as before. Though it became more of an effort, he was careful to hide his fatigue and the tell-tale tremor of his left side from his work colleagues.

He became irritable with little cause at his wife, Sarah, but avoided talking about his illness or feelings to her. He was barely in touch with his feelings in any case. He certainly didn't acknowledge he was scared. Obscurely he found himself angry but without any person he could blame for his predicament. He thought the doctors took a clinical view of his condition without appearing to notice the black pit of despair into which he felt himself to be falling. He dealt with his growing sense of frustration by becoming an expert on his own condition. He got articles off the internet, researching the causes and treatments for Parkinson's disease. He realized it could not be cured and that the disease could progress to a life of dependency. His sense of powerlessness and loneliness turned to depression.

It was at this time that he found his sex life began to suffer. He had lost interest in making love as he became depressed and when now he tried to respond to Sarah's advances he felt unattractive, clumsy and frustrated by his abnormal body movements and stiffness. He found he was unable to get an erection. Impotence, he reflected, was a cruel addition to his other problems.

My experience of John was quite different from his gloomy picture of how others saw him. He was competent and successful in his working life, he was socially adept and charming and he appeared to be minimally handicapped by his Parkinson's disease. It was only after I had heard him talk during several sessions that I realized the extent to which his self-esteem had been effected. And not until he talked to me about the problem he had had in getting an erection, did I realize how important it was to help him overcome this difficulty.

In fact my approach had been a global one intended to help in the broadest way with his situation. I listened when he talked to me. I listened sympathetically because indeed there were many things to be sympathetic about. I checked his general health and found little that needed attention apart from the symptoms of the Parkinson's disease for which he was already receiving treatment elsewhere. After biochemical tests we discussed his nutritional needs and I recommended vitamins and minerals to be taken as supplements to what was otherwise a carefully considered and good diet.

When I did a blood test of his hormonal status I found he had a testosterone level which was at the lower end of the normal range, but which was consistent with his age. When we discussed this John elected to have a trial course of testosterone by mouth. We later changed this to testosterone patches which he replaced himself daily. We found he got better blood levels by this route and I guessed his absorption through the gut wall might be poor because of his 'leaky gut syndrome'. The most noticeable effects of the testosterone was an increase in energy and improved mood. I sometimes use the hormone testosterone to kick start people into a cycle of change.

I had made a bargain with him about his newfound energy: 'If I get you to feel less tired and more energetic, the deal is that you will start a programme of physical exercise'. This often successfully challenges people to start exercising again after years of being sedentary. Once an exercise programme has been underway for a few weeks it gains its own momentum. I truly do rate exercise undervalued as a way to improve mental and physical well-being. With the symptoms of depression it is particularly helpful, maybe due to the brain's production of natural endorphins. Certainly John started to feel he had more energy, and with more physical reserves to draw on, his mood improved and he felt more in charge of his own life.

As regards his sexual problems testosterone supplementation had helped his libido, and boosted his male ego with spontaneous erections when he woke in the morning. So that he could have an erection when he wanted one we decided he try Sildenafil, and after experimenting with the dose we found 50 mg worked reliably. Sarah and John made love in the morning when the Sinemet he was taking gave him the best control of involuntary movements. I advised he continue with Sildenafil on a regular basis so he wouldn't worry about impotence - which might otherwise become self-fulfilling. When he wants to wean himself off the drug and is feeling better about himself he will reduce the dose in small increments.

183

I am reminded again of the importance for men of their ability to make love - and how it remains important even for older men.

John talked to Sarah about the way he needed to make love - about the tremors which he managed better when they lay in a position of 'spooning' so that they could more easily move in rhythm together, and about the stiffness that meant it was easier to climax when she was active on top of him. They talked also of his concern about being unattractive and of his dislike of the sweating and oiliness of his skin. It was a relief for him to talk and her acceptance of his "shame" moved him. What he deemed unattractive about himself seemed of little concern to Sarah, and it certainly didn't put her off love-making. In fact, as it turned out, Sarah had held back, taking his embarrassment for disinterest. She had taken HRT for several years and enjoyed the prospect of their sexual pleasure together.

On the occasions John didn't feel up to sex they were satisfied to hold and stroke one another, distinguishing the tenderness of this contact from expectations that sex would follow.

I think John and Sarah have suffered as a result of his having Parkinson's disease, but I believe they have also been strengthened in their relationship. While John's illness means the future is uncertain, they have learnt life's lesson to live each day to the full and they have discovered resources within themselves to adapt and deal courageously with whatever the future holds. In the end, quality of life is not limited by the degree of disability but by the spirit with which we respond to it.

Editors Notes *For Patients and Healthcare Professionals*

by Lucille Leader *Dip ION* **and Dr Geoffrey Leader** *MB ChB FRCA*

Nutritional Considerations

1. A heavy meal is inappropriate before sexual activity as it may cause people to feel sluggish and uncomfortable. Vegetable soup and fruit are easier to digest.

2. Patients on L-dopa medication are recommended to wait until it "kicks in" before attempting sexual activity.

To ensure optimal absorption of L-dopa before physical demands, if people wish to eat, the following scheme is suggested. However, these are only guidelines, as one has to take into account the fluctuating nature of Parkinson's disease and patient individuality.

a) Take L-dopa.

b) Wait one hour or until the drug has "kicked in" before eating fruit/vegetables.

If a person has eaten any of the dense protein foods (meat, poultry, fish, eggs, dairy, soy, lentils, wheat including couscous and bulgar, rye, oats, barley, spelt, sago, coconut, nuts, seeds, avocado, asparagus and pulses), it is ideal, if possible, to wait at least two hours after eating before taking L-dopa again. This reduces the possibility of exacerbated movement disturbance, which can arise when there is competition for absorption between L-dopa medication and the neutral amino acids found in protein-rich foods[24, 25].

3. Maintaining regular daily bowel movement is essential for a feeling of wellbeing as well as for the optimum absorption of drugs. Constipation causes sluggishness and discomfort.

4. Alcohol may possibly dull the senses and affect balance. It has been recommended that it be avoided by those who take centrally-acting medication[26].

5. Any low-fat diet followed should not exclude the essential fatty acids (Omega 6 and Omega 3) found in nuts, seeds and oily fish such as herring and mackerel. Cholesterol is the precursor of male and female hormones (oestrogen, progesterone and testosterone) and should not be allowed to fall to deficiency levels.

6. Nutritional status should be assessed biochemically. Some nutritional deficiencies can influence energy production[27, 28]. Examples of deficiencies which undermine mitochondrial energy production include CoQ10, NADH, B vitamins, vitamin C, iron, copper, magnesium and manganese. Specific nutrients also act as cofactors in hormone synthesis. Nutritional deficiencies should be addressed by diet and supplements.

7. For a feeling of wellbeing, the daily diet should be well balanced. Energy and blood sugar levels need support. Taking a small snack every couple of hours, which also contains a complex carbohydrate, may be helpful.

8. Anti-oxidant therapy may be prudent if Sildenafil (Viagra) is taken as this drug enhances nitric oxide production[29].

References: Sexuality and Parkinson's Disease: Dr Michael Perring

1. Wise TN. *Sexual dysfunction in the medically ill.* Psychosomatics 1983;24:787-805

2. Brown RG, Jahanshahi M, Quinn N, Marsden CD. *Sexual function in patients with Parkinsons disease and their partners.* J Neurol Neurosurg, Psychiatry 1990; 53:480-486

3. Mutch W, Strudwick A, Roy S, Downie A. *Parkinson's disease: disability review and management.* BMJ 1986;293:675-677

4. Polymeropoulos MH, Higgins JJ, GolbeLI. *Mapping of a gene for Parkinson's disease to 4q21-q23.* Science, 1996;274:1197-1199.

5. Masters WH, Johnson VE. *Human Sexual Response* 1966, Little Brown and Co.

6. Wagner G 1981a. Erection: *Physiology and Endocrinology in Impotence: physiological, psychological, and surgical diagnosis and treatment* (ed G Wagner and R Green pp25-36. Plenum, NY.

7. Robinson BW, Mishkin M 1968. *Penile erection evoked from the forebrain structures in Macaca mulatta.* Achives of Neurology 119: 184

8. Wellings K, Field J, Johnson AM, Wadsworth J. *Sexual Behaviour in Britain: The National Survey of sexual attitudes and Lifestyles,* 1994, Penguin.

9. O'Connell H, Hutson JM, Anderson CR, Plenter RJ. *Anatomical Relationship between urethra and clitoris.* J of Urol 1998;159, 1892-1897.

10. Stewart WFR. *Sex and the Physically handicapped.* Horsham: National Fund for Research in Crippling Disease, 1975

11. Frank EF, Anderson C, Rubinstein D. *Frequency of sexual dysfunction in 'normal' couples.* N Engl J Med 1978;299:111-115

12. Osborn M,Hawton K, Gath D. *Sexual dysfunction among middle-aged women in the community.* BMJ 1988;296:959-962

13. op. cit. n. 2

14. Singer C, Weiner WJ, Ackerman M, Sanchez-Ramos J. *Sexual dysfunction in Parkinson's disease.* Neurology 1990;40 (suppl 1);221

15. op. cit. n. 8

16. Zesiewicz TA: 2000: *Movement Discord:* 15(2): 305-308

17. Riley AJ. Yohimbine in *The treatment of erectile disorder.* BJCP 1994;48 (3): 133-135

18. Clark JT, Smith ER, Davidson JM. *Testosterone is not required for the enhancement of sexual motivation* by Yohimbine. Physiol Behav 1985;35:517-521

19. Morales A, Condra M, Owen J. *Is Yohimbine effective in the treatment of organic impotence?* J Urol 1982;12:45-47

20. Waldinger MD, Hengeveld MW et al. *Paroxetine Treatment of premature ejaculation: a double-blind, randomized placebo-controlled trial,* Am J Psych 1994;151:1377-1379.

21. Wermuth L, Steneger E. *Sexual problems in young patients with Parkinson's disease* acta Neurol scand, 1995;91:453-455

22. Baulieu EE, Thomas G, Legrain S et al. Dehydroepiandrosterone, *DHEA sulphate and aging: contribution of the DHEAge Study to a sociobiomedical issue*, 2000, PNAS,97;8:4279-4284.

23. Welsh M, Hung L, Waters CH. *Sexuality in Women with Parkinson's disease. Movement Disorders:* 12 (6):923-927.

References: Editors Notes: Nutritional Considerations: Lucille Leader & Dr Geoffrey Leader
___

24. *Dietary Reference in the Management of Parkinson's Disease:* P A Kempster MD MRCP FRACP, M C Wahlqvist MD FRACP: Nutrition Reviews, volume 52, 2: 1994.

25. *Parkinson's Disease - The New Nutritional Handbook:* pps.2, 20: Geoffrey Leader MB ChB FRCA and Lucille Leader Dip ION: 1996: Denor Press, London, UK.

26. *ABPI Compendium of Data Sheets and Summaries of Product Characteristics* (1999-2000), p.1610, ISBN: 0-907102-18-2 Datapharm Publications Limited, London, UK

27. *Parkinson's Disease - The New Nutritional Handbook*: p.44: Geoffrey Leader MB ChB FRCA and Lucille Leader Dip ION: 1996: Denor Press, London, UK.

28. *BrainRecovery.com*: p.22: David Perlmutter MD: 2000: Perlmutter Health Center, Naples, Fl, USA

29. *BrainRecovery.com*: p.26: David Perlmutter MD: 2000: Perlmutter Health Center, Naples, Fl, USA

CHAPTER 11

Mercury in Dentistry

*by **Dr Jack Levenson** LDS RCS(Edin)*

There are literally thousands of research papers published in prestigious, peer-reviewed journals on the subject of mercury - a large number with particular reference to mercury amalgam fillings and toxicity. There are some studies which are pertinent to people with Parkinson's disease.

Peralesy Herrero, former Director of the Institute of Occupational Medicine in Madrid, attributed Parkinson's type symptoms to chronic mercury poisoning in his study of miners exposed to mercury[1].

In Singapore, subjects were measured for mercury levels in their blood, urine and scalp hair, in an epidemiological case controlled study of mercury toxicity and idiopathic Parkinson's disease (IDP). There were 54 cases of IDP and 95 matched controls. Subjects with Parkinson's disease had significantly higher mean level of mercury than controls, in all measured areas[2].

Parkinson's disease mortality rates in Michigan[3] were calculated with respect to potential heavy metal exposure. The ecological findings suggested a geographic association between Parkinson's disease mortality and the industrial use of heavy metals.

In another study[4], six diagnosed cases of Parkinson's disease had all been exposed to mercury. The authors recommended further exploration of the possible association between exposure to mercury and Parkinson's disease.

Given the fact that mercury accumulates in brain tissue and affects the central nervous system, combined with measurable electrical current (the battery effect) of dental fillings, it could be expected that there would be some changes in brain activity - itself an electrical organ - when measured by EEG, and this is indeed so[5, 6].

Spurred by these and other case histories, The Brompton Dental and Health Clinic, in conjunction with Julian Campbell of EM DI Ltd, instigated a preliminary research protocol, using computerised equipment to make a record of brain signals using an electroencephalogram (EEG) to test the hypothesis that electricity and mercury from fillings could influence brain wave patterns[7]. Early observations using the EPS Monitoring System[8] have thrown up some interesting ideas and indicate that further research is worthwhile.

In the light of current research, it would seem prudent for dentists not to use mercury in fillings for patients with Parkinson's disease. If old mercury fillings are removed, chelation therapy should be administered[9].

A pre-treatment plan should be designed to improve immune function and place the patient in an improved state of health prior to any dental work being undertaken. Nutritional deficiencies recognised by examination of the mouth, as well as by biochemical tests, should be addressed[10]. Patients are advised to avoid processed foods and to eat fresh poultry, fruit and vegetables - all organic wherever possible - and foods containing sulphur such as eggs, onion and garlic. Fish, both fresh water and from costal areas should be avoided as they usually contain high levels of mercury and other toxins. Small fish such as white bait, sprats and sardines are protected by selenium and are a good source of calcium. Remember, the larger the fish the more mercury is present! Herring, mackerel and salmon are good sources of essential Omega 3 fatty acids. Foods which are salty, sour or eaten at high temperature, increase mercury vaporisation. Refined carbohydrates and sugars should be avoided as the oral bacteria react to produce lactic acid, which increases corrosion of amalgams. Foods, which cause allergic reactions, should be avoided and any desensitisation programmes should be continued.

Most patients with amalgam poisoning are already fatigued and while they should keep mobile, they should not undertake strenuous exercise. The pre-treatment regime may include saliva and urine pH checks and assessment of digestive enzymes and friendly bacteria. Treatment and management of gut dysbiosis, food allergies and constipation should be discussed. Mercury may be retained in the faeces.

Tooth bushing should be confined to the tooth surfaces and friction on the fillings are to be avoided as well as substances containing mercury salts, such as contact lens solutions.

A pre-treatment regime of anti-oxidants is recommended in conjunction with substances which will bind to, and help excrete, mercury. This will include vitamins and minerals, extra selenium and vitamin C powder. Charcoal should be taken half an hour prior to treatment to mop up any mercury vapour which has evaded other precautionary procedures and been swallowed. At the Brompton Health Clinic we have recently introduced intravenous vitamin C[11] with addition of glutathione and sometimes taurine. This procedure may be used before, during or after treatment, depending on presenting symptoms.

Ideally, I think it best for a supplement pre-treatment plan to commence two months prior to treatment. However, many patients are unwilling to wait that long once they have made the decision to have their amalgams removed.

The sensitivity of patients to materials other than mercury used in the mouth should be assessed before use.

Dental Personnel

The removal of amalgam fillings without basic protective precautions is disastrous, as allergic/hyper-sensitive/toxic patients will almost inevitably react adversely to such treatment. *There are protocols for the priority order for removal of fillings, protection of the patient during amalgam removal[12] and post-removal mercury detoxification and chelation programmes[13].*

Precautions are recommended for dental personnel who are working with mercury. Research has demonstrated adverse effects on dentist's health due to mercury toxicity[14, 15, 16, 17, 18]. There is a health risk to the foetus in women dentists and dental personnel who may be pregnant. Substantial published literature exists on the effects of pre-natal exposure to mercury, including behavioural changes[19], alteration of nerve growth factor and its receptors in the foetal brain[20], and adverse affects on motor function, language and memory[21]. Mercury from pregnant females does transfer into the tissues of unborn babies[22] and there is significant association between previous still births and mercury levels in both maternal and cord blood[23].

Tests for Mercury Toxicity

There are a number of tests to indicate mercury toxicity: these include haematology and biochemistry, sweat test for dental metals, electrical measurements on oral metallic restorations, faeces measurement, porphyrins and electro-acupuncture evaluation amongst others. Standard urine and blood tests are of value in cases of acute mercury exposure but not in low level chronic exposure to mercury vapour. Mercury does not live in the transport systems of the body but tends to dump it in tissues and organs.

Cautionary Note

Mercury: Parkinson's disease patients are metabolically compromised. It may not be advisable for them to have all their dental mercury removed and replaced at one time. If mercury levels are too high and treatment needed, dentists should proceed with caution. Advice may be obtained from the British Society for Mercury Free Dentistry[24].

Fluoride[25]: Besides fluoride in toothpaste, fluoride content is increasing in our foods due to the heavy reliance on fertilisers, which are rich in fluoride. Dental fluorosis or mottle teeth can be an indication of fluoride poisoning. The acknowledged safety limit is 3mg per day for fluoride. However, a research project undertaken by Dr Peter Mansfield of the Templegarth Trust in the Fluoridated West Midlands and the non-fluoridated East Midlands in the UK, found that 60% of those tested for fluoride in the fluoridated areas are getting more than 3mg per day, and some up to 20mg per day.

References

1. Perales Y Herrero: Mercury: *Chronic Poisoning in Encyclopaedia of Occ. Health and Safety*: 3rd Edition, Vol. 2: 1983: Ed L Parmeggiani: Int. Labour Office, Geneva: pps. 1334 - 1335

2. CH Ngim, G Pevathasan: *Epidemiological Study on Association between Body Burden Mercury Level and Ideopathic Parkinson's Disease*: Neuroepidemiology: 1989 8: pps. 128 - 141

3. RA Rybick, CC Johnson, J Oman, JM Gorell: *Parkinson's Disease Mortality and the Industrial use of Heavy Metals in Michigan*: Movement Disorder: 8(1): 1993: pps. 87 - 92

4. CG Ohlson, C Hogstead: *Parkinson's Disease and Occupational Exposure to Organic Solvents, Agricultural Chemicals and Mercury - A Case Reference Study*: J Scand: Work Environmental Health 7L: 1981: p. 252

5. Popov L, Gig T, Prof Zabol: *Bioelec Activity of the Brain in Patients with Chronic Occupational Mercury Poisoning*: Russian BCC J.17: 1973: 52(Russ)

6. Piikivi, Tolonen U: *EEG Findings in Chlor Alkali Workers Subjected to Low Long Term Exposure to Mercury Vapour*: Brit J Industrial Medicine 46: 1989: 370

7. *The EPS Monitoring System - Menace in the Mouth*: pps. 252 - 253: Dr Jack Levenson: 2000: Bromptom Health, London, UK

8. *EPS Monitoring System: The Suffolk Enterprise Centre*: Felaw Maltings: Ipswich, IP2 8SJ, UK: Email: campbell@empulse.com

9. *Menace in the Mouth*: pps. 187 - 192: 2000: Dr Jack Levenson, Brompton Health, London, UK

10. *Menace in the Mouth*: pps. 177 - 179: 2000: Dr Jack Levenson, Brompton Health, London, UK

11. Hall G: *The Hall V-Tox Treatment*: Schadow Street 28, Dusseldorf, Germany 40121: Hall: 1995

12. *Menace in the Mouth*: p.184: 2000: Dr Jack Levenson, Brompton Health, London, UK

13. op. cit. n. 9

14. Shapiro IM, Sumner AJ, Spilz LK, Cornblatt DR, Uzzell B, Shipp II, Block P: *Neurophysiological and Neuropsychological Function in Mercury - Exposed Dentists*: Lancet 8282: pps. 1147 - 1150: 1982

15. Ngim CH, Foo SC, Boey KW, Jeyaratnam J: *Chronic Neurobehavioural Effects of Elemental Mercury in Dentists*: Brit J. Industrial Medicine: 1992: 49: pps. 782 - 790

16. Professor P Stortebecker: *Mercury Posioning from Dental Amalgam Through a Direct Nose-Brain Transport*: (Letter) Lancet 27 May 1989: p. 1207

17. Cross JP, Daleim Gooluard L, Lenihan JMA, Smith, Hamilton, *Methyl Mercury in the Blood of Dentists*: (Letter) Lancet 1978: 2: pps. 312 - 313

18. Ahlbom A, Norell S, Nylnder M, Rodvall Y: *Dentists, Nurses and Brain Tumours 4th International Symposium: Epidemiology Occupational Health*, Como, Italy: 1985 (Abstracts): Reported Svenska Dagbladet

19. Frederiksson A, Dencker L, Archer T, Danielsson BR: *Prenatal Co-Exposure to Metallic Mercury Produce: Interactive Behavioural Changes in Adult Rats*: Neurotoxical Teratol 18(2): pps. 129 - 134: March 1996

20. Soderstrom S, Fredriksson A, Dencker L, Ebendal T: *The Effects of Mercury Vapour on Cholinergic Neurons in the Foetal Brain: Studies on the Expression of Nerve Receptors*: Brain Res. Dev. Brain Res: 85(1): pps. 96 - 108: 1995

21. Grandjean P, Weihy P, White RF, Debes F: *Cognitive Performance of Children Prenatally Exposed to 'Safe' Levels of Methyl Mercury*: Environ. Research 77 (2): pps. 165 - 172: 1998

22. Lutz E, Lind B, Herin P, Krakau I, Bui TH, Vahter M: *Concentrations of Mercury Cadmium and Lead in Brain and Kidney of Second Trimester Fetuses and Infants*: J.1 Trace Elem. Med. Biol. 10(20): pps. 61 - 67: 1966

23. Kuntz W P, Pitkin RM, Bostrom AW, Hughes MS: *Material and Cord Blood Background Mercury Levels: A Longtiudinal Surveillance*: Am J. Obs: Gyn: Vol. 143: pps. 440 - 443: 1982

24. British Society for Mercury Free Dentistry, 225 Old Brompton Road, London, SW5 0EA, UK (telephone: +44 (20) 7373 3655.

25. Dr Tony Lees: *The Devil's Element - Fluorine: Menace in the Mouth*: pps. 231 - 239: 2000: Dr Jack Levenson, Brompton Health, London, UK

CHAPTER 12

EDTA
Chelation Therapy

by Dr Rodney Adeniyi-Jones LRCP & SI MRCP (UK)

The brain is critically dependent on an abundant blood flow: "What is good for the heart is good for the head."[1]

Chelation therapy is a non-invasive, non-traumatic way of making major improvements to the cerebral circulation of those patients in whom it is compromised.

Introduction

Some forty years ago it was found that intravenous EDTA treatment caused a remarkable improvement in angina, heart disease and in poor circulation affecting the legs and the brain, as a result of arteriosclerosis. It has since been found to be beneficial in many problems arising from these conditions.

The treatment is called chelation because the active substance is a chelating agent called EDTA. EDTA (a synthetic amino acid called ethylene-diamine-tetra-acetic acid) is given by a 'drip' (also called an infusion) into a vein in the arm over a three-hour period. EDTA has the ability to 'grasp' or 'hook- on' to atoms of calcium, lead, cadmium, mercury, copper, iron and several other minerals in the body by a distinctive chemical process called chelation.[2] The EDTA, together with the metals it is carrying, then passes out of the body through the kidneys and urine.

Definition: Chelation is the incorporation of a metal into a heterocyclic ring-shaped organic molecule.

Arterial Disease in Parkinson's Disease

Arterial disease involves stiffening and narrowing of the arteries, and it can affect many areas of the body. If arteries to the heart are affected, its pumping efficiency declines. If the arteries in the neck are affected, it is harder for blood to get up into the brain. The small arteries actually within the brain can also be affected, making it even harder for the blood to get to the brain tissue that needs it. These problems often coexist in mild forms, but their effect is cumulative, and can leave the brain of the Parkinson's disease patient with a relative deficiency of oxygen and nutrients – fertile soil for further free radical damage.

There is no suggestion that arterial disease is more common in people with Parkinson's disease, but it is a very common disorder, and its prevalence increases with advancing age.

How Chelation Works

The lining of the arteries is a vulnerable tissue, and can be subject to damaging attack from free radicals, toxic metals, infections, deficiencies of critical nutrients, activity of the immune system, hormones and various sources of inflammation.

These influences initiate and accelerate the process of damage to the arterial lining all over the body. They are often called 'hidden risk factors' and serve to compound and aggravate the well-known risks associated with obesity, hypertension, smoking, and diabetes.

It has become clear that EDTA chelation therapy has beneficial effects on many of the damaging factors that attack the arterial walls.

Its effects are thought to include reducing the level of calcium inside the cells and eliminating heavy metals that block enzyme systems. It improves energy production in the mitochondria (the power generating plants of the cells). It stops free radical damage to fat and cholesterol, the so-called lipid peroxidation,[3] and it reduces the 'stickiness' of cells (called platelets) in the blood, so the blood flows more smoothly.[4] This range of effects arrests and reverses the process of damage and inflammation in the walls of the arteries.

During chelation therapy, the fatty, calcium-rich plaque in the walls of the arteries is dissolved slowly and the circulation throughout the body improves. The processes that have caused the plaque to accumulate are reversed, and other dangerous processes that cause instability and spasm of arteries in the heart and elsewhere, are also reversed.

Chelation therapy is widely used for patients with heavy metal poisoning, for example, children or industrial workers with lead poisoning.

How Effective is EDTA Chelation Therapy?

A great deal has been published on the outcomes of EDTA chelation therapy, virtually all of it positive. Herewith an example from Denmark.

Between 1987 and 1993, 92 patients who had been referred for surgery (coronary artery bypass or foot amputation) received EDTA chelation therapy while they were waiting. In 82 of these, the surgeons later cancelled the operations because they were no longer necessary. The estimated saving to the health service was 2 million pounds.

47 of the patients from that study were contacted for review in 1999. Of the 47 patients – all of whom had been told 10 to 12 years earlier that bypass or amputation was inevitable - 34 had still not required surgical intervention and all but one were well. 10 patients had had surgery and 3 patients had died.[5]

Benefits of EDTA Chelation

I recommend EDTA chelation in most cases of arterial disease because it treats all the arteries in the body, not just the problem area. This is important because even though symptoms may appear in one organ, arterial disease always affects the whole of the arterial system – head, heart, aorta and legs to varying degrees. People who have arterial disease of the legs usually die of heart disease, not of gangrene[6].

By removing heavy metals, chelation reduces general free radical activity, which may be beneficial in Parkinson's disease patients. There are case reports of Parkinson's disease patients receiving benefit when chelation was used as an adjunct to their treatment.[7] Fatigue, often a major problem for Parkinson's patients, is reported to improve following chelation[8.]

Doctors and EDTA Chelation

Chelation therapy is an intravenous treatment, and can only be administered by a fully qualified medical doctor. The International Board of Chelation Therapy (IBCT) trains and examines doctors and awards certification to those competent in chelation therapy. The American College for Advancement in Medicine (ACAM) carries out public education and continuing medical education in chelation therapy. It is responsible for the official protocol for the safe and effective administration of EDTA chelation therapy.

Patient Management for Chelation Therapy

Chelation patients follow a programme of non-smoking, diet adjustment, exercise and vitamin and mineral supplements.

Stress management techniques are an important part of the treatment.

'New' risk factors for arterial disease are assessed at the beginning of treatment and monitored during and after treatment.

Supplementary oral zinc, chromium, manganese and vitamin B6 are absolutely essential during chelation, because EDTA accelerates the elimination of these metals from the body and inhibits the action of vitamin B6.

Safety
EDTA Chelation is an extremely safe therapy. In the USA alone, more than 500,000 patients have received over 6 million treatments with no fatalities or serious adverse effects. Thirty years ago high doses of EDTA were often given very rapidly and caused kidney damage, which was severe in some cases. Since then, with modern treatment programmes and with careful monitoring of kidney function, there have been no cases of damage to kidneys or indeed to any other organs.

Duration of Treatment
Most patients with significant arterial disease require 25 - 30 infusions initially. Some patients need more than 30 infusions to achieve maximum improvement in their circulation.[9] Afterwards, a treatment every one or two months is needed to maintain the improvement in circulation.

Side Effects
Slight tiredness is occasionally experienced at the beginning of treatment, but usually disappears over the first three or four treatments. Chelation tends to lower the blood sugar level, an effect which, though advantageous for the diabetic patient, can make others feel a little faint or light headed for a short while. Eating a snack during the infusion prevents this.

References:

1. *Brain Longevity*, p 49, Dharma Singh Khalasa MD, 1997 Warner Books Inc New York USA

2. *The Scientific Basis of EDTA Chelation Therapy*, p5, Halstead & Rozema, 1997 TRC Publishing Landrum, South Carolina, USA

3. *Effect of ethelyenediaminetetraacteate on lipid peroxide formation and succinoxidase inactivation by ultraviolet light.* Barber A A & Ottolenght A; Proc. Soc. Exper. Biol. Med 96 pps 471 – 473 1957

4. *The Scientific Basis of EDTA Chelation Therapy*, p39, Halstead & Rozema, 1997 TRC Publishing Landrum, South Carolina, USA

5. *The Long-Term Effect of Chelation Therapy: A 6 – 12 Year Follow-Up of a 1993 Study;* Hancke C; Clinical Practice of Alternative Medicine p1(3): pps 158 – 163, 2000 Innovision Communications, California, USA

6. *Evidence-based medicine in Practice*, Hampton JR, The Practitioner 243 p 693 1999 Miller Freeman UK Ltd

7. *EDTA Chelation therapy in chronic degenerative disease*, Olszewer E, Carter J, Med Hypoth; 27:41-49 1988

8. *The effect of EDTA chelation therapy with multivitamin/trace mineral supplementation upon reported fatigue*, McDonagh E, Rudolph C, Cheraskin E; Journal of Orthomolecular Psychiatry;13; pps 1-3 1983

9. *The Protocol for the Safe and Effective Administration of EDTA and Other Chelating Agents for Vascular Disease, Degenerative Disease, and Metal Toxicity*, Rozema T, Journal of Advancement in Medicine; 10: pps 5-100 1997

CHAPTER 13

Traditional Chinese Medicine and Parkinson's Disease

by Dr Monika Birkmayer MD

The practice of Traditional Chinese Medicine (TCM) has a long history dating back nearly 5000 years. It was influenced by the philosophy of different times and dynasties. Already in the third and second centuries BC, medicine was based on the laws of nature. In the first century BC, the Huang di Nei Jing (The Book of the Yellow Emperor) was written. It was one of the most important classics in TCM, in which the laws of nature were described for the first time. These are still valid nowadays.

Over thousands of years of practice and empirical experience, a unique medical system developed, with diagnosis and treatment, based on regarding each individual as a whole entity, rather than simply treating a disease.

The Difference between Oriental Medicine and Western Medicine

The fundamental basis of Traditional Chinese Medicine is the concept of "Qi" (internal energy system).

"Qi" is the vital energy of every living organism. "Qi" is invisible and for a long time only its manifestations could be seen or experienced, but there was no material basis. For westerners, who see the world purely in terms of scientifically proven facts, it was hard to believe in its existence. Nowadays however, facilities have been developed to prove the existence of electromagnetic fields so that Traditional Chinese Medicine can also be explained by modern science.

Western medicine is based on natural science. It emphasises the investigation of the structure of matter, which is also the source of diagnosis. Western medicine acts upon cells and chemical substances. It diagnoses and treats the effects of disease.

Oriental medicine diagnoses and acts upon the energy ("Qi") that creates the disease-state.

These two systems can only benefit from each other. One can never substitute the other. Hopefully the commencement of integrating the oriental system into the western world will continue, for the benefit of patients.

The Theory of YIN and YANG (The theory of opposites)

This theory is one of the most important in Traditional Chinese Medicine. It is said that any pathology, physiology and treatment can eventually be reduced to Yin and Yang.

The theory of Yin and Yang is also applicable to western medicine. The body's structure and function is divided into these opposites. For example, the sympathetic nervous system represents Yang whereas the parasympathetic nervous system corresponds with Yin.

Meridian Theory

According to Chinese medicine "Qi" circulates along a system of conduits, the principal ones being the meridians. There is a network of main channels (there are twelve principal bilateral channels) and minor capillaries. The channels connect the surface (skin) with the viscera. A further fine network exists which connects inside with outside and above with below. That explains why stimulating a point on one end of a meridian can have an effect somewhere else.

The Diagnosis

As in every medical system it is also true in Chinese Medicine that the better the diagnosis, the better the treatment. Important diagnostic features include the tongue and pulse.

The Treatment

There are different methods of treatment.

Acupuncture

This is where the acupuncture points on the body are stimulated with a needle. The points selected depend on the diagnosis.

Chinese Herbal Medicine

This part of Chinese medicine is fairly new in the West. In China it covers 80% of Chinese medical treatment and its potential is promising and often astonishing.

To be treated with Chinese Herbs two main things are essential:
1. A well qualified practitioner.

2. Herbs, which are supplied by a recognised supplier, guaranteed for purity and safety and not polluted by pesticides.

There have been reports in the media which warn against taking Chinese herbs as they have been harmful for patients. This happens with bad quality herbs and taking them without seeing a qualified practitioner. Western medicine is also dangerous if taken without proper medical supervision.

If the above advice is followed, Chinese Herbs are safe.

Acupuncture and Modern Science

Most acupuncture points are points of high electric conductance. A model has been proposed by Charles Shang[1]. It presents acupuncture points as organising centres in morphogenesis[2]. Intrinsic electric fields and currents are important factors in growth control, cell migration and morphogenesis. A variety of cells including neurones, myoblasts and fibroblasts are sensitive to electric fields of physiological strength[3]. In most cases there is enhanced cell growth toward cathode and reduced cell growth towards anode in small continuous, pulsed or focal electric fields[4,5]. A change in electric activity correlates with signal transduction and can precede morphological changes[6,7]. For example in frogs outward current can be detected on the site of a future limb bud several days before the first cell grows[8].

The conductance of acupuncture points varies and correlates with physiological change[9] and pathogenesis[10]. Manipulation of the electric field can therefore lead to morphological changes. According to Shinju's model, the network of organising centres retain their growth control function after morphogenesis and communicate with each other to maintain proper functions. Therefore an abnormality inside the network may be detected by measuring the electrical parameters of some points on its surface. Malfunctions of some organs can be preceded by changes of electrical parameters from normal range and treated by manipulation of the connected acupuncture points.

Another study[11] showed that the calcium ion concentration in meridians and acupuncture points in rabbits was significantly higher than in non-meridian and non-acupuncture points. Calcium is involved in various physiological functions. Its electrochemical gradient contributes to the electric potential across the cell membrane. Calcium waves can be elicited by electrical, mechanical, chemical or laser stimulation. Similarly the therapeutic effects of acupuncture can be achieved by various stimuli, including laser, mechanical and electrical. It is suggested that calcium may play an important factor in acupuncture, and may be involved in the activities of the meridian system.

The analgesic effect of acupuncture is explainable by its endorphin effect, which can be blocked by naloxone. This shows an effect of acupuncture on the nervous system. But neither the effect of Auricular Acupuncture nor the fact that a lot of acupuncture points and meridians do not follow the nervous or circulatory system, can be explained by this model.

The Meridian System is a distinct signal transduction system. A combined research project between the departments of Biomedical Engineering, Neuroanaesthesia and Neurointensive Care Medicine, the Department of Anaesthesiaology and Critical Care and the Department of Ophthalmology at the University of Graz, Austria, has shown, with a specially constructed multidirectional ultrasound probe, that stimulating an acupuncture point not only leads to local vasodilation (shown with infrared camera), but also leads to an increased blood flow in certain brain areas. Using the technique of transcranial doppler sonography to monitor blood flow in the supratrochlear and middle cerebral arteries, they demonstrated that acupuncture produced specific reproducable and quantifiable effects on blood flow velocity in arteries to the brain and eye[12].

Traditional Chinese Medicine can play a role in eliminating drug-side effects including constipation, orthostatic hypotension, amongst others, whilst consolidating the effects achieved by western medicine[13].

Clinical Research by Dongyun Liang, Zi Cai Feng, Li Zhong and Chen Dong[14] demonstrated that in 110 cases (70 male and 40 female), a combination of Chinese herbs, acupuncture and massage helped in varying degrees to reduce the amount of medication required by some patients and relieved symptoms.

Conclusion

A combination of Chinese herbs, Acupuncture and Massage can often help to reduce the amount of medication required by the patient. It may relieve some symptoms especially in those with shorter onset of the disease.

Studies demonstrate that Traditional Chinese Medicine together with Western treatment can often have beneficial effects in patients with Parkinson's disease.

References

1. *The Mechanism of Acupuncture* by Charles Shang: Boston University School of Medicine: Website: www.acupuncture.com/Acup./Mech.htm

2. Shang C: *Singular Point: Organising Centre and Acupuncture Point*: Am J Chin Med: 1989: 17: pps. 119 - 127

3. Erickson C A: *Morphogenesis of Neural Crest In*: Browder L W: *Developmental Biology*: 1985: p. 528: Plenum, New York, USA

4. Nuccitelli R: *The Involvement of Transcellular Ion Currents and Electric Fields in Pattern Formation*: Malacinski G M: 1984: *Pattern formation*: Macmillan, New York, USA

5. McCaig CD: *Spinal Neurite Regeneration and Re-growth in Vitro Depend on the Polarity of an Applied Electric Field*: 1987: Development 100: pps. 31 - 41

6. Nelson PG, Yu C, Fields RV, Neale EA: *Synaptic Connections in Vitro Modulation of Number and Efficacy by Electrical Activity*: 1989: Science: 244: pps. 585 - 587

7. Shang C: *Bioelectrochemical Oscillations in Signal Transduction and Acupuncture - An Emerging Paradigm*: Am J Chin Med: 1993: 21: pps. 91 - 101

8. Nuccitelli R: *Ionic Currents in Morphogenesis*: 1988: Experientia: 44: pps. 657 - 666

9. Comunetti A, Laage S, Schiesl N, Kistler A: *Characterisation of Human Skin Conductance at Acupuncture Points*: 1995: Experientia: 51: pps. 328 - 331

10. Saku K, Mukaino Y, Ying H, Arakawa K: *Characteristics of Reactive Electropermeable Points on the Auricles of Coronary Heart Disease Patients*: 1993: Clin Cardiol: 16: pps. 415 - 419

11. *The Study on Calcium Ion Concentration Specificity in Meridian and Acupuncture Point in Rabbit (Chinese)*: by Guo Y, Xu T, Chen J: Zhang C,Jiang P: Chen Tzu Yen Chiu 1991: 16: pps. 66 - 68

12. *Ultrasound-monitored Effects of Acupuncture on Brain and Eye*: Neurological Research, volume 21 June: 1999: Gerhard Litscher, Lu Wang, Nai-Hua Yang and Gerhard Schwarz

13. *Clinical Analysis of Parkinson's disease treated by integration of Trad. Chinese and Western Medicine* (Li Genghe, Central hospital of Honkou District, Shanghai) Journal of Traditional Chinese Medicine 15(3): pps. 163 - 169, 1995.

14. *Treatment by Chinese Medicine Parkinsonism* by Dongyun Liang, Zi Cai Feng (SCCF Acupuncture and Health Center, Miami Beach, USA), Li Zhong (Shan Dong Ji Nan First People Hospital, 250011 China), Chen Dong (Shan Dong Province Chest Hospital 250013 China)

Bibliography

Pomeranz B, Stux G: *Scientific Basis of Acupuncture*: Berlin Springerverlag: 1989

CHAPTER 14

Electromagnetic Field Application in Parkinson's Disease

by Dr Christian Thuile

Electromagnetic therapy is now emerging as a promising new therapeutic application, with ongoing international scientific research.

Hundreds of studies substantiate a wide range of benefits for a large number of clinical conditions including osteoarthritis, rheumatoid arthritis, fibromyalgia, tension headaches, migraines, multiple sclerosis and Parkinson's disease.

One of the major effects of electromagnetic therapy is to decrease muscle spasm. This is the reason why it can have significant effects in Parkinson's disease patients.

Along with the decrease of spasm, weak electromagnetic fields in the picoTesla range provide a general calming effect, probably as a result of the recently discovered magnetism in brain cells. Besides this, studies have demonstrated that high frequency, repetitive transcranial magnetic stimulation is an effective, side-effect-free therapy for depression which may also be associated with Parkinson's disease.

As some patients suffer from increased tremor as first reaction to therapy, starting with extremely low intensities has proven useful.

Studies

1. "The Effects of External picoTesla range Magnetic Fields in the EEG in Parkinson's disease": R Sandyk: International Journal of Neurosci 70 (1-2): pps 85-96: 1993.
   In the case of a 68-year-old male patient suffering from Parkinson's disease over a period of seven years, treatment with external application led to quick improvement with respect to tremor, foot dystonia, gait, postural

reflexes, mood, anxiety, cognitive and autonomic functions. These results were especially remarkable as traditional therapy had brought very little relief.

2) "Transcranial Magnetic Stimulation: A Neuropsychiatric Tool for the 21st Century:" MS George, et al: Journal of Neuropsychiatry & Clin Neurosci, 8(4), pps. 373-382, Fall 1996.
   This article discusses recent studies showing that transcranial magnetic stimulation (TMS) has led to improvements in symptoms associated with Parkinson's disease and depression.

3) "Parkinsonian Micrographia Reversed by Treatment with Weak Electromagnetic Fields:" R Sandyk: International Journal of Neurosci, 81 (1-2), pps. 83-93, March 1995.
   This article reports the cases of two Parkinson's disease patients who experienced improvements in motor symptoms following treatment with external application of very weak electromagnetic fields in the picoTesla range.

Case Experiences

a) A 56 year old male suffering from Parkinson's disease over a period of fours years:
   Therapy with L-dopa quite satisfactory, except for recent increase of tremor. Treatment with very weak electromagnetic fields in the picoTesla range led to a repetitive contemporary disappearance of motoric symptoms.

b) A 64 year old male suffering from Parkinson's disease for six years with increasing immobility and tremor of hands. He also suffered aggravating depression for two years:
   After nine months of treatment with very weak electromagnetic fields in the picoTesla range, motoric conditions improved remarkably. This patient was able to go to the toilet on his own again, and his tremor was reduced to such a degree that he was able to eat and drink independently. At the same time, depressive symptoms disappeared.

CHAPTER 15

The Role of the Psychologist in Parkinson's Disease

*by **Cathryn Burley** MSc PGCE BSc AFBPS*

Introduction

This chapter has been written with different sections - one for patients and the other for psychologists.

For Psychologists

It is as important to recognise the reactions of the person and their family to the diagnosis and the ongoing disease process, as it is to treat the physical symptoms of the condition. In this chapter I hope to encourage the professional reader to focus on what it might be like for the person who is given the diagnosis of Parkinson's disease and has to live with the knowledge of having a progressively deteriorating condition. I shall also describe some psychological interventions with patients, their families and carers. These focus on how to overcome, in a practical way, some of the more common responses to the disease. These interventions will focus on reactions, mood and activity.

The onset of Parkinson's disease is often characterized by a vague feeling that something is not right. This may relate to mood, mobility, grip or to the awareness of tremor. This awareness fluctuates in and out of the conscious and can be ignored for periods of time by the person and their family, in the hope that it is not an illness.

The later stages of Parkinson's disease may be characterized by traditional mask like facial features. What thoughts and feelings lie behind for the person who lives with the condition? There are advances in the management of Parkinson's disease. New drug treatments and potential surgical interventions have given hope to people with Parkinson's disease, their carers and the professionals who work with them. As symptoms develop and professional help is sought, people with Parkinson's disease have probably often thought through all possible scenarios as regards the condition. Sometimes they may imagine the worst possible outcome. The conversation that may be running through someone's mind in the initial phase of Parkinson's disease is likely to include thoughts:

What if? I cannot function normally? Whta if I will not live out my normal life span?

For the professional involved the response might be to rationalise by focusing on thoughts such as:

It is only a mild tremor. We can offer drug treatment. It's not life threatening or terminal.

At this point the person and their professional helper are at very different stages in relation to the disease process. The way in which the investigations prior to the diagnosis are carried out, and the way in which the results are fed back, has important consequences for how people and their families subsequently cope. If the information and help offered support people's thoughts and feelings, the outcome is more likely to be successful for both the person and the professional. At the end of the chapter I shall present some brief case studies and notes for professionals.

• • •

For Patients and their Families

As a clinical psychologist, I work closely with the local Parkinson's Disease Nurse Specialist. She knows that it is important to work with not only the physical symptoms of Parkinson's disease but also to find out how you and your family are feeling. I see people who are at different stages of having Parkinson's disease and we work together to try to resolve their problems.

Clinical psychologists are people who are trained in the study of human behaviour. They look at how you react to your life's experiences, which may be illnesses, as these can sometimes influence the way you think, feel and behave. Psychologists will help you to assess what is happening to you in terms of your mood. Also they will help you to judge whether the way you are thinking about what is happening to you is actually helping you to cope with the situation or not. They are trained to help you to cope with anxiety and depression. They may also talk with your partner or your family to find out how they are feeling. They may ask you to answer some questionnaires to assess your mood, or to perform tests to assess your memory and thinking skills. A small number of people with Parkinson's disease may develop memory problems.

If you have been given a diagnosis of Parkinson's disease recently, you will have had a lot on your mind for some time. You may have been noticing some small changes in yourself and have been anxious about them. Many people say that they have had a feeling that "something is not right". This might be to do with you noticing that you had a tremor; that you did not have the stamina to walk so far or dance so much. It might be that you felt that you could not hold things as well as you used to so that it was difficult to knit or to do repair tasks at home. You may feel less like talking or being sociable and you may have become more withdrawn.

Maybe you are afraid to share your feelings with anyone in case they don't take you seriously. You may become very unhappy and family members may notice that something is wrong but they may not know what to do about it. Perhaps you do not want to see your doctor about something that seems so intangible, as you feel concerned that you may be taking up the doctor's time unnecessarily. You may imagine the worst and wonder whether you have cancer or a brain tumor. Perhaps a family member may encourage you to see a doctor. Sometimes a fall makes it necessary for you to ask for advice.

Hopefully, when you first saw your doctor, he was able to do some tests to confirm whether or not you had Parkinson' disease. He would have explained to you what Parkinson's disease was, the treatments and the help available and the possible outcomes. It is often difficult during this first meeting to feel confident enough to ask all the little questions that have been in the back of your mind. It is helpful if you can get into the habit of writing them down and prioritising them so that you ask the most important questions first. Research suggests that we remember very little of what is told to us if we are anxious, unless it is said very clearly in short sentences and repeated several times – so don't worry if you need to go back and ask the same questions again a few days later.

If you live somewhere where you are able to be assigned to a Parkinson's Disease Nurse Specialist (PDNS) or a District Nurse or a Health Visitor with a special interest in Parkinson's disease, one of these care specialists may call to see you at home and ask if you have any questions. You may prefer to read about things or to use the Internet to find out more information.

When you receive the distressing news of your diagnosis, your initial reaction may be complete disbelief or denial. This is often followed by a huge range of quite unpleasant emotions - grief, fearfulness, anger and despair. At this time you may find that you sit and imagine all sorts of things and ask yourself "what if ?" questions:

What if....?

I become a burden on my family?	I will not live to grow old?... to see my grandchildren?
I cannot drive?	I cannot work?
I cannot care for my husband or wife?	I become dependent?.. dribble?... need a wheelchair?
I need to be fed?	I cannot talk?

This is a completely normal reaction. It is the brain's way of helping you to adjust to some very painful ideas and to make plans for the future. It is unlikely that these very strong feelings of fear, anxiety and panic will last for long as none of the above things are likely to happen quickly, if at all. You are able to adjust and adapt to what is happening now and get on with the process of living day by day.

For many years after the diagnosis you may need very little help other than regular visits to your doctor to review your medication. Day by day, you will find ways of coping with all the small changes and you will develop very successful ways of getting around the problems that you face. Sometimes you may find it more difficult to adjust for a variety of reasons. This may be because several difficult things have happened all at once and you have become stressed. This may be because having Parkinson's disease has affected the kind of work you do, where you live, your income - or because other things have happened to other members of the family at the same time, and you have become overloaded. This can make you panic and behave in a less efficient way.

Some people have a greater ability to cope with change than others - they may be better at problem-solving or have more resources - social, financial or emotional. For those who do not have these resources, for a while, Parkinson's disease can seem very unpleasant. They may completely lose confidence in themselves or they may become anxious or depressed. If this happens, what can you do?

Loss of confidence / Low self esteem

Losing confidence in yourself is something that often happens gradually. Perhaps you try to do something and it doesn't work out as well as usual or, if you are feeling a bit low, you think it doesn't. The next time you try to do the same thing, you remember that feeling of inadequacy and begin to think, even before you start the necessary task, that it will go wrong. You soon let someone else do it for you or you give up all together.

This can apply especially to things like your appearance. As your facial muscles change in Parkinson's disease your features move less and you feel that you are not responding to what other members of the family are saying or doing. If you catch sight of yourself in the mirror, you don't seem to be the same person. You begin not to trust yourself. Other people may say things to you and because your facial response is no longer immediate, they may move on before you have had time to respond. You then feel left out of a conversation and don't try to join in. If you no longer like the look of yourself you may begin to take less care of your appearance, avoid mirrors, stop having your hair done or shaving regularly or wearing make up. It may seem to be too much effort. You may begin to avoid going out.

What might help?
Decide that it is important to you to keep communicating.

Start by doing some exercises every day to keep your muscles working. If necessary ask for a referral to a speech and language therapist who will help you to breathe properly and who will give you exercises that help you to enunciate the words that you are having difficulty with.

Make sure that you look at people when you speak. Keep your head up. Keep eye contact. Smile.

Use touch to show people that you are still listening to them or when you want to join in the conversation.

If your writing is becoming small and spidery, practice it a little each day. Use lined paper and try to make your letters half the size of the lines so they can be easily read. Learn to use a typewriter or computer. Ask someone to write letters or emails for you whilst you dictate if you cannot write or type.

Explain to close family and friends what is happening so they give you time to respond.

Take trouble over your appearance. You will feel better if you know that you are looking good. Shave properly and ask for help with this, if necessary. Wear bright clothes, try new jewelry or make up. Treat yourself to baths or showers with special toiletries. If you look good, you will feel good.

Continue with the activities you have always done and take up new challenges. You will still be able to enjoy walks, concerts, cinema, theatre and other social events!

Depression

It is common for people with Parkinson's disease and their carers to become depressed.

When you were first told that you had this illness you may have become depressed. This is not just a day to day low mood but a clinical condition which can affect your brain metabolism, your eating and sleeping routines, your pleasures in life and occasionally, even your wish to live. If you are depressed you may feel that there is no point in planning for the future any more. You may also feel that it is not worth doing anything, so you stop going out and then you may feel more depressed and worthless. It is very important to see your doctor quickly if you begin to feel so low that you don't feel it is worth living any more and you begin to make plans for how you might end your life. He/she may be able to reassure you and may also suggest a short course of anti-depressant medication or a referral to a counselor in the practice or a clinical psychology department at your local hospital. People cannot read your mind, so, however difficult it is, try to tell them what you are thinking and feeling. Your partner or members of the family may have no idea that you are feeling so lonely and helpless. Try to talk with them. They may suggest ways of helping.

There will be times in your illness when you feel that you have lost control over everything. You may feel that you cannot face all the changes that are happening to you because your life has become so different. However, despite the challenges facing you, you have not lost all the skills and competencies you had for dealing with things earlier. Think about the difficulties you are facing and think about how you can overcome them and where you may need help. List your strengths and your skills. Recognise who you have to support you. Look at the gaps and try to work out where you need additional help and support. Don't be afraid to ask. The worst thing that can happen is that the person you ask says no and you have to ask a second person.

If there is a referral to clinical psychologists, they will probably suggest that you see them for a series of hourly appointments. In that time they will ask you questions about yourself, your life and your family. They may ask you to fill in some questionnaires so that they can rate how severe your depression is and monitor changes over time. They will ask you to keep a diary of how you are feeling and what you are doing so that together you can look at any changes that are happening. You will work together to try to change your thinking and your behaviour. For example, you may be asked to structure your day so that you achieve something small each morning, afternoon and evening. You will be asked to rate how you have done for success (mastery) and enjoyment (pleasure). You will gradually find, that as your involvement increases, your low mood lifts.

Sometimes, when you are depressed, even small things seem to become a catastrophe. It can seem that everything goes wrong all of the time. You may begin to expect failure. You will also be asked to look at the negative spiral your thought patterns get into and to try to change negative thoughts for more positive ones.

I can't face going abroad on holiday. I'll never manage to walk along all those corridors at the airport. How will I climb the steps to the plane?

Could be changed to:

I am concerned about going on holiday this year but with a little help and preparation I am sure I will be able to manage it. Airports provide wheelchair services and take you directly on and off the aircraft.

You may also find it harder to concentrate on things that you had previously enjoyed, for example, writing, gardening, reading. You may find that your attention wanders. By breaking down what you have to do into small steps, which are achievable, things will improve. For example, try to read a magazine instead of a book. Set yourself small targets. Recognise your successes.

Anxiety

Bad news can often feel quite overwhelming. Before you were given your diagnosis, think back to what you knew about Parkinson's disease and what you now know. Your thoughts may relate to your understanding of what Parkinson's disease is and how it may progress. Try not to think about people you knew who had Parkinson's disease when you were younger as both treatment and expectations have changed since then. Try not to only listen to family, friends and neighbours or other sufferers but ask your doctor or other professionals for their understanding too. You may also get information from a Parkinson's Disease Society or support group.

This is especially important in relation to medication. If you are prescribed medication talk with the doctor about it so you are sure why you are taking it and what the benefits might be. Many people do not take medication as they are instructed because they fear that it may be addictive, or they take too much or they do not realise the need to take the same dose at the same time each day so that the chemicals give the body the optimum dose.

Do not take too much or too little or stop suddenly or you may get side effects. If you think the medication is causing you side effects, keep a diary of what these are for a few days so you remember the time of onset and nature of your symptoms. You can then discuss them with your doctor or pharmacist (see the chapter 'The Patient's Diary').

Anxiety, like depression, is a word that has both an everyday and a clinical meaning.

In everyday terms, anxiety is a mild state of worry, which passes when you solve the difficulty, which was facing you. In clinical terms, anxiety can mean that feeling of being completely overwhelmed or almost paralysed with fear. It can lead to very unpleasant physical feelings - breathlessness, heart palpitations, sweaty palms, a need to go to the toilet frequently, a feeling of nausea, the development of a rash. There is a surge of adrenaline through your body because it fears a threat (which may or may not be physically real). This state of fear can result in what is called the "fight or flight" reaction. You may become aggressive, irritable and bad tempered or you may feel like running away from the situation, your responsibilities, the illness. At worst, the avoidance may mean that you are paralysed with fear and only want to stay in a safe place, your bed or the house and not confront the real or imaginary dangers at all. As a result, all your muscles tense up ready to fight or to run away. If this state of tension continues for several hours without the opportunity to relax your mind and your body, you may switch into panic as a coping mechanism. You may then learn to dread waking up or facing things over the day because this feeling seems to happen almost automatically. Strangely, the more you avoid things, the worse they may become.

Psychologists would help you to try to understand how this state of extreme arousal has come about. They would help you to learn breathing and relaxation exercises which would teach you to notice when your body was tense or relaxed. They would also help you to challenge your "what if?" thoughts and to face the things that you feared, step by step. By trying a problem solving approach and taking things little by little, you might then be able to go to town again or go on holiday. By setting up a ladder (or a hierarchy) of activities to achieve step by step, you will regain your confidence. Planning is useful. Worrying and anxiety are a fruitless waste of energy.

Reaction to illness
Think about how you have reacted to this illness. Has it completely overwhelmed you? Do you see it as a challenge to be mastered and overcome? For some people, knowing they have an illness can turn them into a patient. They can feel out of control and they can become over-reliant on others to do things for them.

Sometimes partners or family members may collude with this and take over things you used to do for yourself. Although this may be helpful when you are feeling overwhelmed initially, if it continues you may become less and less likely to take responsibility for yourself. You may feel smothered and powerless. This can lead to you feeling very angry and frustrated. Your family may feel that you are not grateful for the help. They become resentful of the time they are spending on the role they have taken on for you even though they have never asked your permission to do so. Conversely, if you see the illness as a challenge and try too hard to do everything for yourself, you may distance friends and family who would like to help you with practical tasks. Try to find a middle path. If your family do too much for you try to stand up to them and suggest that you try for yourself first and then ask for help later, if necessary.

What else can you do?

Do part of a job at a time – tile the kitchen in sections or do a little ironing each day.

Ask for help with high areas or big items.

Ask your family to attend a carers' group so they can talk with others in the same situation.

Talk to other people with Parkinson's disease yourself so that you share what you are going through.

If you notice that your partner is getting over-tired and low in mood, talk together about getting additional help in the house or the odd respite break or support from specialised societies.

Changes in thinking and memory.

Some types of Parkinson's disease cause changes to your brain, which affect your thinking and memory. It is important to check whether these changes are due to anxiety or depression, or whether they are due to a loss of brain cells. Your doctor may ask you to see the psychologist who will do some tests with you which will look at which areas of the brain may be affected and how you can use your remaining abilities to overcome your weaknesses. The assessment will help you and your doctor to plan together the help you may need later. Initially you may have a slight difficulty searching for words or phrases, or remembering what it is that you are doing. By talking it through together, you may come up with helpful strategies to compensate for this.

What else can you do?

Use lists or diaries or memory boards, clocks and timers or electronic aids. You may need to do this more frequently and in a more structured way.

Keep things to a regular (but not inflexible) routine.
Exercise your mind with puzzles, quizzes, crosswords.

Use music or diagrams to help you to remember if you find words difficult.

Delegate financial matters to someone else.

Case studies

Betty: Betty's husband Daniel had retired 6 months before Betty began to feel unwell with Parkinson's disease. He had held a very responsible role as a director of a company and had traveled extensively leaving Betty to work as a teacher and to care for their two sons. When he retired they moved from their home in Birmingham to rural Suffolk to be near one of their sons.

For some time Betty had been feeling that something was not right. She felt a bit depressed and although she knew she should be enjoying her retirement and looking forward to having time with her husband and grandchildren, she did not feel like doing anything. She was finding it harder to sew and knit and to do the housework but couldn't explain why. Daniel began to take over jobs in the house and the garden. Gradually, Betty made excuses not to visit friends and became more withdrawn. She had noticed that it was harder to do up buttons or undo jars and thread needles. She was worried that she might have a brain tumour - especially when she began to develop a tremor. She did not want to go and see the doctor in case he confirmed her suspicions.

After some months, Betty's other son visited. After that he telephoned his father to ask what was wrong. Daniel asked Betty how she was and for the first time she shared her feelings with him. They went to see their doctor who told them that Betty probably had Parkinson's disease and would need to be on tablets for the rest of her life. Both of them were very shocked. Betty continued to do less and less. Daniel continued to do more and more. They did not trouble their doctor again because they thought that there was nothing he could do.

When their son next visited he was even more worried at the changes in his parents as his father was becoming more and more tired. He went to see their doctor to ask about Parkinson's disease and to see if further help was available. Betty was referred to the Parkinson's Disease Nurse Specialist but did not want anyone to visit the house. She did agree to attend the clinic at the local hospital where she met the psychologist.

Betty was very nervous about her first appointment. She felt that she was taking up time unnecessarily and that nothing could be done. The psychologist asked her how long she had been feeling unwell and what she had been thinking. Betty told her of her worries about having a brain tumour and then about how sick she had felt when she received the diagnosis. She has a close friend whose husband had Parkinson's disease and had heard the friend talk about how embarrassed she was that her husband was never still, that he could not talk without dribbling and always drew attention to himself in public. Betty said that she wished that she was dead because she did not wish to put her family and friends through that. She felt that she was letting her husband down by spoiling his retirement, and her sons, by not being a proper grandmother. She would not be able to have her grandchildren to stay.

From the psychologist, Betty and her husband learned more about Parkinson's disease and the drug treatments available. The psychologist explained about a therapy called Cognitive Behaviourial Therapy, which works with anxiety and depression. It looks at what people are avoiding and tries to see how their feelings influence their thoughts and stop them from doing things. The psychologist encouraged Betty to talk about her fears and to recognise that her illness would not necessarily be the same as that of her friend's husband. She explained to Betty that problems like dribbling could be helped with both drugs and exercises.

She also suggested that it was better to go out for a meal than not to go out at all and that there were ways that she could make herself less noticeable, if that was what was worrying her. For example

a) she could sit with her back at a 45 degree angle to the room

b) choose food from the menu with careful consideration - foods which are easier to manage such as soups, ratatouille and risotto, which are presented in soft, small pieces

c) ask for help with cutting food, if necessary, ask for small portions

d) have one fewer course than other people so that she could start and end at the same time

They also talked about what being a proper grandmother meant to Betty. She also admitted that for her the most important thing about being a grandparent was to spend time with the grandchildren - and Parkinson's disease did not stop her doing that. Together they worked out when the grandchildren could visit and what kinds of things they could still do together easily. She also came to recognise that her friend was embarrassed about keeping up appearances and needed psychological support herself in order to cope. Betty began to feel much less out of control. She was less depressed.

Ann and Philip: Ann and Philip lived alone in a small Lincolnshire village. Ann had an ulcer and more recently mobility problems due to Parkinson's disease. At 76 Ann had never driven. She shared many interests with their daughter who Lucy had emigrated to Canada eight years earlier. Philip had been a hard worker and a good provider, well respected who worked with him. While Ann was responsible for organising the finances and the running of the home he did the practical tasks and fetched the shopping. He developed memory problems. When Ann met the psychologist she did not think that she could be helped. She found it difficult to talk about her feelings. She found it very distressing that her husband couldn't talk with her anymore, but she would not talk to anyone else. With regular visits she began to talk about how much the loss of her daughter had meant to her and how the Parkinson's disease and then her husbands memory problems had seemed too difficult to share with anyone. She felt that she had to keep going alone. With some persuasion she rejoined a church group and made contact with a school friend. She began to share her feelings, a little and to feel less isolated.

Robert: Robert had been suffering from Parkinson's disease for several years. His had a shuffling gait and his balance was affected. His speech was whispery. His wife May was very hard of hearing and had her own physical problems due to a previous back operation which had gone wrong. She had no family or friends in the small market town where they lived. She became very exasperated with Robert and with the restrictions in her own life. When Robert began to attend a Day Hospital he quickly made friends who enjoyed his sense of humour. Speech therapy and physiotherapy helped his confidence and the staff visited his wife to explain how to help him walk through doorways without shuffling or freezing, by looking up and ahead or by singing a marching song. May joined a carer's group, and listened to others, but did not join in. The tension between them eased.

Notes for Professionals

"Stand in the shoes" of the person with Parkinson's disease and their family. Ask what they are thinking or feeling.

Ask what they already know about Parkinson's disease.

Ask how they normally cope with sickness and ill health.

Ask what their expectations of life and retirement had been.

Ask what other responsibilities they have.

Discover their fears, however small. If someone is sitting silent, allow them time to think before they speak. Do not be too alarmed if they cry or are angry.

The Team

Do you know what resources exist in your area and what kind of role each professional has and what they can offer.

Keep a folder of information relevant to Parkinson's disease.

Find out about the clinical psychology service. Do they have a waiting list? How long is it. Will they visit people at home. What therapies do they offer.

Loss of confidence

Try not to overwhelm with too many suggestions

Encourage people to do more of what they are already doing.

Look at how people present themselves – what else could they do?

Comment on successes.

Depression

Use the Beck Depression Inventory, The Hospital Anxiety and Depression Scale or Geriatric Depression Scale to monitor mood.

Listen for fears about suicidal thoughts.

Try to encourage compliance with medication.

Increase activity then challenge thoughts.

Give small achievable tasks to do between sessions.

If they are unable to record things, do it for them.

Anxiety

Teach breathing and relaxation exercises and keep records.

Look for natural relaxation and reinforce it (eg singing).

Teach people how to cope with panic.

Break tasks down into small parts.

Expect some setbacks and help people learn to set new targets from these.

Explain that Parkinson's disease is a fluctuating illness and some symptoms will come and go.

Reaction

This happens throughout the illness.

Check how someone is feeling now and what they are thinking will happen next.

Help with practical problem solving.

Memory

Recognise when someone needs specialist help to cope with memory loss and refer on.

Help to plan additional care.

Encourage the use of memory skills, daily. Suggest using lists, notice boards, calendars, timers, clocks and watches with alarms.

Encourage making notes to help with key points but only to use them as a prompt, if necessary.

Notes of topics to cover

Reaction to diagnosis, perception, meaning.

Feelings about medication.

Changes in mood - anxiety, panic, poor relaxation, avoidance, tension, suicidal thought, self harm, living wills fear of madness.

Challenging negative thoughts.

Recognise competencies.

Grief, loss.

Developmental skills.

Goal setting.

Managing outcomes, planning.

Compliance.

Low self-esteem, poor self image.

Lack of ability to view self as positiv, mask like features, poor writing, poor emotional reaction.

Stress management - interplay of physical, emotional and biochemical factors

Illness behaviour - avoidance - what if?

Partner/spouse collusion - smothering, over-protecting carers.

Partner/spouse low mood.

Reaction to disability - coping strategies - who cares? - networks.

Changes in cognition - assessment of memory and thinking.

Sensory engagement.

Bibliography

Anxiety And Parkinson's Disease; Pps. 383-392; Irene Hegeman Richard MD, Randolph B. Schiffer MD, Roger Kurlan MD; June 1995; *The Journal Of Neuropsychiatry And Clinical Neurosciences* 1996.

Behavioral Analysis Of The Freezing Phenomenon In Parkinson's Disease: A Case Study. Pages 241-7; Macht, M., Ellgring, H., *Journal Of Behaviour Therapy And Experimental Psychiatry*. 1999 Sep; 30(3).

Behavioral Dysfunction In Parkinson's Disease. Pps. 87-93; Friedman, J.H., 1998; *Clinical Neuroscience* 5(2).

The Correlation Of Depression With Functional Activity In Parkinson's Disease; Pages 493-498; Chia-Yih Liu, Shuu-Jiun Wang, Jong-Ling Fuh, Cheng-Huai Lin, Yong-Yi Yang, Hsiu-Chih Liu; January 1997; *Journal Of Neurology* (1997).

Depression In Parkinson's Disease: A Quantitative And Qualitative Analysis; Pages381-389; A-M Gotham, RG Brown And CD Marsden; 1985; *Journal Of Neurology, And Psychiatry* 1986.

Do Ya Think I'm Sexy? February 26, Volume 23, No. 9, 1997 *Nursing Times*.

Expressions - Understanding The Language Of Parkinson's Communication; January 1998; Bridget Mccall, Information Manager Parkinson's Disease Society; *Parkinson's Disease Society Of The United Kingdom*

Measuring Symptom Change In Patients With Parkinson's Disease. Pages 41-5; Harrison J.E., Preston. S., Blunt S.B., *Age And Ageing; Age Ageing*. 2000 Jan; 29(1).

Mind Over Mood: A Cognitive Treatment Manual For Clients. Greenberger, D. Padesky, C.A. 1995 Guilford Press New York

*Parkinson's Disease: Drug-Induced Psychiatric State*s. Pages 115-38. Factor, SA., Molho. ES., Podskalny. GD., Brown. D., 1995. *Advance In Neurology*. 65.

Parkinson's Disease In The Elderly Special Interest Group Conference Proceedings Supported By The British Geriatric Society; Mark Greener; Macmillan Magazines

Psychological Effects Of Structured Cognitive Psychotherapy In Young Patients With Parkinson's Disease: A Pilot Study; Pages 217-221. 1999; Dreisig, -Hanne; Beckmann, -Jorn; Wermuth, -Lene; Skovlund, -Soren; Bech, -Per. *Nordic Journal Of Psychiatry* 1999; Vol 53(3).

Therapy Of Behavioral Disorders In Parkinson's Disease; Pages149-153; F. Valldeoriola, J. Molinuevo; 1999; Biomed & Pharmacother 1999

Treatment Of Behavioural Disturbances In Parkinson's Disease; Pages 175-204; F. Valldeoriola, F.A. Nobbe And E. Tolosa; 1997; *Journal Of Neural Transm* (1997).

Treatment Of Parkinson's Disease (Letter; Comment). Pages 643-4. Grieger. TA., Cozza. K., Armstrong. S., 1994. *The New England Journal Of Medicine*, Mar 3; 330(9).

Understanding The Challenges Of Parkinson's Disease Website: http://www.nursinghome.org/closeup/cupdocuments.cu120.htm

CHAPTER 16

The Role of the Parkinson's Disease Nurse Specialist (PDNS)

by Carolyn Noble RGN

The development of the role of the Parkinson's Disease Nurse Specialist (PDNS) has been shown to have a significant contribution to the quality of life of those affected by Parkinson's disease. It raises awareness of the difficulties imposed by the condition upon the individual, their relatives or carers and for health professionals involved in their care[1].

Most Parkinson's Disease Nurse Specialists have considerable nursing experience with a background in neurology or community nursing and have experience in teaching and counselling skills. Whilst all Parkinson's Disease Nurse Specialists undergo further training to up-regulate their practice, their most important asset is the empathic approach to those experiencing difficulties resulting from Parkinson's disease.

The first Parkinson's Disease Nurse Specialist was appointed in 1989 and a few years later in 1994 the Parkinson's Disease Nurse Specialist project was launched by the Parkinson's Disease Society together with the pharmaceutical industry[2]. There are currently seventy-eight Parkinson's Disease Nurse Specialists in posts in the UK, employed in a variety of settings including specialist centres, acute hospitals and in the community. Almost all Parkinson's Disease Nurse Specialists work alongside a consultant neurologist or geriatrician with an interest in Parkinson's disease, providing a service to people in the hospital environment and the community.

Some Parkinson's Disease Nurse Specialists are involved primarily with research, others work with people undergoing neurosurgery and a number play a major role in facilitating clinical drug trials. Although there are variations within the different roles, the Parkinson's Disease Nurse Specialists share a common aim: to improve quality of life for those with Parkinson's disease and for those who support them by promoting a higher level of understanding through education.

At the Point of Diagnosis

Early referral to the Parkinson's Disease Nurse Specialist can ensure alleviation of some of the distress experienced by the patient and their relatives around the time of the diagnosis[3].

It is well recognised that people receive the diagnosis of Parkinson's disease in situations far from ideal. Not all health professionals are skilled at breaking bad news and recognising the distress that this can evoke.

On receiving the diagnosis, a person may have difficulty assimilating complex information. However, it is important to understand what is happening. The diagnosis of Parkinson's disease is a life-altering experience, which can threaten many aspects of quality of life. When people have had the opportunity to come to terms with the news of the diagnosis, they can then reflect on its personal meaning and be ready to receive further information. The Parkinson's Disease Nurse Specialist can offer individual support, re-inforce and clarify any information provided in the clinical setting and elicit hope at this very difficult time.

Continuous support and information will enable newly diagnosed people to work towards acceptance of the diagnosis and by encouraging them to ask questions, they will be able to make choices and become involved in the management of the condition. It is very important to enable people to regain control over the situation and to regain their identity.

Personal Identity is all about 'holding on to who we are'

Identity is threatened by:

- Loss of skills
  - *in the workplace*
  - *driving*
  - *difficulties with personal care*

- Loss of social roles
  - *coping with role reversals and transferring tasks that one was once responsible for, to one's partner*
  - *changes to social life and social networks*
  - *communication with others (threat to identity comes from changes in the way that others react to the person and also the way in which the person perceives himself/herself)*

■ Threat of future change - *views on life and the life that is to come*
- *concern about the disease itself and its progression*
- *worry about the future, "who will care for me?"*

For younger people, anxieties concerning work, finances, relationships, pregnancy, younger children and changing lifestyles can create uncertainties regarding the future.

When Parkinson's disease is diagnosed in later years, the anxiety focus is around loss of independence and increasing dependence on others.

KEYNOTE FOR PROFESSIONALS

GPs rarely see more than a few people with Parkinson's disease. The presentation and progression in each case may be quite different.

- *Ensure that the patient is referred to a specialist for confirmation of diagnosis.*

- *Refer to the PDNS to provide support and information and enable the person to come to terms with the diagnosis[4]*

Individual with Parkinson's disease and their partners or carers may react to the diagnosis in different ways and subsequently will come to terms with the impact of the diagnosis at differing times. People cope with the impact of major changes in their lives by passing through a series of phases that will gradually lead to an adaptive adjustment to the change.

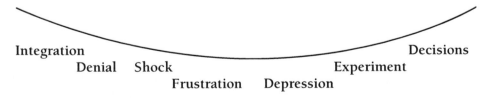

Integration   Decisions

Denial   Shock   Experiment

Frustration   Depression

The usual reaction to bad news is one of disbelief, followed by resistance to acknowledge the information or to seek out further information. The next stage includes a period of exploration when information is actively sought and people feel ready to tell others about their condition in a less inhibited way. Finally, the last phase is one of decision making or acceptance of change.

Difficulties can arise when people with Parkinson's disease and their partner or carer are at different stages within the process of change. For example, people diagnosed with Parkinson's disease may remain in a phase of denial, whilst their partners/family or carers may have reached the 'experimental' phase and may be actively seeking information.

The Parkinson's Disease Nurse Specialist is skilled at recognising conflicts and providing support for all of those involved by encouraging good communication to enable people to progress through the period of change.

The Parkinson's Disease Nurse Specialist is skilled at assessing individual needs and referring to other professionals within the multi-disciplinary team for early advice.

As the condition progresses the complexities of treatment and deterioration in functioning can create difficulties. The Parkinson's Disease Nurse Specialist can supervise changes to drug regimes under the direction of the consultant. Side effects can be monitored and changes to medication can be initiated following liaison with the consultant or GP. It is often the Parkinson's Disease Nurse Specialist who explains how the medication may work and enables the person to use it to their best advantage.

Risk assessment is an important part of the role of the Parkinson's Disease Nurse Specialists. As the condition progresses, the risk of falls and hospital admission increase. Identification of those at risk can sometimes help to prevent unnecessary stays in hospital, which can be extremely distressing for someone with Parkinson's disease. For those admitted to hospital, the Parkinson's Disease Nurse Specialist can liase with the ward staff and advise on timing of medication and self-medication programmes if available.

During the later stages as the condition progresses, the carer requires a great deal of support and it is often the Parkinson's Disease Nurse Specialist who arranges day care, respite care and personal care packages. Recognising carer strain is an important role for the Parkinson's Disease Nurse Specialist who may introduce the carer to support groups and the local branch of the Parkinson's Disease Society.

The role of the PDNS can be defined as follows:

- Counsellor

- Advocate

- Educator

- Facilitator of individualised care

- Enabler

- Expert practitioner

- Researcher

The role of the Parkinson's Disease Nurse Specialist is extremely challenging and rewarding and is a service, which is greatly valued by those affected by the condition.

The Parkinson's Disease Society in the UK is working towards a target of facilitating the appointment of 240 Parkinson's Disease Nurse Specialists to ensure greater coverage of services throughout the UK.

KEYNOTE FOR THOSE AFFECTED BY PARKINSON'S DISEASE

- Find out if there is a Parkinson's Disease Nurse Specialist in your area by contacting the Parkinson's Disease Society (UK Helpline Tel: Freefone 0808 800 0303 or other similar support groups.

OR

- Enquire at your local Doctors surgery or hospital clinic, if there is a specialist Parkinson's disease nursing service available.

References

1. MacMahon. D. G, Thomas. S. *Practical Approach to Quality of Life in Parkinson's disease: The Nurses Role.* J. Neurol. (1998) 245 (suppl. 1) p 519 - 522.

2. Baker. M, Roy. S. (1997) *The Development of the Parkinson's Disease Nurse Specialist, PDS.* London p. 2:

3. Primary Care Task Force for PDS. UK. (1999) *Parkinson's Aware in Primary Care, PDS* London p. 1:

4. Op. cit. 3

Bibliography

Parkinson's Disease Nurse Specialist Association.

The Developing Role of the PDNS (1998) RCN, PDS, London.

Parkinson's, The Nurse (1999) PDS, London, UK

On Death and Dying: E Kübler-Ross: 1970: Tavistock, London, UK

On Death and Dying: E Kubler-Ross: 1969: MacMillan Publishing Company Inc., New York, USA

CHAPTER 17

Communication
The Role of the Speech and Language Therapist

---

by S Christine Glover MCSLT

Introduction

Communication between people generally breaks down barriers, enhances the quality of life, and extends social interaction. Many people with Parkinson's disease find that the problem can create barriers leading to isolation and withdrawal, depression and a disconnection from society.

Communication is about much more than speech. The mechanics of speech cannot be isolated from the overall purpose of language and communication, and the social implications linked to them. Communication is a lifeline, a two-way interaction requiring effort and acceptance on both sides. A person with Parkinson's disease is battling, not only with the symptoms and frustrations of the disease, but also with the attitudes, responses and general reactions of other people. Communication is a social skill, and the way we communicate tends to determine how we are perceived by other people.

When people have difficulty communicating with each other, for whatever reason, both sides tend to become embarrassed. Embarrassment upsets the communicator who may well withdraw. Family and friends may then wrongly get the impression that the person with Parkinson's disease is no longer able or does not wish to maintain contact. Because they lack understanding of what is really happening, family, friends and colleagues at work do not know how to handle the changed circumstances and may come to the completely erroneous conclusion that the person with Parkinson's disease has changed personality and is not the same person as before. He/she then loses the will to talk, will avoid social situations, and become further isolated and depressed.

For these reasons, it is an important role of the Speech and Language Therapist to help the family, the patient and any other carers to accept changes in behaviour, to keep alive the desire to communicate, and to include the patient in decision making, giving him/her time to offer opinions, make choices, and be angry. Maintaining self-esteem and confidence is very important in maintaining the will to live life to the full despite any difficulties.

Something over 50% of all people diagnosed with Parkinson's disease will develop problems with one or more aspects of communication at some time, and of these, nearly all will experience some difficulty with swallowing, and many also with drooling.

Involvement with a Speech and Language Therapist at an early stage, even before such symptoms develop, will enable simple strategies to be learned which will help delay the onset and progression of speech and swallowing difficulties and can minimise their severity significantly. It is more effective to delay or diminish the onset of these difficulties than to try to remedy them once they become established. Early referral is, therefore, to be strongly recommended. Referral may be made by the General Practitioner or any member of the multi-disciplinary team. The patient, however, can also refer him/herself to the Speech and Language Department of the local hospital (applies in the UK only). At the initial appointment with the Speech and Language Therapist, a full assessment of present and incipient problems will be discussed and the patient will be encouraged to become aware of and monitor any changes as they occur. If appropriate, regular appointments for advice on remedial or preventive strategies will be offered over some weeks, followed by review appointments at regular intervals of, say, three months, with the proviso that the patient may ask for an earlier date if they feel the need. In this way, a relationship of trust develops between the therapist and the person with Parkinson's disease, which encourages him/her to ask for help and express fears as they arise, and become more confident that many of their difficulties can be tackled successfully. If the Speech and Language Therapist is a member of a multi-disciplinary team involved with the person referred, he/she will be able to liaise closely with other professionals and work with them to combine expertise.

Non-verbal Communication

Throughout life, we communicate in many ways in addition to speech. In fact, even within speech, the words we use are only 7ure, facial expression, and posture all reinforce the content and meaning of what we are saying. To some extent, we can all communicate with people whose language we can neither speak nor understand, by all these non-verbal means. We use hand movements, smiles, frowns, etc, but all body language is affected by Parkinson's disease. Facial expression is diminished by rigidity, slowness of movement (bradykinesia), poor co-ordination or stiffness of the facial muscles, and by difficulty in making and retaining eye contact. Smiling and frowning become difficult, muscles do not respond to emotion and people who do not understand the cause of this gain the wrong impression, misunderstand and ignore or retreat from further contact. Likewise, loss of body language like waving, pointing or shrugging, beckoning, etc, again causes confusion and misunderstanding on both sides. The involuntary and uncontrolled movements of dyskinesia, often associated with the taking of drugs, can affect any part of the body, including the face. This contributes a further hazard in distorting speech or making eating and drinking more difficult.

Fluctuation of symptoms from day to day or even from hour to hour is very difficult for people to understand, and can lead to irritation when, for instance, 'freezing' occurs at a socially inconvenient moment.

Social Interaction

Social interaction tends to be inhibited because conversation generally requires an immediate response. In people with Parkinson's disease response may be delayed. There is often difficulty in initiating speech - a 'trigger' is required. Speech flow may also 'dry up' in mid-sentence if the person loses the thread of what they are saying. Oral muscles may freeze in mid-sentence so the speaker is unable to continue even though they know exactly what they wish to say. Poor eye contact makes concentration difficult. Observers may have difficulty in recognising humour, anger or other nuances, especially in the absence of subtle changes of intonation, which can affect meaning.

Speech

Let us look more specifically then at the problems which may occur with speech and what may be done about them. Various aspects need to be considered including respiration, phonation, articulation and expression (including rhythm, pitch/speed, change, stress, intonation etc).

Respiration and Phonation

Respiration is the first and most important function of the speech system. Up to 87% of people with Parkinson's disease have decreased lung function and shallow breathing, which is uncoordinated with speech. There may be weak, hoarse, strained or tremulous voice, fading, volume and difficulty in initiating voice. Reduced capacity and control of the air stream leads to poor breath support for the voice and poor synchronisation with phonation. Breathing and breath control exercises begun at an early stage can be very effective and have other benefits in promoting feelings of well-being, especially when combined with relaxation exercises.

Articulation

Weakness and reduced range of the oro-facial muscles may contribute to poor articulation, particularly reducing the contrast between sounds in longer words, which tend to 'run together' and sound slurred (dysarthria). Exercises to increase strength, flexibility and range of movement in these muscle groups, practised for a few minutes at regular intervals, can help both to improve the clarity of articulation and to maintain variety and ease of facial expression.

Co-ordination / Prosody

Because of difficulties co-ordinating the rate of speech and getting the rhythm right, emphasis and variation tend to disappear, leading to speech which sounds flat and monotonous, giving the impression of apathy, boredom and even low intelligence. A common problem is the inability to control the speed of speech, which may start off at a normal rate but speeds up (or festinate) to a point where it 'runs away' and becomes unintelligible. Alternatively, the opposite may be the case and speech may become abnormally slow and laboured. Again, strategies and exercises can be learned to help to counteract this.

Cognitive Impairment / Dementia

Research shows that there is likely to be some cognitive impairment associated with Parkinson's disease. This can vary in severity and may be noticeable in slowness of recall and response, forgetfulness, some high-level comprehension deficit and high level word-finding difficulty. All people with Parkinson's disease are different but a comprehensive assessment and individually planned programme of therapy for all affected areas can make a big difference to the quality of life. Dementia can be difficult to diagnose accurately in Parkinson's disease as symptoms such as have already been described, combined with depression, can confuse the diagnosis. However, the possibility of it occurring increases with age and the length of time since the onset of the disease.

Communication Aids

If speech fails completely, or is very variable according to the person's general state of health, reaction to drugs, tiredness, etc, a range of communication aids is available to cater for different abilities. These include amplifiers to increase the volume of speech, communication boards or folders tailored to individual needs, and a variety of small speech-output computer aids. The Speech and Language Therapist will be able to arrange a full assessment to determine the best aids for any particular individual, and will offer support and guidance in getting the best use from them. Help with funding for these aids can sometimes be arranged, through charitable foundations or voluntary groups.

Group Therapy for Patients and Carers

The opportunity for Group Therapy will be offered where appropriate. There is often much benefit to be gained if patients who have similar problems and anxieties can exchange views and experiences and enjoy socialising together in a non-threatening atmosphere. For similar reasons, support groups for carers either separately, or in tandem with the patients' groups, are helpful.

Eating, Drinking and Swallowing

Eating and drinking should be a pleasurable social activity and, when problems occur, the results are distressing both for the people with Parkinson's disease and their relatives and friends. Weakness and/or poor co-ordination of the muscles involved in swallowing give rise to fear and tension, and to a reluctance to eat, especially in front of others. This reluctance can also be caused by poor head control, poor posture of the upper body, poor attention span, forgetfulness and dementia.

Over 50% of Parkinson's disease patients will, at some time, have problems with swallowing (dysphagia), which can vary from mild and occasionally to severe regular disruption of the swallowing mechanism when the swallowing may become unsafe and life-threatening, possibly leading to aspiration pneumonia.

Problems may arise at any of these stages of swallowing: the oral stage, whilst food is still in the mouth, the pharyngeal stage, whilst the food is in the upper part of the throat, or the oesophageal stage, when the food is carried down to the stomach. Only the first stage is voluntary. Once the food arrives at the back of the throat, the automatic or reflex action of the muscles takes over, and we have no further control.

Lips, tongue, jaw and palate all play a part in preparing the bolus of food to be directed towards the pharynx. The lips provide a seal to prevent the food falling out of the mouth, the jaws move up and down and rotate sideways to chop the food (chewing). The tongue then manipulates the bolus into a suitable consistency, mixing it with saliva until it is soft enough to be swallowed. It then pushes it towards the roof of the mouth, pressing and squeezing it onto the palate, and the reflex swallow is initiated. The larynx (voice box) is raised up to meet the epiglottis to form a tight seal, which prevents food from going into the airways down to the lungs or "going down the wrong way". Should this happen, coughing or choking occurs in an attempt to expel the food or drink from the airway. If the coughing mechanism fails and food reaches the lungs, aspiration pneumonia may follow and may be fatal. In stage three, the food is propelled down the oesophagus into the stomach by a combination of gravity and reflex muscle action. Since between 30 and 40 muscle movements are involved in a complete swallow, it is easy to see how weakness or lack of co-ordination at any stage can disrupt it.

The problems of swallowing are complex and individual and can affect both eating and drinking:

- Tremor or rigidity may make it difficult for the person with Parkinson's disease to get food to the mouth, or need so much effort that fatigue sets in and leaves no energy for chewing and swallowing. In this case, it may be appropriate for the patient to be fed by a carer, or the Occupational Therapist may be able to suggest adaptations to cutlery, crockery, or head/arm supports to ease the problem.

- Poor lip seal results in anterior leakage, and food falling from the mouth.

- Difficulty with chewing (poor jaw/tongue movement or ill-fitting dentures) may cause the person to swallow food pieces whole, before they are soft enough and ready to be swallowed.

- Delayed triggering of the swallow reflex leads to food staying in the mouth, and a build-up, or 'pocketing' of food. The patient may 'forget' and lose concentration and need frequent reminding and encouraging to swallow.

- If eating becomes slow and effortful, patients lose interest in food and may become malnourished. The Speech and Language Therapist will liaise with the Dietician or Nutritionist so that adequate nutrition can be achieved, while appropriate consistencies for safe swallowing can be maintained.

- There may be delay at the pharyngeal stage of swallowing. Delayed or poor lift of the larynx, and inadequate closure of the epiglottic seal, may cause food to escape into the airways.

Dysphagia needs detailed and specific assessment by a Speech and Language Therapist. Other assessment tools, including Videofluoroscopy, may be employed to explore problems with swallowing which cannot be identified by other means. Following full assessment, advice on strategies for coping with dysphagia are offered, and will include attention to posture and head control, lip closure, chewing action, controlling the quality of food per mouthful, the texture and consistency of food and liquid, the need for concentration, allowing plenty of time and encouraging extra swallows between mouthfuls, and the importance of ensuring a completely empty mouth at the end of each meal. If swallowing fails completely, it may be necessary to consider alternative, non-oral feeding methods such as tube feeding. Decisions about this have ethical implications and will be made jointly by medical staff, the Speech and Language Therapist, the patient and his/her family.

Drooling

Drooling is the leaking of saliva through a poor lip seal, and is another embarrassing symptom leading to withdrawal from the company of friends. Rigidity may make the automatic swallow less reliable, causing pooling of saliva in the mouth which builds up and spills over. Reduced oral sensation contributes to the delay in swallowing saliva as the patient is unaware of its accumulation. We generally swallow saliva two or three times a minutes, and the person with Parkinson's disease should be encouraged to keep the head up, practice holding the lips together, and swallow deliberately every 20 - 25 seconds to re-establish the habit.

General Advice for Carers

Since no two people with Parkinson's disease have identical communication difficulties, it is inappropriate here to give specific advice on exercises. However, here are a few tips to help carers communicate with people with Parkinson's disease.

- Allow plenty of time for the patient to respond.

- Try to gain and maintain eye contact to help concentration.

- Encourage short phrases to preserve energy.

- Try to maintain a quiet atmosphere.

- Listen and do not interrupt.

- Do not finish their sentences for them.

- Do not pretend you understand when you don't. Ask the patient to repeat key words or to put it in another way.

- Always face the person when speaking or listening.

- Include the patient in family discussions and decision-making, especially those, which directly affect him/her.

Note:

If the speech problem is really bad, make a set of cards with a key word or phrase on each individual card so that the person with Parkinson's disease can use these for communication.

Conclusions

The way forward for Speech and Language Therapists dealing with Parkinsonism is positive and multi-faceted. Their role includes:

- Raising awareness with other professionals of the benefits of early referral and ongoing involvement with Speech and Language Therapists.

- Optimising all aspects of the communication function for people with Parkinson's disease through planned programmes of appropriate relaxation, breathing and muscular exercises, and offering strategies to help overcome specific problems in daily situations, monitoring and reviewing changes as they occur.

- Helping raise confidence and self-esteem in the patient and encouraging participation in suitable hobbies and social activities.

- Offering support and suggestions to family members and carers to help them understand the true nature of the communication difficulties experienced by people with Parkinson's disease.

- Offering support and suggestions to help maintain pleasure and safety in eating and drinking and giving explanations for advice given.

- Where necessary, facilitating access to or providing appropriate communication aids, and advising on their use.

- Offering, where appropriate, the opportunity for Group Therapy and Support Groups for carers.

- Using all opportunities to raise awareness, amongst the general public, of the nature of the communication problems faced by people with Parkinson's disease.

Conclusion

With early intervention, advice, regular monitoring and support, many people with Parkinson's disease will be able to function at their maximum potential for a long period. In my experience, people who are seen soon after diagnosis and who then adopt appropriate strategies which they have been taught, learn to be aware of any slight changes as they arise and then ask for further guidance. In many cases, their condition (providing they are on an appropriate drug regime) can be stable, and their lives fulfilling and purposeful for many years.

CHAPTER 18

Osteopathy in Parkinson's Disease

by John Bird DO

O steopathy focuses on the diagnosis and treatment of musculoskeletal dysfunction. Defects in the musculoskeletal system cause a serious impediment to the daily lives of those affected, which in turn may reduce quality of life.

The main aim of osteopathic treatment is to restore optimal musculoskeletal function and reduce pain.

The musculoskeletal system comprises of over 60% of the human body. It is the primary machinery of life and is therefore of major importance in terms of dysfunction and treatment.

Often the primary cause of musculoskeletal dysfunction is neurological. Parkinson's disease is characterised by musculoskeletal manifestations - tremor, rigidity, stiffness and poverty of movement.

Parkinson's disease is one of the most common neurological diseases and as such assumes an important place in the development of osteopathic treatment.

The osteopath assesses skeletal alignment, the function of muscle tissue and joints and functional disorders. Osteopathic management may include treatment to soft tissue, articulation, low velocity manipulation, muscle energy, visceral, counter strain and functional techniques. This indirectly influences associated vascular and neural elements and may help relieve stiffness and stress rigidity.

Rehabilitation exercises should be prescribed for long-term benefit together with medical advice and treatment, providing an integrated approach in the overall management of the patient. This approach is particularly appropriate in Parkinson's disease, which has diverse and multifaceted manifestations and symptoms.

Osteopathic treatment may help to relieve some of the musculoskeletal symptoms associated with Parkinson's disease, such as stiffness and rigidity. Patient collaboration (the willingness of patients to undergo treatment and do remedial exercise) is a vital ingredient in any treatment plan. This can positively influence the patients overall mobility and ability to perform the "activities of daily living", which is so important in living an independent and fulfilled life.

It is best not to have eaten a large meal before treatment. If patients are on L-dopa therapy, it can be helpful for them to present for treatment when their drugs have "kicked in". Patients should be aware of drug-nutrient interaction[1,] which may undermine drug absorption and impair motor control. (See details of *L-dopa "Sinemet" and "Madopar" with Protein*, in the section "Optimising Function by Nutritional Manipulation", on page 235 by Lucille Leader, in the chapter Nutritional Management.)

References

1. *Parkinson's Disease - The New Nutritional Handbook*: p.2:
    Dr Geoffrey Leader and Lucille Leader: 1996: Denor Press, London, UK

Bibliography

Principles of Manual Medicine (2nd edition): Philip E Greenman DO FAAO: 1996: Williams and Wilkins, Baltimore, USA

The Manual of Osteopathic Practice: Dr Alan Stoddard MB BS DO MRO: 1986: Hutchinson and Company Limited, London, UK (reprinted 1993)

Physical Examination of the Spine and Extremities: Stanley Hoppenfeld MD: 1976: Appleton Century Cross, a publishing division of Prentice Hull Inc, Norwalk, USA

CHAPTER 19

The Role of the Physiotherapist in Parkinson's Disease

by Pam Stanbridge MCSP Grad DipPhys SRP

Chartered physiotherapists are uniquely placed to treat Parkinson's disease having learnt to analyse human movement both biomechanically and neurologically (understanding the problems of increased and decreased muscle tone and the interplay of these areas upon one another and with the surface upon which they rest). With knowledge of the disease process and its effects, they can work with patients towards agreed realistic functional goals and achieve more efficient, useful movement in its appropriate setting.

This can be done as part of the hospital environment, in a dedicated area with specific equipment either in a ward or as an outpatient. The treatment can also be given in the community, workplace or fun environment. By seeing patients in their own environment, however, their whole situation can be analysed from a functional angle and help to make life as physically easy as possible. A specific exercise programme can be set up using home furniture (safely), or that environment, as equipment. For example, the difficulty of sitting to standing - by breaking down the movement of sitting to standing into its constituent parts and working on these separately, or by using different exercises to enable better strength or ease of movement of the muscles and joints concerned, the whole action can be noticeably improved.

The chair used at home may be too low or cushioning inappropriate. It can be raised and the cushioning re-arranged with pillows to achieve the best starting position to enable easier standing. As a last resort, a new chair may need to be purchased. All furniture used by the patient should be considered from a functional angle. Often furniture is detrimental to posture and ease of movement.

General Problems

Physiotherapy will not change the course of the disease, but presents strategies to make life easier and maintain greater ease of movement.

Each patient is different with the Parkinson's disease problem superimposed on a body that is unique in the way it moves.

There may be other problems allied to or completely separate from Parkinson's disease that can be managed by physiotherapy. Pain originating from joints and muscles, caused by poor posture or by extra stressing can be addressed using electrical modalities such as ultrasound or appropriate joint mobilisation techniques.

Carers and Family

It may be necessary for physiotherapists to give advice to relatives and carers on how to move the patient with minimum stress to themselves. As it is the family who relates to the patient, it is important that they enable the patient, by their actions and words, to make the best of the situation. As an observer of the relationship between patient and carers, physiotherapists may observe stresses and strains developing. Although not specifically trained in counselling, advice from a trusted outsider may help diffuse tensions.

Ideally each patient needs individual careful physiotherapy assessment, with perhaps a home visit to see the situation as a whole. A treatment plan can be drawn up to deal with the multiple problems identified.

Some strategies that I have found to be very useful for common problems:

ROOTED TO THE SPOT ("FREEZING")

This occurs in the standing position perhaps when a movement is being initiated or when going through a doorway or narrow space, or it just occurs at any time.

"Freezing" happens because body weight is equally distributed between both feet. It is impossible to move one's foot in these circumstances. The weight needs to be shifted to one side to 'free up' a weightless foot in order to step forwards.

| Weight is shifted to the left to allow the right heel to lift | Weight acts downwards through both feet | Weight is shifted to the right to allow left heel to lift |

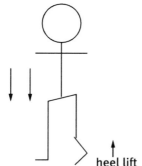
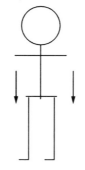
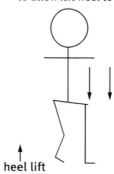

heel lift

heel lift

The way to achieve this is to start a side to side rocking movement of the body through the hips, shifting the weight to the right to allow the left heel to lift; shifting the weight to the left to allow the right heel to lift.

As the rocking develops, more and more weight can be shifted from side to side, until the whole foot can be lifted and then stepping and walking can be started.

The rhythm of the rocking or weight transference needs to be continued into the walk to help maintain the forward momentum of the body weight onto the next step. Steeping needs to be small initially, and rhythmic.

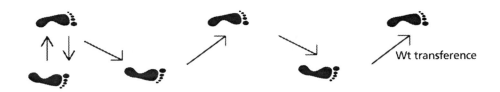

WALKING (HEEL AND TOE)

Part of the 'rooted to the spot' problem is the lack of movement through the foot when walking. Normal walking involves the heel hitting the ground first followed by contact with the outer side of the foot with the ground, and then pushing off through the ball of the foot and the big toe.

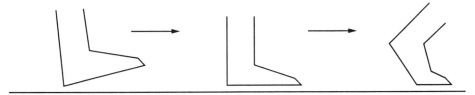

People with Parkinson's disease lose this technique with only a forefoot contact with the ground.

Strategy

Practise 'heel to toe to push off', first whilst sitting, then standing, and eventually walking, practising particularly with the foot that gets more rooted. This will bring back some mobility into the foot.

Say "heel and toe" as you perform each practise stage, using the same tone and rhythm on each occasion.

DIFFICULTIES GETTING UP FROM A CHAIR

The most difficult part of getting up from the chair is the initial lifting of the buttocks from the seat.

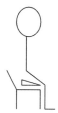

A wedge shaped cushion placed on the chair can help this as it raises the buttocks above the level of the knees, for the starting position. This cushion should be covered in a heavily textured material rather than plastic to prevent it slipping to the floor.

Getting up

It is helpful to have chair arms that extend forwards to enable the person's arms to push down and back.

Place the feet directly under the knees.

Move the hips forwards on the chair to bring the weight closer to the feet.

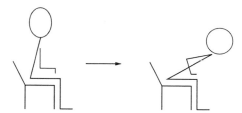

Lean forwards so that the head is over the feet.

Keeping the head forwards, push down and backwards with the hands in order to lift the hips up.

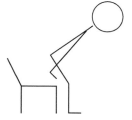

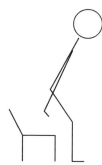

Then still keeping the head forwards, bring the hips up and in and tuck the bottom in to stand up.

If your head is far enough over your toes, your weight will be over your feet and you can let go with your arms.

POSTURE

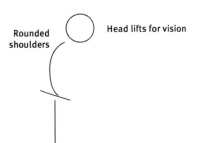

Rounded shoulders

Head lifts for vision

As every one ages there is a tendency to stoop forwards with rounded shoulders and a poking chin. This is the result of a heavy bone box, the skull, acting on the length of neck. The head then lifts for vision and results in a poking chin.

Patients need to see a physiotherapist on an individual basis for exercises to align the spine and exercise postural muscles.

Once you have learnt to align your spine, every time you pass a mirror or a shop window, cast a sideways glance and straighten up from the base of the spine through the upper back. Tuck the chin in and STRETCH UP tall.

The temptation, for those with a walking frame, is to get up and rush off to the task in hand without finally straightening up.

In sitting

Starting from the base of the spine, push the hips slightly forwards, then gradually uncurl the spine so that each vertebra sits squarely on top of the one below, leaving the head dropped forward until the last moment.

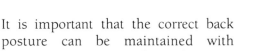
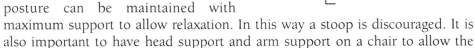

It is important that the correct back posture can be maintained with maximum support to allow relaxation. In this way a stoop is discouraged. It is also important to have head support and arm support on a chair to allow the

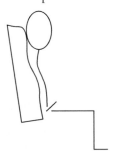

neck and shoulder muscles to relax and 'let go' from their job of holding the upper body in position. The arms need a wide, soft but firm support so that they don't fall off the chair arms. A wing chair will give the spine lateral support and prevent falling sideways. The bottom needs to sit in the angle of the chair, the thighs be firmly supported and the feet in firm contact with the floor. It may be necessary to incline the back of the chair backwards to allow full head support.

If one spends several hours a day sitting in the same chair, in the same wrong posture, the body will take up the shape that the chair gives it. This posture has to be corrected on standing upright again or the stoop will be maintained in walking and other activities.

CALF MUSCLES

There is a tendency for the calf muscles to shorten in people with Parkinson's disease. As a stoop develops, the heels tend to lift making it difficult to keep weight acting through the heels. The gait becomes faster and faster and more unmanageable. The calf muscle attaches from behind the knee joint through the Achilles tendon to the heel bone. To maintain its full length and prevent shortening, it is important that it is regularly stretched with a gentle sustained stretch (no bouncing) to feel a tension in the muscle without forcing it past its limit (for a stretching exercise see the chapter The Role of the Podiatric Surgeon in this book).

BALANCE EXERCISES

Balance tends to fail when the body weight acts too far away from its base (the feet on standing; bottom and thighs and feet on sitting).

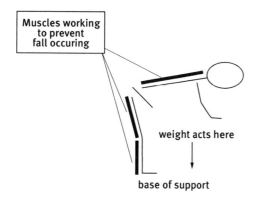

If the muscles behind are too weak, a fall forward may occur. The example above illustrates this. Falls can occur in any direction if the body weight cannot be controlled beyond the base of support.

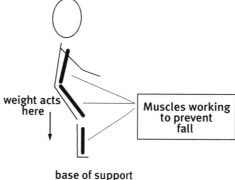

In the example right, the weight is acting behind the base, so that the fall may occur backwards if the muscles at the front cannot counteract this force.

Muscle weakness occurs around the back, thigh, and lower leg muscles. The balance problem is analysed by the physiotherapist who will then recommend a series of exercises to challenge these muscles, always within their range of control. The range of control is extended as strength develops.

Ideally the balance problem is analysed, then a series of exercises set up to challenge these muscles; but within their range of control and then the range extended as the strength develops.

RHYTHM AND MOVEMENT

Doing exercises and walking or moving to a strong musical beat sets a pace for performance and enhances the activity.

Marching 1-2, 1-2 helps with maintaining the quality of the walk for a longer period than perhaps before, and a longer distance is achieved.

A strong tune alerts the mind and allows automatic movements to occur more freely.

HALLUCINATIONS - A STRATEGY

Carers and families have said that the best way to deal with hallucinations (often a side effect of drugs) is not to argue about their presence.

Recognise them as if they are real - for example, snakes or monkeys in the room. Chase them out, clapping hands. Shut the door noisily, saying "That has got rid of them!" Apparently this works. In case hallucinations are a result of pharmaceutical side effects, the medical advisor should be contacted with a request for a drug management review.

GENERAL ACTIVITY

To maintain general health it is important to keep moving. A certain amount of strength is required to keep the bony skeleton in alignment, and to move the body weight around against gravity.

When activity declines, strength and fitness waste away because of lack of muscle support. This leads to greater difficulty in movement and a likelihood of bony injury from falls or joint problems.

It is thus important for people with Parkinson's disease to keep going at all times and if on drugs, to take full advantage of the better movement enhanced by them.

Little things can make all the difference - regular walks around the house or garden, standing up to switch over the television channel, going to the upstairs toilet, leaving the installation of a chair lift or recliner/riser chair as long as possible.

Body movement also contributes to circulation of the blood by the pumping action of the muscles (particularly the calves), kidney function and drainage and movement of food through the gut.

It is now recognised that the prolonged bed rest that used to be recommended for low back pain causes as many problems as the original pain, due to decreased muscle strength. The present recommendation is three days maximum.

Space travellers now perform regular strenuous workouts in space as it was found that the weakness generated by lack of activity against gravity necessitated the use of wheelchairs on landing back on earth. Their muscles couldn't cope with gravity.

Notes for Healthcare Professionals

Parkinson's disease can be an exhausting disease especially for those whose muscles are kept in a state of abnormal tension. This requires extra energy and effort to overcome.

The lack of facial mobility and difficulty with movement may suggest a general slowness but the intelligent person remains within, dealing with the frustrations caused by the difficulties of the disease. Therefore, any strategy or exercise routine should be properly explained and understood by both patient and carer.

It is a very easy mistake for family and carers to move at their own pace rather than at that of the patient, causing avoidable stress.

I have found that slow explanations can make all the difference. Often patients have lost trust in their own body reactions and have become withdrawn and passive. They need to regain an element of control and renewed confidence.

Bibliography

Parkinson's Disease Physiotherapy July 1986: vol 72 no7: pps.4 - 29

Neurological Rehabilitation: Optimising Motor Performance: Carr J Shepherd R: 1998: Butterworth Heineman, London UK

A Motor Relearning Programme for Stroke:Carr J Shepherd R: Butterworth Heineman, 1987: Oxford, UK

Information Pack for Physiotherapists: Felicity Handford, Chair of the PDS Physiotherapy Working Party: *Papers on Parkinsons Disease, Motor and Psychological Factors affecting Physiotherapy, Physiotherapy and Parkinson's Disease, Information for Physiotherapists to give to Patients and further information*: Ref.B26 Literature/Booklets for use by Professionals: Available from the Parkinson's Disease Society, London, UK. Tel: 020 7931 8080.

CHAPTER 20

Remedial Exercise

by Adrianne Golembo Dip Mass DWR GICFFI Dip IPTI
Nutrition Notes by Lucille Leader Dip ION

Experience has shown that the benefits of regular exercise, in particular stretching and joint mobility movements, help to maintain function more optimally and for longer in people with Parkinson's disease. Building stretching and gentle muscle strengthening exercises into your everyday routine will help to alleviate stiffness, reduce muscle tension and improve the circulation. Because flexibility is a problem in Parkinson's disease, it is essential to work on methods of improvement.

It is important to expect bad days as well as good days and treat these bad days as temporary setbacks. On some days you will feel like exercising, whilst on others it may be more difficult. However, remember that exercising every day really does make a difference!

Starting an Exercise Programme

- Select a regular time every day to do your exercises. The length of time you exercise may vary depending on your capabilities that day. Start with 3 – 10 minutes and build up to twenty minutes a day if possible.

- Don't exhaust yourself to the point that you dread exercising. The idea is to feel better and look forward to exercising again the next day.

- If you are under pressure or stressed it will be more difficult to exercise, so do your relaxation techniques before starting.

- When stretching, always work within comfortable, pain free limits.

- "Stretching will not only increase your flexibility and minimise your chances of pulling or tearing muscles, but it will also improve your performance. A flexible muscle reacts and contracts faster, and with more force, than a non-flexible muscle. Flexibility also increases your agility and balance."[1]

■ Put on some music when doing your exercises. Choose something that is both rhythmical and relaxing so that it becomes a pleasure to exercise whilst listening. The rhythm in music has been found to be helpful to co-ordination in people with Parkinson's disease[2].

■ For additional motivation encourage others in your home to get involved in doing the exercises too. They will benefit by reducing stress and improving physical function.

■ Physiologically, exercise will give you a sense of well being and as you progress and find yourself more in control, the benefits will accumulate.

■ It is essential to adopt a positive attitude and not become despondent as a result of fluctuations in performance. This fluctuation is symptomatic of Parkinson's disease and it is important to understand that there are bad and good days. Simply do what you can, and take one day at a time.

■ Some amount of soreness will almost always be experienced by individuals that have not stretched or exercised much in the last few months.

■ Remember that Parkinson's disease does not exclude you from taking the responsibility to do your exercises on a regular basis!

■ Some medication will affect your ability to exercise so take this into account when planning. Whichever drug you take which optimises your movement, wait for its beneficial effects before exercising.

Nutritional Considerations for Patients when Exercising

by Lucille Leader Dip ION

■ Do not exercise after having a large meal.

■ If you take L-dopa medication, wait for it to "kick in" before you start to exercise. This way you will have more control over your movements. If L-dopa tablets ("Sinemet", "Madopar" or equivalent) take a long while to give you any benefit, ask your doctor to consider prescribing "Madopar" dispersible to take before your exercise session. This is L-dopa in liquid form and it is rapidly absorbed[3].

■ Avoid protein-rich foods (such as wheat, rye, oats, barley, spelt, meat, chicken, fish, dairy, eggs, avocado and asparagus) within one hour of taking your L-dopa. Rather have a small carbohydrate snack (fruit, vegetables, rice, buckwheat, millet) This will limit your side effects.

Notes for Professionals *by Adrienne Golembo and Lucille Leader*

The following exercises have been selected as they are simple to follow and may be gradually increased once stamina, strength and mobility have improved.

Whilst the prescribed exercises provide a basic structure to mobilise, stretch and strengthen the body, there are many additional exercises which may be introduced once the above have been mastered.

Stability and strengthening of the abdominal muscles is essential and should be taught on an individual basis by the professional to ensure that these are done correctly.

The posture needs to be addressed and corrected as appropriate. Any other remedial requirements should be assessed.

There is a real problem of enthusiastic, able patients tending to overdo any form of exercise. This can lead to problems of over-use and exhaustion and they should be cautioned.

As stress tends to exacerbate symptoms, relaxation techniques can be used to calm the patient.

It is necessary to guide patients to exercise at a time appropriate to their drug regime.

If they take L-dopa medication, ("Sinemet", "Madopar" or equivalent) they must wait for it to "kick in" before starting to exercise. This way they will have more control over their movements.

If L-dopa tablets take a long while to give any benefit, we recommend discussing with the doctor the possibility of prescribing "Madopar" dispersible. This L-dopa in liquid form is much more rapidly absorbed.
To obtain the best environment to exercise with your patient it is necessary to understand the relationship between protein rich foods and the drug L-dopa.

In order for L-dopa to be optimally absorbed with the least amount of side effects (typically dyskinesia which makes it difficult to work with the patient), the following protocol is recommended.

1. Protein rich foods (gluten grains - wheat, rye, oats, barley, spelt, meat, chicken, fish, dairy, eggs, avocado and asparagus) should not be eaten for two hours after L-dopa medication has been taken.

2. Carbohydrates (fruit, vegetables, rice, buckwheat, millet) are most suited in combination with L-dopa. Patients usually need to wait 45 minutes before eating these after L-dopa has been taken.

3. Large meals should generally be avoided prior to exercise.

4. If dyskinesia or stiffness are a problem even after the recommended nutritional manipulation (thus making exercise difficult) it could be that the levels of L-dopa are too high or too low. Review of the dosage regime is recommended and communication with the patient's doctor essential.

5. Good bowel function is essential for well-being and comfort in order to exercise.

See page 248 for the Remedial Exercises.

Exercises

Whenever performing strengthening exercises do not overdo it. Start slowly with the minimum amount and let your body guide you as to what is right for you each day. When performing stretching or mobilising exercises it is essential that you do not overstretch or over-extend the body. Always work within comfortable, pain-free limits. Stretch slowly and never bounce. Breath normally, relax and concentrate.

STRETCHES

STARTING POSITION:
Standing Neutral | Seated Neutral

Starting Position

OBJECTIVE:
Stretch and mobilise the neck, reducing tension in neck and shoulders

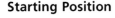

- Return head to neutral position after each movement. (see figures in starting position)

- Take each movement to the comfortable limit of your range. Stop if you feel pain

- Hold each movement for 3 seconds

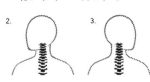

1. Lower the chin down towards chest

2. Turn as far as possible to right without overextending

3. Turn as far as possible to left without overextending

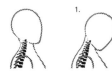

4. Lower the right ear down towards shoulder (side bend)

5. Lower the left ear down towards shoulder (side bend)

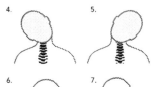

6. Protrude chin forward, stretching the neck

7. Pull chin back towards the neck

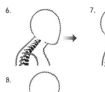

8. Lower chin down towards chest and protrude chin downwards stretching the neck. Repeat sequence twice

SHOULDER SHRUG

STARTING POSITION:
Standing Neutral | Seated Neutral

Starting Position

OBJECTIVE:
Mobilise shoulder girdle and relieve tension in upper back and neck

■ The shoulder girdle constitutes the shoulder blade, the shoulder joint the collar bone and the muscles that connect them

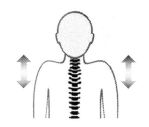

Shrug the shoulders by slowly raising them up and then slowly releasing down. It is essential to perform this movement slowly and rhythmically. Repeat x 3

SHOULDER CIRCLES

STARTING POSITION:
Standing Neutral | Seated Neutral

OBJECTIVE:
Mobilise shoulder girdle and relieve tension in upper back

Starting Position

■ When performing this sequence, ensure you are circling just the shoulder joint and not the shoulder blade as well.

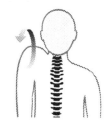

1. Circle right shoulder forwards x 3.

2. Repeat with left shoulder

3. Circle right shoulder backwards x 3.

4. Repeat with left shoulder

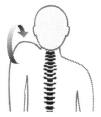

SHOULDER BLADE SQUEEZE

STARTING POSITION:
Standing Neutral | Seated Central

OBJECTIVE:
Mobilise shoulder girdle & thoracic spine. Relieve tension between shoulder blades

Starting Position

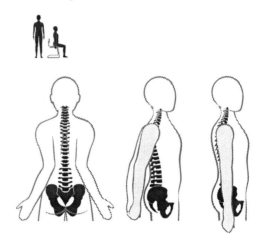

1. Keep the head upright and squeeze the shoulder blades together

2. Keeping the squeeze, take the hands back and clasp gently behind the back. Do not lock elbows.

3. Hold for 4 seconds

4. Relax shoulders and return to neutral position

5. Go straight into next exercise - Shoulder Blade Stretch

SHOULDER BLADE STRETCH

STARTING POSITION:
Standing Neutral | Seated Central

Starting Position

OBJECTIVE:
Mobilise shoulder joint and relieve tension across the upper back

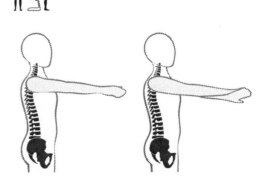

1. Raise the arms forward to chest level (about 4 inches below the level of the shoulders)

2. Cross over hands with palms touching

3. Drop head down towards chest

4. Stretch forwards from shoulder joints. NB Do not bend lower back

5. Hold for 4 seconds

6. Return to STARTING position then repeat Shoulder Blade Squeeze exercise

■ Repeat 2 sets of alternating Stretch & Squeeze

SHOULDER JOINT STRETCH ABOVE HEAD

STARTING POSITION:
Standing Neutral | Seated Neutral

Starting Position

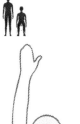

OBJECTIVE:
Mobilise shoulder joint, upper thoracic spine and stretch the triceps

1. Raise right arm straight up

2. Bend elbow lowering hand behind the neck

3. Place left hand on right elbow

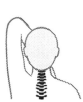

4. Gently pull right elbow towards the head taking care not to over stretch

5. Hold for 4 seconds

6. Release and return to STARTING position

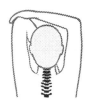
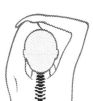

■ Repeat this sequence with left arm

■ Repeat x 2

Alternative

If you are unable to perform step 3, place your left hand on the inside of the right arm and gently push your right arm up and back. This will help to stretch the triceps, and mobilise the shoulder joint. Eventually you may be able to perform the exercise as stated above, but if not, don't worry, just persevere with what is comfortable for you.

LATERAL ARM RAISERS

STARTING POSITION:
Standing Neutral - Set| Seated Neutral - Set

Starting Position

OBJECTIVE:
Strengthening shoulders and upper arms

1. Arms relaxed at sides

2. Raise arms slowly till parallel with the ground and return slowly down to sides.

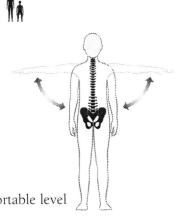

- Repeat x 3 for the first 2 weeks

- Increase by multiples of 3 each week to a comfortable level

As this is a strengthening exercise it is designed to put a strain on the muscles. In order to release this tension we now repeat several mobilising exercises.

- Repeat one set of Neck Stretches (page 248) Shoulder Circles and Shoulder Shrugs (page 249)..

LATERAL ARM MOVEMENTS

This exercise should only be attempted once you are able to do at least 10 repetitions of the previous exercise comfortably.

STARTING POSITION:
Standing Neutral - Set | Seated Neutral - Set

Starting Position

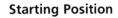
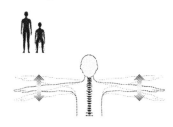

OBJECTIVE:
Strengthen shoulders and upper arms

1. Raise arms to shoulder level parallel with the ground

2. Lower and raise arms approximately 3 inches to create small bounces x 4

3. Small circles forward x 4

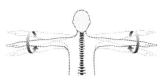

4. Small circles back x 4

5. Repeat no 1 then one set of Shoulder Shrugs (page 249).

CALF RAISERS

STARTING POSITION:
Standing Neutral - Set

OBJECTIVE:
Strengthen calf muscles

Starting Position

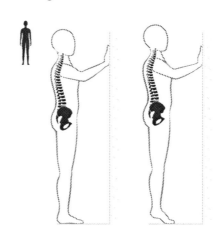

1. Elbows flexed, palms against the wall

2. Stand with feet 4 – 6 inches away from wall, with the shoulders directly above hips and the back straight

3. Raise heels up and lower down.

- Repeat x 6
- Build up to as many repetitions as you can

As this is a strengthening exercise it is designed to put stress on the calf muscles and you should feel the muscles getting tense. After completing the exercise, shake your legs.

RELAXATION POSITION

The body is generally given very little opportunity to relax completely.

This position allows the entire body, but most specifically, the muscles supporting the neck, back and the entire spine to totally relax. It is essential that the entire length of the spine is flat on the floor. If you cannot achieve this with the pillows, please elevate your legs on a chair or couch as indicated in the last picture. Let the knees relax outwards away from the body once in this position.

OBJECTIVE:
To relax all the muscles of the body, particularly the muscles of the back and reduce pain and tension.

- This position is best done on the floor but for those who are unable perform these movements, try lying on your bed with pillows in the same supportive positions as in the drawings

To get down into Relaxation Position: **Starting Position**

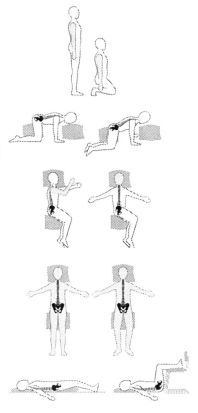

1. Standing with feet hip distance apart and at the base of the pillows, keep the back straight and bend onto he knees.

2. Go down onto hands and knees. Keep knees and hands hip distance apart. Ensure that the knees are in line with the top of the pillow.

3. Sit the buttocks down towards the pillows and lie down on your side. Ensure that the top pillow is comfortably under your head and neck

4. Roll the top of the body slowly over, then roll one leg then the other over the pillows, tightening the abdominal muscles as you move.

5. Straighten the body so your spine is in alignment and you feel comfortable.

6. Relax the legs on the pillows and then drop the knees outwards.

7. The spine should now be flat on the floor - (if not, you require additional pillows under the legs or elevate legs onto a chair or couch (see last figure)

To get up from Relaxation Position:

1. Roll over onto your side with knees bent and off the pillows.

2. Raise the top of the body by pushing up with your hands

3. Roll over onto hands and knees with arms shoulder distance apart and knees hip distance apart.

4. Sit back on your heels and straighten the back

5. Place one foot flat on the floor and stand up using the thigh muscles. You can hold onto something if your thigh muscles are not strong enough to help to level up.

SHOULDER JOINT MOBILISING

STARTING POSITION:
Relaxation

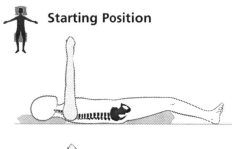

Starting Position

OBJECTIVE:
Mobilise the shoulder joint

- Do not over stretch – raise only from the joint and not the shoulder blade

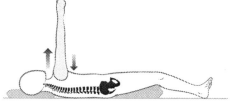

- Keep arms straight throughout the movements

- Release the joint slowly, do not bang down

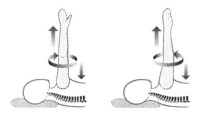

1. Raise right arm up in line with the right shoulder

2. Raise the right shoulder joint slightly upwards and gently release down Repeat x 4 Repeat with left arm

3. Shoulder joint rotation inwards –Raise joint as in 2. Rotate joint towards body then rotate back to central position and gently release down Repeat x 4. Repeat with left arm

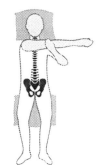

4. Shoulder joint rotation outwards – same as 3 but turn joint away from the body. Repeat x 4 Repeat with left arm

5. Raise the right shoulder joint upwards and stretch arm across the chest NB do not bend the elbow. Place opposite hand above the elbow and gently push downwards - hold for 5 seconds then release and return to central position above shoulder, lower joint down, lower arm down. Repeat with left arm

Once you are comfortable with all the movements you may do the entire sequence from start to finish first with the right arm, then with the left.

FOOT SEQUENCE

STARTING POSITION:
Sitting or Lying with leg raised and hands supporting the knee

OBJECTIVE:
Mobilise foot, ankle and toes

Starting Position

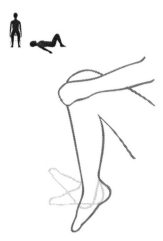

1. Circle right ankle x 4 in both direction

2. Alternately point foot towards floor then pull up towards ceiling repeat x 4 in each direction

3. Alternately turn ankle inwards then outwards repeat x 4 in each direction

4. Wiggle toes

5. Repeat no 1

■ Repeat with left foot

HAND SEQUENCE

STARTING POSITION:
Standing, Sitting or Relaxation Position with elbows bent

Starting Position

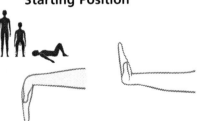

OBJECTIVE:
Mobilise wrists and hands

1. Circle both hands from the wrist 4 times in each direction.

2. Point hands towards the floor then raise towards the ceiling x 4

3. Turn wrists away from body, then towards the body x 4

4. Wiggle fingers if possible for 5 seconds

5. Relax hands from the wrist and shake hands loosely

6. Repeat no 1.

THIGH STRENGHTENING

STARTING POSITION:
   Relaxation Position or Lying on bed with pillows under the knees

OBJECTIVE:
   Strengthen thigh muscles

Starting Position

Straighten the right knee, pointing toes towards head.
Keeping the back of the thigh in contact with the pillow, raise the calf and lower.
Repeat x 5

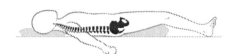

■   Repeat with left leg

■   Build up to 2 sets of 5 gradually over a few weeks

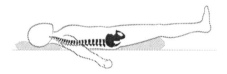

HIP ROTATION IN

STARTING POSITION:
   Lying on floor or bed with knees bent

Starting Position

OBJECTIVE:
   Mobilise hip joint

1. Shuffle legs wider apart.

2. Lower right knee slowly inwards towards the floor and return to neutral position

3. Repeat x 4

Repeat with left leg

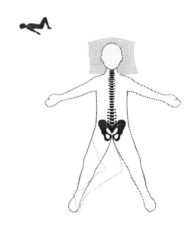

STANDING or SEATED LEG RAISE

STARTING POSITION:
Standing Neutral or Seated Neutral

Starting Position

OBJECTIVE:
Strengthen hip flexors and thighs

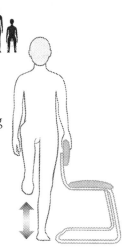

- NB Do not attempt this exercise when standing if balance and dizziness is a problem. It can be performed when sitting.

1. Holding onto chair with left hand, bend right knee, raising the leg so the thigh is parallel with the ground

2. Return to floor and touch with flat foot. Do not bang down

3. Repeat x 5

4. Repeat with left leg

Build up to 10 and increase gradually over the weeks.

BACK EXTENSION – Shoulder lift

Starting Position

STARTING POSITION:
Flat on Stomach with arms at sides and legs hip distance apart, head facing left

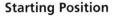

OBJECTIVE:
Stretch the whole spine and muscles of the back.

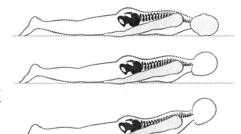

- Ensure the chin is kept tucked in throughout exercise and move very slowly so as not to get dizzy

Level 1
Breathe in and raise shoulders slightly and turn head to the right. Then lower head and shoulders down, keeping head facing right. Repeat turning head back to left Repeat x 4 in each direction.

Level 2
Same as level 1 but now raise the shoulders higher within comfortable limit of range. Do not over-lift.

ABDOMINAL STRENGTHENING

STARTING POSITION:
   Standing or Seated

OBJECTIVE:
   Strengthen abdominal muscles and stabilise lower back

1. Sit in a comfortable position (or stand). Take a breath in and exhale. Then pull the lower abdominal muscles in towards the spine.

2. Now push the muscles away from the spine.

Repeat x 4.

This exercise can be repeated at least 3 times a day.

CHAPTER 21

Hands
Maintaining Muscle Tone & Flexibility

*by **Dr Geoffrey Leader** MB ChB FRCA, **Esther Roos-Lohner** Dip Phys.
& **Lucille Leader** Dip ION*

Because of tremor or stiffness, patients may under-utilise their hands. According to a small assessment of hand function of patients with Parkinson's disease at The London Pain Relief and Nutritional Support Clinic by Mr Ian Winspur, Consultant Hand Surgeon, there was nothing intrinsically wrong with their hands other than the effects of the lack of dopamine. It should be possible to do specialised exercises to ensure continuing muscle function. In those who rely on L-dopa medication for control of movement, exercises are best done after the effects of the drug have "kicked in".

If people have specific skills involving fine movements of the hands including playing a musical instrument or typing, they should be encouraged to continue practising hand exercises and maintain any specialised activities for as long as possible.

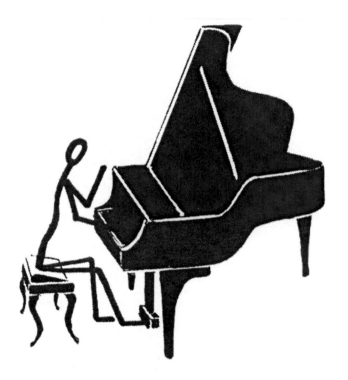

ILLUSTRATION DR PIET ADMIRAAL

Special Notes for those who wish to play a musical instrument, compute or type

It is good to keep up playing an instrument if you have done so before Parkinson's disease has been diagnosed. Doing gymnastics for the hands and postural muscles before you begin to play or type, will help with flexibility and a feeling of vitality. Playing slower pieces or typing slowly can still give pleasure, as can doing the exercises at a pace which you can manage rather than frustratingly trying to move at an inappropriate speed.

If you have never learnt an instrument before, perhaps now is the time to give yourself the challenge of learning something new. This will not only stimulate you mentally and emotionally but help to maintain physical co-ordination. Percussion instruments of various types may suit those who cannot execute fine movement. Rythm is helpful with coordination. Doing the exercises in this chapter, twice a day, for a few weeks before you start lessons, will prepare your muscles for playing an instrument or learning to type.

Relaxation, Concentration and Breathing

a.

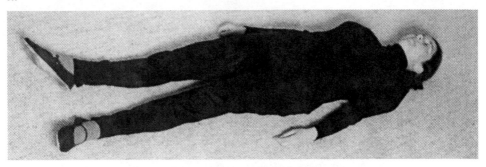

b.

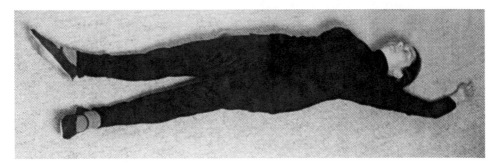

c.

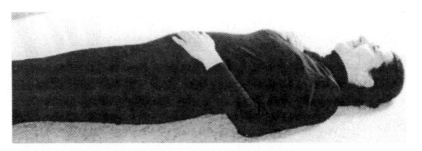

Description of the Movements	Analytical Comment
a. Relaxation Lie on your back, totally relaxed. Relax your lower jaw. Breathe naturally. Duration 3 minutes	a. Lying reduces tone because the muscles do not have to work against gravity. More blood flows to the brain in the horizontal position.
b. Breathing and Concentration I. Lie in the relaxed position, arms at your sides as in the first exercise. II. Breathe in through the nose upwards and placing it behind you. III. Return your arm slowly to it's original position at your side whilst breathing out and making a gradually diminishing hissing like sound - "sss....." Repeat twice with each arm	b. Hissing whilst breathing out creates resistance and encourages a subsequent deeper inspiration. Lifting the arm also increases the volume of the thorax. Accentuated breathing regulates emotional and muscle tension via a bio-feedback mechanism whilst lifting your right arm
c. Abdominal breathing Lie on your back with one hand on your chest and the other on your abdomen. Inhale slowly so as to feel especially the abdomen rising up against your hand. Then passively allow exhalation. Do not inhale so deeply as to significantly move the hand, which is on your chest.	c. Abdominal breathing allows reduction of tension in the upper thorax and shoulder girdle. This in turn facilitates freedom of movement of the arms and hands.

Toning and Relaxing the Muscles of the Back and Neck

a.

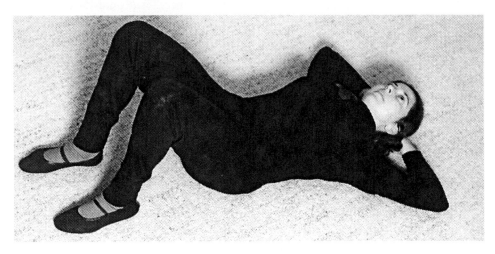

b.

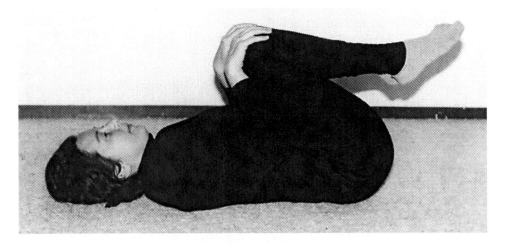

Description of the Movements	Analytical Comment
a. Toning the muscles of the back and neck I. Lie on your back with your knees bent, feet flat on the floor and your hands, palms upwards, under your head. II. Press your lower back gently downwards, flattening it against the floor whilst allowing your buttocks to rise slightly. III. Still holding position II, press your elbows gently downwards onto the floor. IV. Still holding positions II and III, press your head gently downwards into the floor, as it were. V. Slowly relax all the positions and breathe in. *Note:* Take a breath in before starting this exercise and breathe out in one continuous slow breath during steps II, III and IV. Repeat three times	**a.** The muscles of the back and neck play a major role in supporting the skeleton in the correct position for keyboard skills. This exercise strengthens them. The position flattens the lumbar lordosis. Muscle contraction occurs in the abdominal muscles, the buttocks and the back, especially between the shoulder blades.
b. Relaxing the muscles of the back and neck I. Lie on your back with your knees bent up over the abdomen. II. Close your eyes, relax your jaw and small, place your hands on your knees. III. Initiate a small rocking movement of the knees by alternately pulling your knees not more than ten centimetres towards your chin, and then releasing. Keep your hands on your knees throughout this exercise in order to maintain the rocking position. Let your head and neck follow your movements in a pleasant wave-like rhythm. Keep your body as relaxed as possible during this exercise. Continue this exercise until the desired effect of relaxation is experienced.	**b.** This is a very helpful exercise. It relaxes your neck and back muscles. Because of hip flexion, the lower back makes contact with the floor-but without muscle contraction. The extensor muscles of the back, which are frequently in spasm, are encouraged to straighten and become relaxed through the rocking motion. Rythmical tilting of the pelvis causes a wave-like movement in the spine. This in turn, passively rocks the head and also allows relaxation of the neck muscles.

Toning the Leg Muscles and Flexibility of the Ankles

a.

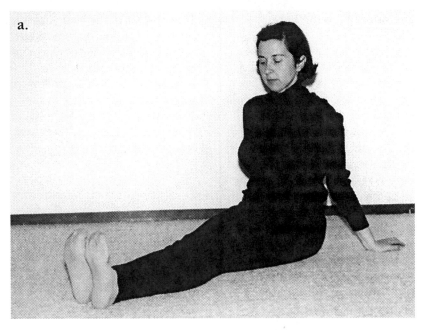

b.

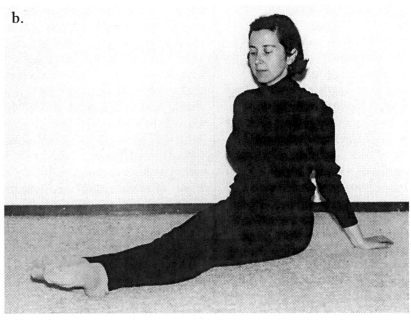

Description of the Movements	Analytical Comment
a. Sit on the floor with your legs stretched parallel before you. Bend your feet upwards towards your face whilst keeping your legs flat on the floor.	The lower leg muscles are exercised by moving the ankle joint throughout it's whole range of flexion and extension.
	Fixing the knee in extension causes the frontal muscles to contract and the rear muscles to be passively stretched. Alternatively, the peroneal and calf muscles are contracting.
	Changing the work of agonist and antagonist works the "muscle pump" for the return flow of venous blood. This improves circulation.
b. Continuing from exercise a. Point your toes downwards, away from you.	

Sitting Posture at the Keyboard

a.

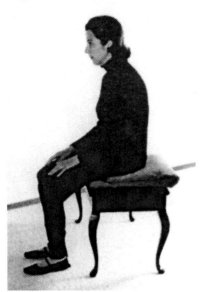

b.

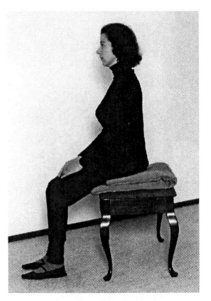

c.

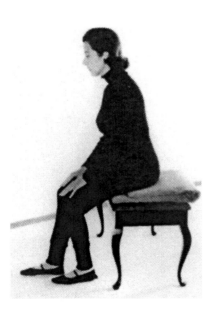

Description of the Movements	Analytical Comment
a. This photograph illustrates sitting in a drooping position. The spine is not stretched. This results in a heavy feeling both in the body and spirit.	Correct posture enables you to "play" with maximum ease. Bad posture hampers breathing and free movement of the arms. The feet flat on the floor and one's position on the "sitting bones" help to provide a solid support for the spine. Sitting on a slightly forward-sloping pillow makes it easier to transfer one's weight forward. The angle of the hip joint may vary between 120° and 90°. Less than 90° puts too much pressure on the hip joint. By leaning towards the keyboard with a foot forward, one's centre of gravity is transferred forwards. This is the basis of balance and control at the keyboard.
b.1 Sit on your "sitting bones" with approximately a 90° angle between thighs and lower legs. II. Press your feet flat on the floor, simultaneously allowing your back and neck (spine) to elongate upwards. Feel the ripple of energy within yourself. Notice how much lighter you seem compared with the drooping position a. NB: Keep your shoulders relaxed throughout this posture c. The right foot is placed forward. The straight back is leaning slightly forward towards the keyboard.	

Depressing Piano Pedals

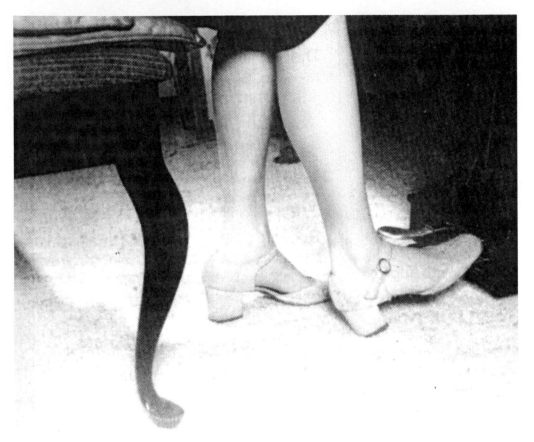

Description of the Movements	Application to Pianists
	Using the pedals is part of piano playing. If you depress the pedals using only ankle movements, you might become stiff and experience muscle cramp.
I. Sit at the piano, the ball of your right foot on the pedal and your heel on the floor. Your left foot is flat on the floor.	Keeping your weight forward, thus utilising it to depress the pedals, and using an appropriate heel, facilitates economical physical movement whilst pedalling.
II. Leaning forward, keep your right heel on the floor and transfer body weight onto the ball of your right foot. As a result, the pedal will be depressed.	**Analytical Comment** Leaning forward displaces the centre of gravity of the body, causing the foot to put pressure on the pedal.
III. Relax back into position I.	The foot pivots downwards from the heel and the calf muscles have only a minimum of work to perform.
Advice: It is best to wear a shoe with a fairly wide heel, the same height as the pedal is from the floor. **Repeat** exercise 12b three times.	To release the pedal, slight relaxation of the calf muscle suffices.

The Relaxing Position for the Hand

a.

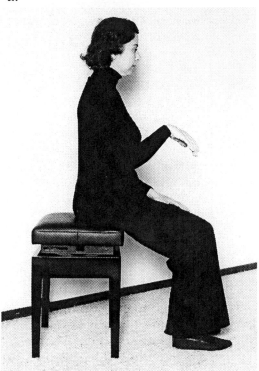

b.

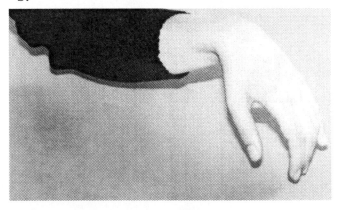

Description of the Movements	Analytical Comment
	This movement is a **natural** and important **way to reduce muscular tension and lessen muscle tone**. It is an essential element in the art of optimal movement or flexibility of the keyboard.
Position yourself exactly as in the photograph. Bend at your elbow, allowing your hand to drop down from the wrist. Your upper arm must hang, totally inert, from the shoulder. Your hand, with all it's fingers, must be as loose as possible.

Pay particular attention to the relaxation of your thumb (see detailed close up of hand in photograph b). | The flexor muscles of the elbow are more dominant than the extensors, so that the arm naturally tends to bend at the elbow. During flexion at the elbow, the hand progressively flexes at the wrist under the influence of gravity. |

Flexibility

a.

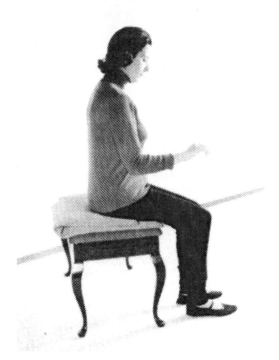

b.

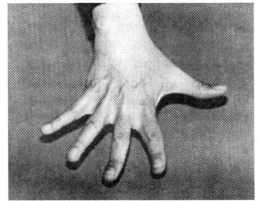

d.

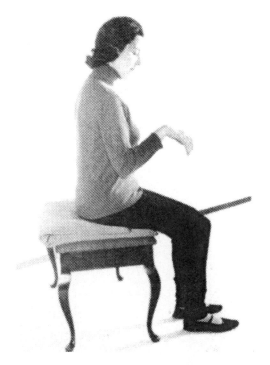

c.

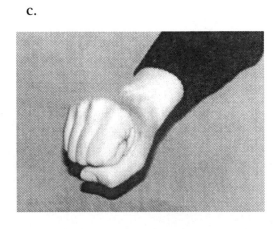

Description of the Movements	Analytical Comment
a. Position yourself as in photograph a.	This exercise is an invaluable aid to promoting muscular flexibility of the hand. By contracting the extensor muscles one is lengthening the flexor tendons. This facilitates flexor muscle contraction and closure of the hand.
b. Stretch and spread all your fingers as in photograph b.	The exercise also promotes flexibility of the small joints of the fingers. During the spreading of the fingers, the small spreading muscles (interossei) are brought into play. All flexor muscles contract to produce a good fist.
c. Continuing from this stretched position, clench your hand as in photograph c.	
d. Flowing from the clenched position, drop your wrist into the "relaxing position" (which is the same as you learned in the previous exercise). See photograph d. **Repeat** this exercise five times with each hand.	

Muscle Toning (conditioning)
This exercise may be more suitable for those who have tremor rather than stiffness

a.

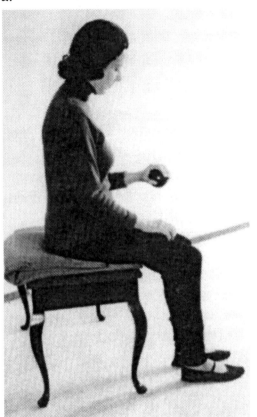

b.

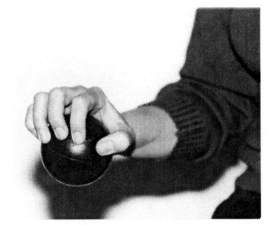

c.

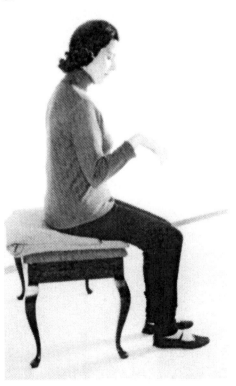

Description of the Movements	Analytical Comment
a. Sit as in photograph a, a tennis ball comfortably and loosely held in your left hand.	This exercise trains the small intrinsic flexor muscles of the fingers to **maintain the natural grasping position of the hand**, used for economic finger work. Note that the wrist is slightly dorsiflexed.
b. Slowly squeeze the ball, keeping all your knuckles rounded as in photograph b. Hold this position for about three seconds. Then, slowly release your "squeeze", returning to a gentle comfortable hold on the ball whilst keeping your fingers rounded.	
Note: Be aware of these two relative states of muscle use - the feeling of **tension** when squeezing the ball and the feeling of **lesser tension** when loosely holding the ball.	
Repeat this exercise three times.	
c. After the last repetition, drop the ball and assume the "relaxing position".	
Repeat this exercise series with the opposite hand.	

Finger Movement Training

a.

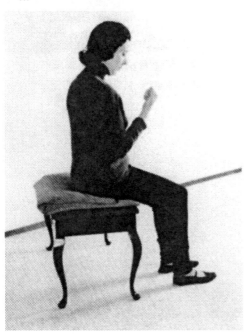

b.

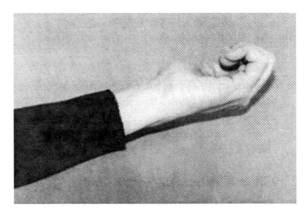

c.

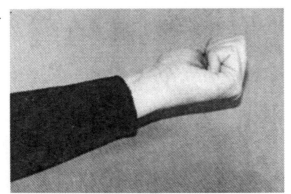

d.

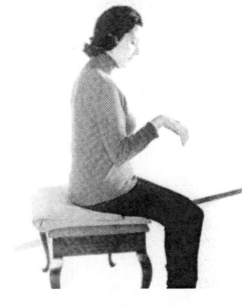

Description of the Movements	Analytical Comment
	This exercise trains your fingers to move with equal effort.

The most important movement in this exercise takes place at the metacarpo-phalangeal joints. This especially trains the small hand muscles (the lumbricals). |

a. Sit as in photograph a, your hand forming a loose "fist" position. Your fingers rest lightly on the palm of your hand, your thumb gently rounded.

b. Lift your fingers slowly and simultaneously about one centimetre above the palm of your hand. Keep your thumb rounded and as relaxed as possible, as in photograph b.

c. Continuing from b, slowly replace your fingers back onto your palm, as in a.

Repeat this finger "lifting and placing" exercise twenty times. When you have control over these movements, practise them faster if it is possible.

If speed increases, your fingers should barely lift up from your palm.

d. Turn your hand over and assume the relaxing movement as in photograph d.

Repeat this exercise series using the opposite hand.

Note: Each week increase the number of repetitions by twenty.

Thumb Training

a.

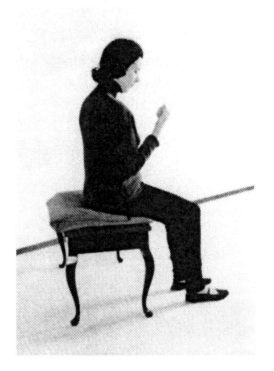

b.

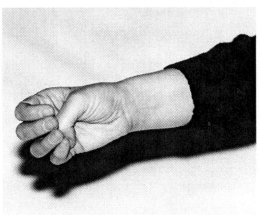

d.

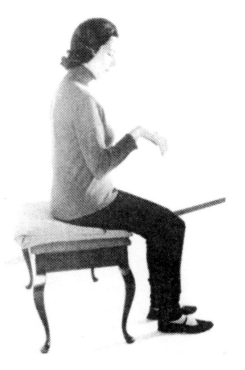

c.

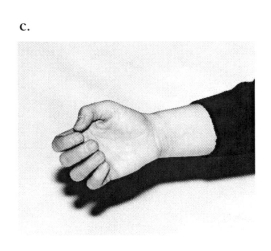

Description of the Movements	Analytical Comment
	Opposition of the thumb takes place at the carpo-metacarpal joint by means of the flexor opponens and the long flexor muscle. Reposition is done primarily by the long extensor muscle.

a. Sit as in photograph a, your hand held loosely rounded with minimal tension in your thumb. The palm of your hand faces you. For detail see photograph c.

b. Place the tip of your thumb at the base of your 5th finger as in photograph b.

c. Return to the starting position a. Repeat this exercise five times.

d. Turn your hand over and let it assume the "relaxing position" as in photograph d.

Repeat this exercise series using the opposite hand.

Sideways Stretching of the Fingers

a.

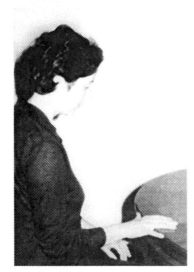

b. and c.

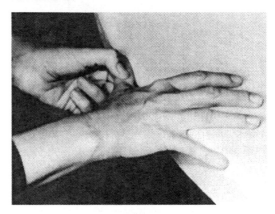

dɪ.

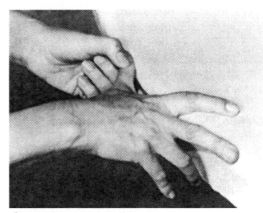

e.

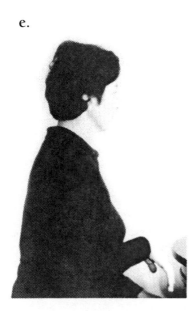

dɪɪ

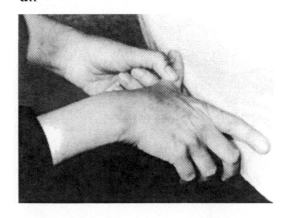

Description of the Movements	Analytical Comment
a. Place your thumb and fifth finger of your right hand along the edge of a table, as in photograph a.	Stretching the metacarpo-phalangeal joints gently sideways is important in order to maintain flexibility of the hand.
b. Grasp your right thumb between the thumb and second finger of your left hand, as in photograph b.	The metacarpo-phalangeal joints are moved slightly sideways and their surrounding ligaments are gently stretched.
c. Keeping your right hand as soft and loose as possible, gently slide your right thumb leftwards along the table edge so as to increase the distance between the tips of the thumb and fifth finger. The thumb and second finger of the left hand help by gently pulling on the right thumb (photograph c).	

Note: Do not hold this stretched position for more than five seconds, and thereafter relax the whole hand. During the exercise, keep your jaw, shoulders and arms as relaxed as possible.

d. Repeat this entire exercise, combining the thumb successively with the fourth, third and second fingers. Photograph d1, demonstrates the combination of the thumb and the third finger. Photograph d11, shows the stretch between the thumb and the second finger.

e. Conclude this exercise sequence by flowing into the "relaxing position" as in photograph e.

Note: Breathing out slowly whilst assuming the "relaxing position" aids the feeling of relaxation.
Repeat the entire exercise sequence from a to d placing your left hand along the edge of the table.

CHAPTER 22

Muscles and Movement
An Overview of Helpful Suggestions

by Lucille Leader Dip ION *and Dr Geoffrey Leader* MB ChB FRCA

- All movements should be performed at a pace that the body will comfortably permit.

- Sufficient time should be allowed between thinking about a movement and attempting its execution. Moving to a rhythm can be helpful.

- Patients should try to "accept" whatever pace suits them.

Getting up in the morning
A physiotherapist or remedial movement therapist can provide appropriate stretching, toning and mobilising exercises to be done in bed before getting up. This routine might be helpful in increasing circulation and benefiting stiffness.

Whirlpool / Jacuzzi
A regular jacuzzi is wonderful for the circulation and can sometimes benefit stiffness. If the budget allows, have a jacuzzi or a whirlpool bath installed at home and everyone can use it! If the size of the bath permits, appropriate exercises can be executed under the warm water.

Bathing and Showering
Warm water helps with muscle relaxation, circulation and a feeling of wellbeing. If lying is a problem, a "walk-in" type of "sitting-bath" bath is available. Shower cubicles can be supplied with seats.

Hydrotherapy
Movement is facilitated when limbs are supported by warm water. Referral to a physiotherapist for hydrotherapy and specialised exercises (done in a warm hydrotherapy pool) can be beneficial.

Kneipp Therapy
This is an effective German therapy for the enhancement of the circulation. It encompasses the use of warm and cold showers, baths and wraps.

Swimming
Swimming in a heated pool, ALWAYS WITH SOMEONE PRESENT, enhances wellbeing, muscle flexibility and circulation.

Massage

Referral by the GP to a recognised, qualified masseur/masseuse - massage gives a sense of well being, relaxation, improves circulation and can be helpful with muscle spasm.

Exercise

Regular appropriate exercise makes people feel good, increases energy, improves circulation, helps peristalsis (bowel function) and helps maintain flexibility and bone integrity but must not be overdone. If standing is a problem, exercises can be performed sitting or even lying.

Exercises should include toning and stretching of muscles, mobilising of joints and suitable aerobic movement. Special attention should be given to the postural muscles and the entire body must be taken into account when a remedial programme of exercises is designed. It is sensible for patients to have their exercise programme created for them on a one-to-one individual basis, as each patient's physical status and movement potential differs.

Hands and Feet

It is important to do exercises to stretch, tone and mobilise these parts in the interests of functional maintenance.

Facial Exercises

It is vital to do specialised facial exercises to maintain flexibility of muscles, if possible, and to enhance circulation.

Occupational Therapy

Occupational therapists will help patients find a way to achieve the movements necessary for their daily functions. They will also assist in directing patients to acquire helpful aids such as specialised bath equipment, kitchen and eating utensils.

Speech Therapy

A speech therapist can provide specialised exercises to help maintain function of the vocal chords and flexibility associated with the oral cavity. Problems of communication can be sorted out by the speech therapist who will provide strategies for times when speech is inadequate.

Music Therapy

This specialised subject can help not only with emotional expression but also with co-ordination, sense of rhythm and circulation. Relaxation and happiness are generated at sessions with a music therapist.

Dancing

Moving gently in rhythm with another person, often assists with co-ordination and balance. Dancing with a partner is good for physical exercise and emotional well being. Choose music of a suitable tempo. Remember that slow dancing is romantic!

Walking

Walking should be enjoyed at a speed which suits the individual. Do not try to walk at a pace which is an effort but choose, instead, to walk at a slower speed which you can comfortably control. It is sometimes helpful to walk to the rhythm of a song or poem. You can also practice swinging both arms to the rhythm, whilst standing still. When comfortable with both, try to combine walking with arm swinging - and a song in your heart or on your lips!

Tai Chi Exercises

If bradykinesia (slow movement) is a problem, exercise activities such as Tai Chi, are ideal. This system of exercises is performed very slowly and helps with centring, balance and circulation. There are many movements in Tai Chi, and only those appropriate to patient potential can be selected by the teacher.

Standing from Sitting

There a various techniques for this manoeuvre. The authors find that the following technique works well.

1. Sit, if possible, on a wedge shaped cushion, (slightly sloping downwards towards the knees). This can be bought at a specialised "back shop". Try to choose a chair which will allow you to have at least a 90° angle or more between your trunk and thighs.

2. When wanting to stand up from a sitting position: -

Movement	Associated Breathing
Move your strongest foot forward	Normal
Stretch your back up	Breath in
Bring your trunk forward so that your head is over the foremost knee, and get up	Breath out

(either bring your hands forward to over your knees
or push down from the chair - **see the chapter Physiotherapy**)

Freezing

There are many different ways to "unfreeze". The authors find that the following routine can be helpful.

If you freeze:

1. Say to yourself: "Am I frozen? NO I am NOT!"

2. Breathe out long and slowly whilst thinking "My neck and shoulders are heavy, I am relaxed"

3. Lean your body weight onto your stronger leg whilst simultaneously allowing your other knee to bend slightly, thereby releasing its tension.

4. Then almost simultaneously, push your pelvis forward whilst taking a step forward with your relaxed leg (the leg which is not carrying your weight). Do this whilst saying "and one", stepping on "one." Glide forward slowly.

Note: All the movements must flow rythmically into each other. Do not stop between the steps otherwise you might loose momentum.

Incontinence (Bladder / Bowel)

This subject is best discussed with the General Practitioner, a Physiotherapist and the Parkinson's Disease Nurse Specialist. They will have helpful recommendations.

Bibliography

Eva Fraser's Facial Workout: 1992: Penguin Health/Medicine, London, UK.

CHAPTER 23

Autogenic Training

Relaxation which Promotes Stress Control in Parkinson's Disease

*by **Vera Diamond** Dip AT MBAS MNCP*

Autogenic Therapy (AT) is a self-help method which brings about profound relaxation and relief from stressful effects of many kinds. "Autogenic" means "generated from within", and this technique mobilises our innate systems for healing, recuperation and re-balancing.

AT consists of a series of easily learned mental exercises which link mind and body together in a specific way, in association with deep relaxation. This is very enjoyable. There are up to six Standard Exercises, which are generally taught in once weekly sessions, for six to eight weeks. During this time many subtle or dynamic processes may come about, influencing different body systems. Several of these are particularly helpful in Parkinson's disease. During the process of training the mind to calm itself, there is a natural switch which gradually becomes automatic when we learn to use the AT tools to switch from the sympathetic nervous system to the parasympathetic, on self-command.

The practices begin during a state of calm observation known as "Passive Concentration" and includes the ability to become the "Passive Observer" of oneself. One also becomes more self-aware as the exercises flow through feelings of heaviness and warmth, to experiences of a calm steady heartbeat, a gentle natural breathing technique, pleasant soothing warmth in the solar plexus region, and a cool clear head. The exercises end with a positive personal formula and a deepening sense of peace within.

These exercises are a valuable "Toolkit" to be used by Parkinson's patients. Each exercise formula seems to reduce stress and tension throughout the system. When the system of exercises is mastered and used regularly, there is a positive response, which promotes a feeling of emotional cohesiveness and balance. Autogenic Training may act synergistically together with the other therapies in this book.

How can Autogenic Training benefit Parkinson's Disease Patients?

- The hormones noradrenaline and adrenaline are released in the body during stress. These hormones are metabolised from dopamine. As dopamine may be deficient in Parkinson's disease one could postulate that it is essential to spare adrenaline. This has been the reason that The London Pain Relief and Nutritional Support Clinic (Dr Geoffrey Leader and Lucille Leader) decided to introduce Autogenic Training into its management protocol for patients with Parkinson's disease. If one reduces the levels of these stress hormones by regular and enjoyable AT practice, this results in less need for adrenaline.

- Tremor and movement disturbance can be exacerbated by stress. Using an AT technique to promote deep mind and body relaxation, at times of conscious stress, may alleviate stress related symptoms.

- This form of deep relaxation improves sleep.

- By letting go of tension, systematically throughout the body, relaxation seems to be gained at a deeper level, which helps to reduce tremor.

- Exercises promoting sensations of "heaviness and warmth" improve circulation. Improved blood flow is helpful for the transport of drugs and nutrients in the body. This specific form of relaxation, while working through the body, also increases communication between the two halves of the brain, which consequently improves co-ordination between the brain and limbs. This is one of several reasons why both the Russian and American NASA astronauts use AT to help them cope with weightlessness and preparation for re-entry to the earth's gravitational pull. It helps them to remain calm and better co-ordinated.

- AT reduces tension-related symptoms such as headaches, high blood pressure, joint pain, The Irritable Bowel Syndrome, colitis, asthma, phobias or panic attacks and may influence the regulation of heart rate.

- Gentle abdominal warmth in the solar plexus region further reduces stress chemistry diminishing tension at gut level, sometimes alleviating constipation and improving intestinal function. These benefits work well with improved nutrition.

- Continuing practice of AT results in improved control of anxiety.

Blocked Emotions

Autogenic Training also provides important exercises to review our feelings. Blocked emotions have to go somewhere and may need releasing safely, so that less energy is expended, keeping them locked up inside.

There is frequently a need to discuss sexual problems confidentially. Perhaps there is a need to improve personal relationships, or to have support in renewing a sexual relationship, which all too frequently, has remained lost in silence. Competent, sympathetic counsellors and therapists can help individuals and couples to renew and enjoy the sexual part of their lives. Sexuality in relation to Parkinson's disease rarely seems to be mentioned by doctors. The nature of the disease causes so many to lose confidence all round, so that I suspect many give up in despair. As people experience a growing sense of well being, it is not surprising when their love and sex lives improve too. The deep mind and body relaxation achieved by Autogenic Training techniques, is an ideal prelude to intimacy.

Note for the Therapist

Because of the nature of this debilitating disease, it is important to realise, when working with a Parkinson's disease sufferer, that special qualities can help whilst teaching AT or working in any capacity with this situation. We need to make patients feel welcome and comfortable whatever stage they are at. Patients have spent so much time trying to control tremor, and appear "normal", whilst actually feeling "out of control", along with mixed feelings of anger, resentment and fear. I often use supportive cushions when positioning patients for exercise, and encourage them to allow their limbs to move as they will, whilst we begin to relax.

It is important to use calm speech, slow down, and even repeat instructions carefully, so that they can be absorbed without making the patient feel awkward or further demoralised. My instructions are written down on sheets to be taken away for everybody who wishes to learn AT, so that they have an ongoing programme to refer to.

With an AT "Toolkit", a reduction in symptoms can gradually be achieved in combination with other therapies or medication. The ability to "switch off" regularly, applying a state of peace to the autonomic nervous system, is experienced as trustworthy and automatic.

At The London Pain Relief and Nutritional Support Clinic, we realised that partners and carers or supportive family members who shared the same stress load, would also benefit from this training. It is a very positive technique for carers and patients to learn together with a qualified trainer. This has resulted in improved, shared-relationships, understanding and strategies for gaining energy and providing an escape or release from tension whether personal or professional.

It's early days, we need further AT research, and it will be interesting to see whether practising it will continue to contribute to improved control of symptoms and feeling of well-being.

Many patients have commented that being equipped with new "tools" enables them to try to gain control over stressful situations. This therapy helps people to calm down within moments. As stress does exacerbate movement disturbance with people with Parkinson's disease, this is a bonus.

Case History

I recently received this letter from Mr Joe Colfer, who lives in Wateford, Ireland, and who studied Autogenic Training with Liz Norris in Dublin.

He writes: "I like walking and walk quite often by the sea. I feel very much at one with the sea, as it never stops moving, somewhat like my tremor - this is not a complaint. My feelings about the sea and I are good. While walking, I use my Autogenic Training, swinging my arms and feeling very much an important part of creation. In this situation my tremor stops.

I should tell you that I absolutely love and enjoy my life. I feel very much at one with creation. My philosophy with regard to Parkinson's disease is - that I have Parkinson's disease, but it does not have me… I am in control. I do AT exercises every day using plenty of "heavy and warm" phrases quite often, and IT WORKS".

Joe Colfer works at a Personal Development Centre teaching teenagers and adults how to build confidence and self-esteem.

For a list of Autogenic Training Therapists in the UK:

The British Autogenic Society, The Royal London Homeopathic Hospital, Great Ormond Street, London, WC1N 3HR

Website: **www.autogenic-therapy.org.uk**

CHAPTER 24

Depression and Stress

by Lucille Leader Dip ION

Depression often affects people with Parkinson's disease. In addition to pathophysiological reasons, it would be unnatural if people were not depressed by their symptoms. However, depression may sometimes be exacerbated as a side effect of certain drugs and a review of these could be helpful. There are also many psychological reasons for depression - some carried through from the past and others arising because of interpersonal changes in relationships as well as life style due to the onset of the illness. Professional help by a counsellor, psychologist or psychiatrist should be sought, as this will be of comfort and support. In some cases, medication may be indicated together with psychological counselling.

Many people with Parkinson's disease find that their symptoms of motor disturbance are exacerbated by stress. This is not surprising when one realises that adrenaline, the hormone released in response to stress, is metabolised from dopamine! Stress also affects gastrointestinal function, pH levels, glycaemic control, cortisol elevation and the immune system.

Therefore, if stress control, relaxation and co-ordination of mind and body are problems, it would be wise to seek help from appropriate specialists including:

- Psychologist, Psychiatrist or Sexual Therapist.

- Autogenic Training Counsellor (Autogenic Training teaches deep mind and body relaxation. It is an invaluable technique for symptom control as well as the lowering of blood pressure and the control of heart rate and is of great benefit to patients/partners and carers.)

- Teacher of Biofeedback techniques. Muscle tension can be monitored and relaxation techniques implemented.

- Occupational Therapist, Speech Therapist, Physiotherapist, Osteopath, Dentist and Dental Hygienist, Music Therapist, Nutritionist and other therapists who offer support of stressful conditions.

The following recommendations can be helpful:

- Exercising, walking, singing, laughter therapy (comedy videos, joke books avoiding of depressing subjects), attending entertainment, visiting friends and inviting people, developing religious faith, if so inclined.

- Avoid stress in the kitchen by having liquids prepared in thermos flasks - especially easy are those with a pump mechanism. Straws will make drinking easier and less stressful. Occupational Therapists can direct you to specialised utensils which may be easier to use and control. If people are on their own, buying and preparing food can be stressful, especially if movement is difficult. The General Practitioner may well be able to recommend organisations which can help. A delivery of ready-made foods from shops is also a possibility. If movement is a problem, a microwave oven, whilst not ideal for health, might be of assistance as it allows economy of movement and avoids the risk of burning arms.

- Turning in bed can be an effort and stressful. Using silk sheets and pyjamas facilitates turning.

- Bathing and showering may present difficulties and be stressful. An occupational therapist should be consulted for solutions.

- Partners and Carers may also be suffering from stress and depression. They should be encouraged to seek the support and guidance of the appropriate counsellor. Autogenic Training techniques are ideal for relaxation as well as regular breaks to maintain interests, hobbies and contact with friends.

CHAPTER 25

Patients' Self-Esteem

by Lucille Leader Dip ION and Ruth Robbins

Self-esteem is a very personal and broad concept, which is handled by counsellors, psychologists and psychiatrists. It is imperative that this subject be managed on an individual basis as each person's experiences, feelings and relationships are unique. In this chapter, therefore, we will only present some strategies, which people have used to "stay on track" and assist them in keeping a reasonable measure of self-esteem.

Of course, everyone is shocked and horrified at the diagnosis of Parkinson's disease. One person, however, who has survived chronic illness magnificently for many years, told us the following story which had helped her to keep "centred" and appreciate her own character:

When her doctor pronounced the shattering diagnosis in the surgery, her big strapping husband who was with her and who had always been the "strong one" in their relationship, fainted! At that moment, because she loved him so much, she realised that she would have to "be strong for two" or they both would sink. She had to convince herself and her husband that there was still so much that she and they could do, that she was exactly the same person with the same intelligence and emotional capacity as before and that she herself was quite capable of negotiating her treatment plan with her medical advisors. She then realised that tremor or stiffness did not necessarily mean that she was "dying." She was actually still "living" with these conditions and able to enjoy sights and sounds, company, books, walking, hugs and kisses, reading and many other activities! And so, you see that caring about someone else besides yourself, whether a partner or some other person or interest, can keep you involved. You will then be able to appreciate your own efforts which in turn will help you to retain your self-esteem.

There is much help available for people with Parkinson's disease, as the other chapters in this book do illustrate. You can feel brighter if your nutrition is appropriate and bowel function is well managed. Appropriate nutritional management can also support cellular energy. Your posture and muscle function can be optimised. Communication need not be a problem and counsellors offer a broad spectrum of help, if necessary. Intelligent drug management, which is kept to an appropriate dosage in order to give provide self control without uncomfortable side effects, can alleviate some symptoms and so can new surgical technique. Decide together with your doctor on a drug treatment plan that does not undermine your health and cause side effects, which can be more uncomfortable than Parkinson's disease itself.

You will feel worthy by being kind and caring of others. This can take the form of a gesture, word or deed. You can insist that those who support you also have *your* support for their needs (be that for a break, counselling, other social needs and hobbies, performing any tasks that you still can, or by just being a good listener). Remaining as active as possible either mentally, physically or both, keeps you feeling alive.

Feelings of self-esteem will be enhanced if you continue to dress well and remain interested in your appearance. Ladies, keep your hair well styled and nails and make-up attended to. Make the most of your looks - they are still there, as before! Gentlemen, attend to shaving / beard and hair. You can still feel proud of how you look. Loved ones will feel so happy to see you looking good and consider it as a compliment to them. This is important in maintaining relationships with others.

If you remain withdrawn after your diagnosis, this will affect your inter-personal relationships. Other people might interpret this as a lack of interest in them. This could initiate a cascade of rejection which would adversely affect your self-esteem. Reassurance from others that you are still loved unconditionally is necessary for your spirit to survive. However it is equally important for you, with the illness, to re-assure your partner or supporters that your feelings for them are unchanged by your illness and that you will continue to give them your love and moral support as before. Your partner will then have the confidence and strength to re-affirm feelings for you. This is a vital and worthwhile task for the person with Parkinson's disease and must not be under-estimated. It can be undertaken with or without disability.

Sexual problems may occur as a result of depression, drug treatment or the illness itself. This can cause loss of self-esteem. Reticence about this problem is counter-productive and immediate help should be sought from a sexual therapist. It is vital to remember, however, that expression of warmth can be demonstrated in many beautiful ways other than intercourse - the giving of gifts and loving looks, words of appreciation, touch, holding hands, hugs and kisses. These gestures of love must always be made so that there is reassurance of continuing affection. Self-esteem should not have to suffer because of sexual problems. As Dr Michael Perring writes in his chapter on Sexuality, "the mindset" love and affection are most important.

Some other points, which undermine self-esteem, are as follows and need to be addressed by the appropriate counsellor:

- not dealing with other people's unrealistic expectations

- not being able to forgive yourself and others

- dwelling on your problems and inadequacies

- having a complex about how you "appear"

- inability to work, loss of income and ego

- not dealing with fear of health deterioration of self and carer

By remaining pro-active and caring within your relationships, having good communication with your neurologist about supportive drug therapy, specialised nutritional management, help from appropriate specialists and counsellors, exercise and speech therapy and attending to your physical appearance and interests, you should be able to "stay on track" and maintain a reasonable measure of self-esteem. You will be able to list and admire your strengths in this way, realising that they out-weigh your weaknesses.

Do not dwell on your faults for they will consume you. But if you think of your strengths you will become courageous. If you still love yourself after the diagnosis then this will mean that it is worth making a great effort to help yourself, as you really deserve it.

The great philosopher, Mahatma Gandhi, said that no one can take away one's self-respect unless one gives it to them. This statement gives much food for thought!

Bibliography

Creating Confidence, The Secrets of Self-Esteem: R Johnson, D Swindley: 1994: Element Books Limited, UK

Voices from the Parking Lot: Parkinson's Insights and Perspectives: Compiled and Edited by Dennis Greene, Joan Blessington Snyder and Craig L. Kendell: 2000: The Parkinson Alliance, Princeton, New Jersey, USA www.parkinsonalliance.net

CHAPTER 26

Carers

by Lucille Leader Dip ION

Caring for a loved one at home is a very demanding vocation. Watching someone suffering physically, mentally and emotionally can be very draining. Due to the illness of one family member, there may be a need for an exchange of roles within the family unit. For instance, someone who has previously been "cared for" will now have to become the "active carer". This is a very difficult adaptation and carers would be well advised to seek the support of a professional counsellor to guide them with the realignment, as it were, of the cornerstones of their lives.

Carers also have personal rights! They often tend to forget this in their constant devotion to the needs of their charges. In addition to carers sometimes doing tasks unnecessarily for patients, ill people can easily become unreasonably dependent, giving up movements which they are still quite capable of performing. This situation should be avoided at all costs, both in the interests of the patient's self-esteem as well as for the carer, and should be sensitively negotiated between them.

Carers should realise that they must care for themselves physically, mentally and emotionally if they are to remain stable, well and capable of helping their loved ones to the best of their ability. Regular respite care should be organised so that carers can have time and space to relax and re-load physical and emotional energy, exercise, follow interests and have social contact which may be difficult if those they care for are very ill. Outings can also include visits to counsellors for management of general problems, which may include sexuality. They will return home revitalised and be able to express their loving care in a happier way.

Very dependent patients are usually difficult to placate, as they are genuinely afraid that no one else is as trustworthy as their own family or close friend. It is imperative, however, for healthy family members to maintain balanced contact outside the home where they can move and express themselves freely. Carers need to express their needs, gently but firmly, to those for whom they care, whilst reaffirming their love and concern. If they do not attend to all aspects of their own health, carers run the risk of developing health problems themselves.

In some cases, imagining a reversal of roles with the ill person might also help in providing a more accepting and tolerant attitude in very difficult situations.

It is quite understandable that carers should feel very angry and disappointed at their lot in life. Healthcare professionals do observe this in some instances in the clinic where partners present together. Carers need counselling to enable them to express their anger, fear or other emotions as "bottling it up" can result in them unconsciously "taking it out" on their charges (for instance carers expressing impatience with the patient's disability in the presence of a third party). This causes excruciating humiliation to patients. Whilst this is understandable because of the unremitting stress and frustration experienced, it demonstrates that all good intentions can easily be undermined if well-meaning and devoted carers are unsupported and emotionally exhausted.

Carers should not loose pride in their physical appearance and presentation - weight, hair, nails, face and clothes. This is essential for their self-esteem.

There are support groups for carers. Parkinson's Disease Societies should be able to direct carers to these groups. Counsellors can usually be recommended by a carer's doctor.

Some recommended activities for carers

- Count the blessings that you still have and appreciate yourself as a worthy and loving human being who is capable of a very special job

- Autogenic Training sessions for deep mind and body relaxation

- Dancing Classes / Gym / Swimming

- Playing a musical instrument

- Joining a library

- Joining a religious affiliation, if so inclined

- Yoga or Tai Chi exercise classes

- Cinema / Shows / Concerts

- Group therapy

- Counselling

- Hypnoanalysis and Hypnotherapy

- Keeping social contact and regularly inviting friends / family

- Enjoy a laugh each day - rent a comedy video, acquire a book of jokes and also have a chuckle with the patient

- Do something loving towards yourself each day - the simplest gesture is rewarding such as using a beautifully fragrant oil in your bath, watching your favourite TV programme, munching something delicious whilst dipping into a delightful book, exercising to jolly music, contemplating a beautiful flower

- Regular visits to the hairdresser and/or beautician

- Regular massage and facials

- Keeping the home environment comfortable and pleasant

- Finding travel organisations who cater for disabled people so that appropriate holidays or short breaks may be taken

The following presentation is from The Parkinson's Resource Foundation in the United States. I have included it in this chapter as I have found their president and founder, Jo Rosen and her team, to be innovative, enthusiastic, and very impressive in their pursuit of any new knowledge, which would help carers. I originally came to know of them under the name Children of Parkinsonians (COPS). In 1984 Jo's mother was diagnosed with Parkinson's disease. Subsequently, in 1989, her husband was diagnosed with it. Jo is committed to educating families who know very little or nothing about Parkinson's disease and to informing doctors and healthcare professionals on how they can better serve the Parkinson's disease community. COPS, which is now The Parkinson's Resource Foundation, have built an organisation that thousands of people with Parkinson's disease, *around the world*, have come to depend on.

A WORD TO CAREGIVERS FROM THE PARKINSON'S RESOURCE ORGANISATION

On a regular basis, a caregiver should remind himself/herself of what the cabin attendants on an airline say before a flight, namely, "In case of an emergency the oxygen masks will fall. If you are travelling with a child or someone who needs your assistance, please place the mask on yourself first and then help the person in need of your assistance with their mask". It definitely makes sense! If you are no longer around to take care of the person needing your assistance, the chances are they will fail. The same goes when caring for another person with Parkinson's disease. If you give all of your emotional and physical strength to them, there is nothing left for you. When your immune system declines from taking care of you, you risk the chance of becoming ill. When you are sick, your ill partner cannot take care of you and you certainly cannot take care of your partner. With this, you are NOT doing good for either of you. Take care of yourself first, it is an UNSELFISH act!

The Parkinson's Resource Organisation *is a non profit, charitable organisation dedicated to disseminating information, providing funds for respite care, and giving emotional comfort to families of people with Parkinson's Disease.*
**Telephone: (760) 773-5628 email: info@parkinsonsresource.org
website: www.parkinsonsresource.org**

Other US Caregivers' Support Associations include:
**Michael J Fox Foundation Tel no (212) 604 9182 email: info@michaeljfox.com
National Parkinson's Disease Caregivers' Information www.parkinsons-care.com
American Parkinson's Disease Association Inc. Tel no (718) 981 8001
National Parkinson's Disease Foundation Inc. Tel no (305) 547 6666**

UK Carers Associations include:
**The Princess Royal Trust for Carers Tel no 020 7480 7788 email: info@carers.org
Tel no 0141 221 5066   email: infoscotland@carers.org
UK Younger Alert Parkinsons, Partners and Relatives Tel no 01485 578592
The Carers National Association UK   Tel no 020 7490 8818
Parkinson's Disease Society UK Helpline Tel: Freefone 0808 800 0303
European Parkinson's Disease Association email: lizzie@epda.demon.co.uk**

A CARER'S VIEWPOINT

My husband has Parkinson's disease. As a loving carer, I have suffered all the stresses associated with this situation. I was fortunate enough, however, to eventually find a team of healthcare professionals who offer us an integrated (multi-disciplinary) approach to the management of his illness. My husband and I were recommended to learn autogenic training techniques, *together*, which we can use for deep mind and body relaxation. Physiotherapy and remedial exercise optimise his musculoskeletal function. Speech therapy, drug therapy and nutritional management round off "our" support and I do try to take a regular break. I also have a healthcare professional whom I can approach without inhibition, at any time, and with whom I can speak about my husband's condition and my own concerns. This moral support keeps me "on track" and gives me strength. It is important for us to know that someone really cares about pointing us in the right direction in order for us to adjust and cope along the way. I do hope that this type of management will become routine for all sufferers and carers. *If it does not come your way, do ask for it!*

Dorothy Churchman, 2001
Saffron, UK

CHAPTER 27

A Patient's
Point of View

by Tony Leather

When I was first diagnosed with Parkinson's disease in 1996, I was utterly distraught. I had always been a loving family man, keen sportsman and successful businessman. My anxiety about the implications of the disease was acute and coupled with the slight tremor and stiffness that had manifested itself, I had also lost much weight. The latter of was of great concern to me and my GP. My energy was severely impaired.

Coincidentally, I came upon an article written by a medical doctor about an integrated approach in the management of Parkinson's disease, which was being pioneered in London. This included nutritional management on a cellular level as well as attention to musculoskeletal problems, stress relief and support of carers. This clinic worked by medical referral and having spoken to the Clinic Director who explained the nature of the team approach to management, my General Practitioner was happy to write me a letter of referral.

My life changed positively from the time of that first consultation. My psychological needs were supported. I learnt autogenic training techniques in order to control stress and thereby symptoms, which typically of Parkinson's disease, are exacerbated by stress. Bowel function was optimised and after extensive nutritional biochemical tests demonstrating a lack of digestive enzymes, increased gut permeability ("leaky gut") and many nutritional deficiencies, I very soon put on weight and my energy improved. Intolerances to specific foods, drugs and nutrients were demonstrated and substitutes recommended. My stiffness was alleviated by osteopathic manipulation, daily swimming (during my lunch break) and exercise to include feet and hands (computer skills maintained). I also went for acupuncture, which relieved symptoms. I returned to playing racket sports and golf and continued with my work.

I met other Parkinson's disease patients and their partners during my sessions at the hospital when we were receiving intravenous nutritional support.

Seeing fellow patients doing well, with no signs of dyskinesia (because of proper instruction in drug-nutrient interactions) was very comforting, especially when I noted that some patients had suffered from Parkinson's disease for many years and were now in their mature years. It was encouraging to see partners or carers invited to sit with patients in the individual cubicles where intravenous nutritional administration was taking place. I noticed how supported carers and patients felt and how friendly and approachable the staff were.

I remained from 1996 to the end of 2000 without the use of L-dopa medication. Now that I am on it, I have been instructed how to "time" the taking of L-dopa in relation to food containing the competing amino acids. As such, my dose remains modest, I am comfortable, in control and have no side effects.

I wholeheartedly recommend fellow "travellers" to request a multi-disciplinary approach to the management of their illness. A secure partnership with one's doctors and healthcare advisors is the only way forward down a long winding road!

Tony Leather, 2001
Bledington, UK
email: Tony@tonyleather.co.uk

TONY LEATHER B ED (HONS) qualified in Education and went on to become Education Director of the dynamic company, Young Enterprise, UK. He retains an interest in sport and cultural events and is comitted to working in the interests of those with Parkinson's Disease. Tony now works in Marketing and as a teacher of computer studies. He considers himself to be a "teacher, learner and bigger than Parkinson's"!

Some International
Parkinson's Disease Organisations
and Helpful Addresses

EUROPE
European Parkinson's Disease Association www.epda.eu.com
Email: Lizzie@epda.demon.co.uk   Tel/fax: +44 1732 457683

UNITED KINGDOM

The Parkinson's Disease Society UK Tel: (020) 7931 8080 Freefone: 0808 800 0303
Email: enquiries@parkinsons.org.uk

UK Carers' Associations (see page 300)

UNITED STATES OF AMERICA

Michael J Fox Foundation Tel: (212) 604 9182 Email: info@michaeljfox.com

American Parkinson's Disease Association, Inc. Tel: (718) 981 8001   www.apdaparkinson.com

National Parkinson's Disease Foundation Inc. Tel: (305) 547 6666   www.parkinson.org

USA Carers' Associations (see page 300)

The Parkinson's Web List of Parkinson's disease Resources www.pdweb.mgh.harvard.edu/

The Parkinson's Web www.neuro-chiefe-e.mgh.harvard.edu/parkinsonsweb/Main/PDmain.html

The Parkinson's Disease Menu
www.demonmac.mgh.harvard.edu/neurowebforum/ParkinsonsDiseaseMenu.html

Functional Neurosurgery at Massachusetts General Hospital/Harvard
www.neurosurgery.mgh.harvard.edu/fnctnlhp.htm

AUSTRALIA

The Parkinson's Association of Western Australia Tel: (08) 9322 9322 Email: pawa@cygnus.uwa.edu.au

Parkinson's Australia c/o Parkinson's New South Wales, Concord RG Hospital, Building 64,
Hospital Road, Concord, New South Wales 2139

NEW ZEALAND
The Parkinson's Disease Society of New Zealand Email: parkinsonsnz@xtra.co.nz

ITALY
The Italian Parkinsonian Association (AIP) www.parkinson.it/aip

CANADA
The Parkinson's Foundation of Canada www.parkinson.ca

SOUTH AFRICA
The Parkinson's Association of South Africa Tel: (11) 787 8792 Email: parkins@global.co.za

MISCELLANEOUS

World Parkinson's Disease Association (WPDA) www.wpda.org

Parkinson's Disease Books at www.wellnessbooks.com

Comprehensive books on Parkinson's Disease www.findwhat.com/bin/findwhat.dll

Web Resources for the Brain Sciences Red Reef Publications offers unique learning resources for the
brain sciences including human brain models, neuroanatomical charts, study guides, new and used books,
software, and videos. www.findwhat.com/bin/findwhat.dll

Index

Lightning Source UK Ltd.
Milton Keynes UK
28 August 2009

143130UK00001BC/95/A